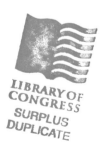
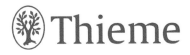

Ophthalmic Plastic Surgery

Tricks of the Trade

Suzanne K. Freitag, MD
Associate Professor of Ophthalmology
Director
Ophthalmic Plastic Surgery Service
Co-Director
Center for Thyroid Eye Disease and Orbital Surgery
Department of Ophthalmology
Massachusetts Eye and Ear Infirmary
Harvard Medical School
Boston, Massachusetts

N. Grace Lee, MD
Assistant Professor of Ophthalmology
Department of Ophthalmology
Massachusetts Eye and Ear Infirmary
Harvard Medical School
Boston, Massachusetts

Daniel R. Lefebvre, MD, FACS
Assistant Professor of Ophthalmology
Department of Ophthalmology
Massachusetts Eye and Ear Infirmary
Harvard Medical School
Boston, Massachusetts

Michael K. Yoon, MD
Associate Professor of Ophthalmology
Department of Ophthalmology
Massachusetts Eye and Ear Infirmary
Harvard Medical School
Boston, Massachusetts

Thieme
New York • Stuttgart • Delhi • Rio de Janeiro

Library of Congress Cataloging-in-Publication Data

Library of Congress Control Number:2019950105

© 2020 Thieme Medical Publishers, Inc.

Thieme Publishers New York
333 Seventh Avenue, New York, NY 10001 USA
+1 800 782 3488, customerservice@thieme.com

Thieme Publishers Stuttgart
Rüdigerstrasse 14, 70469 Stuttgart, Germany
+49 [0]711 8931 421, customerservice@thieme.de

Thieme Publishers Delhi
A-12, Second Floor, Sector-2, Noida-201301
Uttar Pradesh, India
+91 120 45 566 00, customerservice@thieme.in

Thieme Publishers Rio de Janeiro, Thieme Publicações Ltda.
Edifício Rodolpho de Paoli, 25º andar
Av. Nilo Peçanha, 50 – Sala 2508,
Rio de Janeiro 20020-906 Brasil
+55 21 3172-2297 / +55 21 3172-1896
www.thiemerevinter.com.br

Cover design: Thieme Publishing Group
Typesetting by Thomson Digital, India

Printed in The United States of America
by King Printing Co., Inc.   5 4 3 2 1

ISBN 978-1-62623-897-8

Also available as an e-book:
eISBN 978-1-62623-898-5

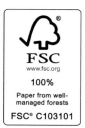

To Lotus, Thelonius, Peebert, Princess, Mr. Scrabbles, Anastasia and Svetlana

Suzanne K. Freitag, MD

To my family: Leo Kim, Eva Bomee, and Everett Julian (making an entrance right in the nick of time)

N. Grace Lee, MD

To my parents Dean and Kathleen for supporting me in all my pursuits with love
and encouragement from childhood to today

Daniel R. Lefebvre, MD

I have been fortunate to have worked with and learned from so many teachers, colleagues,
and friends through my career. Through their friendship and generosity, this book is made
possible. I would also like to express gratitude to my patients for trusting in me to care
for them. Lastly, I recognize my family whose love and patience has fueled me
throughout my professional life.

Michael K. Yoon, MD

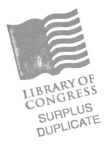

Contents

Part X Miscellaneous

Preface

We were inspired when Thieme approached our ophthalmic plastic surgery team to compile and edit a practical textbook on the most common procedures performed in the periorbital area, including eyelid, orbit and lacrimal surgery. We were particularly enthusiastic to tackle this project because we feel that there is a dearth of currently available ophthalmic plastic surgery textbooks that serve as practical how-to guides for procedures.

This book was designed with a dual purpose in mind. First, by nature of its structured format, it is a concise surgical atlas targeted for residents and fellows – the type of book that can be reviewed efficiently the night before surgery by trainees in order to have an understanding of the basic principles and steps of the surgery. The second purpose and strength is that each chapter is written by an author who is an expert in the field, providing advanced tips and pearls based upon years of experience performing the procedure. Hence, the book is pertinent for more experienced surgeons with the goal of improving technique and outcomes as well. The text is most directly targeted for ophthalmic plastic surgeons, but the material is useful for any surgeon performing procedures in the periorbital area, including ophthalmologists, otolaryngologists, facial plastic surgeons, plastic surgeons, dermatologists and maxillofacial surgeons.

We have recruited authors who are experts in the field from across the United States and around the world. The book is divided into 10 parts with a total of 46 chapters. The first chapter is a detailed overview of the anatomy of the eyelids, orbit and lacrimal system. The second chapter discusses fundamental principles of periorbital surgery. The following 44 chapters discuss a wide range of topics, including: eyelid trauma, lower eyelid, upper eyelid, eyebrow, lacrimal system, aberrant last management, tarsorrhaphy, orbit surgery, anophthalmic socket, and temporal artery biopsy.

Like Thieme's other Tricks of the Trade series of textbooks covering a wide range of surgical subspecialties, each chapter is subdivided into the same logical sections that include: goals, advantages, expectations, key principles, indications, contraindications, preoperative preparation, operative technique, tips/pearls/expert suggestions, what to avoid, complications/bailout, postoperative care, and references. The chapters contain numerous figures, illustrations and photographs to demonstrate the salient points. The procedures are presented in a step-by-step fashion for ease of understanding.

We hope that surgeons of all levels of experience will enjoy reading and utilizing this textbook as much as the editors enjoyed designing and compiling it. We hope that this book will serve as a standard for disseminating concise useful information about the core procedures in the ophthalmic plastic surgery armamentarium.

Suzanne K. Freitag, MD
N. Grace Lee, MD
Daniel R. Lefebvre, MD, FACS
Michael K. Yoon, MD

Videos

A selection of videos is available on MedOne illustrating the concepts and procedures covered in this book.

Contributors

Vinay K. Aakalu MD, MPH
Associate Professor
Division of Oculofacial Plastic and Reconstructive Surgery
Department of Ophthalmology and Visual Sciences
University of Illinois at Chicago/Illinois Eye and Ear
    Infirmary
Chicago, Illinois

Blair K. Armstrong, MD
Private Practice
Armstrong George Cohen Will Ophthalmology
Assistant Professor of Ophthalmology
Sydney Kimmel Medical Center of Thomas Jefferson
    University
Clinical Faculty
Wills Eye Hospital
Oculoplastics and Orbital Surgery Service
Philadelphia, Pennsylvania

Anne Barmettler, MD
Assistant Professor of Ophthalmology
Director of Oculoplastic Surgery
Montefiore Medical Center, Albert Einstein College
    of Medicine
Bronx, New York

Arpine Barsegian, MD
Resident
Department of Ophthalmology
SUNY Downstate Medical Center
Brooklyn, New York

Mica Y. Bergman, MD, PhD
Staff Physician
Oculoplastic Surgery/Ophthalmology
Sansum Clinic
Santa Barbara, California

Wenya Linda Bi, MD, PhD
Assistant Professor of Neurosurgery
Department of Neurosurgery
Brigham and Women's Hospital
Dana-Farber Cancer Institute
Harvard Medical School Boston, Massachusetts

Benjamin S. Bleier, MD
Associate Professor
Department of Otolaryngology
Massachusetts Eye and Ear Infirmary
Harvard Medical School
Boston, Massachusetts

Lucas Bonafede, MD
Resident
Wills Eye Hospital
Philadelphia, Pennsylvania
Fellow
Duke eye Center
Durham, North Carolina

Alison Callahan, MD
Associate Professor
Tufts/New England Eye Center
Boston, Massachusetts

Ashley A. Campbell, MD
Assistant Professor of Ophthalmology
Wilmer Eye Institute
Johns Hopkins University School of Medicine
Baltimore, Maryland

Christopher B. Chambers, MD
Associate Professor of Ophthalmology
Associate Professor of Plastic Surgery
University of Washington
Seattle, Washington

Emily Charlson, MD, PhD
Resident Physician
Gavin Herbert Eye Institute
Department of Ophthalmology
University of California, Irvine, School of Medicine
Irvine, California

Shu-Hong (Holly) Chang, MD
Clinical Associate Professor
University of Washington Eye Institute
Seattle, Washington
Pacific Oculofacial Plastic Surgery, PLLC
Bellevue, Washington

Christina H. Choe, MD
Oculoplastics Surgeon
Carolina Ophthalmology
Asheville, North Carolina

Catherine J. Choi, MD, MS
Clinical Instructor
University of Miami
Bascom Palmer Eye Institute
Miami, Florida

Liza M. Cohen, MD
Resident
Department of Ophthalmology, Massachusetts Eye and
    Ear Infirmary
Harvard Medical School
Boston, Massachusetts

Omar Dajani, MD
Resident Physician
Tufts/New England Eye Center
Boston, Massachusetts

Kristen E. Dunbar, MD
Clinical Instructor
Department of Ophthalmology
New York University, Langone Medical Center
New York, New York

Ian F. Dunn, MD
Associate Professor of Neurosurgery
Center for Skull Base and Pituitary Surgery
Brigham and Women's Hospital
Harvard Medical School
Boston, Massachusetts

Kian Eftekhari, MD
Assistant Professor of Ophthalmology
Department of Ophthalmology
University of North Carolina at Chapel Hill
Durham, North Carolina

Alexandra T. Elliott, MD
Ophthalmologist
Department of Ophthalmology
Children's Hospital Boston
Boston, Massachusetts

Suzanne K. Freitag, MD
Associate Professor of Ophthalmology
Director
Ophthalmic Plastic Surgery Service
Co-Director
Center for Thyroid Eye Disease and Orbital Surgery
Department of Ophthalmology
Massachusetts Eye and Ear Infirmary
Harvard Medical School
Boston, Massachusetts

Roxana Fu, MD
Assistant Professor of Ophthalmology
Wilmer Eye Institute
Johns Hopkins University School of Medicine
Baltimore, Maryland

Joseph Giacometti, MD
Ophthalmologist
Wills Eye Hospital
Wayne, Pennsylvania

Lora R. Dagi Glass, MD
Assistant Professor of Ophthalmology
Edward S. Harkness Eye Institute
Columbia University Irving Medical Center
New York, New York

Kyle J. Godfrey, MD
Assistant Professor of Ophthalmology
Department of Ophthalmology
New York Presbyterian Hospital-Weill Cornell
Weill Cornell Medicine
New York, New York

Mithra O. Gonzalez, MD
Associate Professor
Departments of Ophthalmology, Otolaryngology,
    and Dentistry
Flaum Eye Institute
University of Rochester Medical Center
Rochester, New York

Seanna Grob, MD
Clinical Instructor
Division of Oculofacial Plastic and Orbital Surgery
Irvine Department of Ophthalmology
University of California
Irvine, California

Larissa H. Habib
Oculoplastic Surgery Fellow
Department of Ophthalmology
Massachusetts Eye and Ear Infirmary
Boston, Massachusetts

Natalie Homer, MD
Resident
Massachusetts Eye and Ear Infirmary
Harvard Medical School
Boston, Massachusetts

Sanjai Jalaj, MD
Cornea/Refractive Fellow
Cole Eye Institute
Cleveland Clinic
Cleveland, Ohio

Juan C. Jiménez-Pérez, MD
Private Practice
San Juan, Puerto Rico

Daniel R. Lefebvre, MD, FACS
Assistant Professor of Ophthalmology
Department of Ophthalmology
Massachusetts Eye and Ear Infirmary
Harvard Medical School
Boston, Massachusetts

Bradford W. Lee, MD, MSc
Assistant Professor of Clinical Ophthalmology
Division of Oculofacial Plastic and Reconstructive Surgery
Bascom Palmer Eye Institute, University of Miami
  Miller School of Medicine
Palm Beach Gardens, Florida

N. Grace Lee, MD
Assistant Professor of Ophthalmology
Department of Ophthalmology
Massachusetts Eye and Ear Infirmary
Harvard Medical School
Boston, Massachusetts

Gary J. Lelli, Jr., MD
Associate Professor of Ophthalmology
Department of Ophthalmology
New York Presbyterian Hospital – Weill Cornell
Weill Cornell Medicine
New York, New York

Shu Lang Liao, MD
Head of Orbit and Oculoplastic Section
Department of Ophthalmology
National Taiwan University Hospital
Professor
National Taiwan University
Taipei, Taiwan

Catherine Y. Liu, MD, PhD
Assistant Professor of Ophthalmology
Division of Oculofacial and Plastic Surgery
Shiley Eye Institute
The Viterbi Family Department of Ophthalmology
University of California, San Diego
San Diego, California

Honglei Liu, MD, PhD
Director
Center of Oculoplastic and Orbital Disease
Vice President
Eye Hospital of Shaanxi Province
Hospital of Oculoplastic and Orb
Head
Orbit and Oculoplastic Section
Deaprtment of Ophthalmology
The Fourth Hospital of Xi'an City
Professor
Guangren Hospital
Xi'an Jiaotong University
Xi'an City, PR
China

Peter W. MacIntosh, MD, BSc
Assistant Professor of Ophthalmology
University of Illinois
Chicago, Illinois

Nicholas Mahoney
Assistant Professor of Ophthalmology
John Hopkins University School of Medicine
Baltimore, Maryland

Jason S. Mantagos, MD, PhD
Assistant Professor of Ophthalmology
Boston Children's Hospital
Harvard Medical School
Boston, Massachusetts

Sonul Mehta, MD
Assistant Professor of Ophthalmology
Co-Director
Division of Oculofacial and Orbital Surgery
Scheie Eye Institute
Hospital of the University of Pennsylvania
Philadelphia, Pennsylvania

Michael E. Migliori, MD
Professor of Surgery
Clinician Educator
Warren Alpert Medical School of Brown University
Providence, Rhone Island

Sarina K. Mueller, MD
Medical Doctor
Department of Otolaryngology
Massachusetts Eye and Ear Infirmary
Harvard Medical School
Boston, Massachusetts
Department of Otolaryngology, Head and Neck Surgery
University of Erlangen-Nuremberg
Erlangen, Germany

Tieu Vy Nguyen, MD
PGY-5 Ophthalmology Resident
Boston Medical Center
Boston University
Boston, Massachusetts

Julius T. Oatts, MD, MHS
Clinical Fellow in Pediatric Ophthalmology and Strabismus
Boston Children's Hospital
Harvard Medical School
Boston, Massachusetts

Osiris Olvera-Morales, MD
Ophthalmologist
Specialist in Surgery of Orbit, Eyelids, and Tear Ducts
Institute of Ophthalmology, "Conde de Valenciana"
Mexico City, Mexico

Chau Pham, MD
Oculoplastics Fellow
Illinois Eye and Ear Infirmary
University of Chicago
Chicago, Illinois

Do Eon Rok, MD
Board Certified Plastic Surgery
Chief Director
1mm Plastic Surgery Clinic
Seoul, Korea

Javier Servat, MD
Oculofacial Plastic Surgeon
Oculofacial Plastic Surgeons of Georgia
Assistant Clinical Professor
University of Georgia School of Medicine
Atlanta, Georgia

Pete Setabutr, MD
Associate Professor of Ophthalmology
University of Illinois
Director
Oculoplastic & Reconstructive Surgery Service
Illinois Eye and Ear Infirmary
University of Chicago
Director
Millennium Park Eye Center
Chicago, Illinois

Neil Shah, MD
Resident
Loyola University Medical Center
Maywood, Illinois

Roman Shinder, MD, FACS
Assistant Professor of Ophthalmology
Department of Ophthalmology
SUNY Downstate Medical Center
Brooklyn, New York

Nora K. Siegal, MD, PhD
Acting Instructor
University of Washington
Seattle, Washington

Brittany A. Simmons, MD
PGY-3 Resident
Department of Ophthalmology
Flaum Eye Institute
University of Rochester Medical Center
Rochester, New York

Victoria Starks, MD
Oculoplastic Surgery Fellow
Department of Ophthalmology
Massachusetts Eye and Ear Infirmary
Boston, Massachusetts

Jeremiah P. Tao, MD
Professor of Ophthalmology
Chief of Oculofacial Plastic and Orbital Surgery
Gavin Herbert Eye Institute
University of California, Irvine
Irvine, California

Livia Teo, MD
Adjunct Assistant Professor
Singapore National Eye Centre
Singapore Eye Research Institute
Duke National University of Singapore Medical School
National University of Singapore Yong Loo Lin School
  of Medicine
Singapore

José Luis Tovilla-Canales, MD
Director
Orbit and Oculoplastics Department
Instituto de Oftalmologia
Mexico City, Mexico

Ann Q. Tran, MD
Fellow in Oculoplastics
Bascom Palmer Eye Institute
Miami, Florida

Michael Tseng, MD
Resident
Montefiore Medical Center
Bronx, New York

Adam Weber, MD
Resident
Cullen Eye Institute
Baylor College of Medicine
Houston, Texas

Bryan J. Winn, MD
Associate Professor and Vice Chair
Department of Ophthalmology
University of California, San Francisco
Ophthalmologist-in-Chief
San Francisco Veterans Affairs Medical Center
San Francisco, California

Edward J. Wladis, MD, FACS
Professor and Chairman
Department of Ophthalmology
Lions Eye Institute
Albany Medical College
Albany, New York

Natalie Wolkow, MD, PhD
Fellow
ASOPRS Ophthalmic Plastic Surgery
Ophthalmic Plastic Surgery Service
Mass Eye and Ear
Department of Ophthalmology
Harvard Medical School
Boston, Massachusetts

Prashant Yadav, MD, FRCS, FACS
Staff Physician
Ocular Oncology Service
Wills Eye Hospital
Assistant Professor
Thomas Jefferson University
Philadelphia, Pennsylvania

Michael T. Yen, MD
Professor of Ophthalmology
Cullen Eye Institute
Baylor College of Medicine
Houston, Texas

Michael K. Yoon, MD
Associate Professor of Ophthalmology
Department of Ophthalmology
Massachusetts Eye and Ear Infirmary
Harvard Medical School
Boston, Massachusetts

Hunter Yuen, MBChB, FRCOphth, FRCSEd, MRCSEd, FCOphthHK, FHKAM (Ophthalmology), DipClinDerm (London)
Consultant Ophthalmologist
Hong Kong Eye Hospital
Head
Oculoplastic Surgery and Orbital Service
Honorary Professor
Department of Ophthalmology and Visual Sciences
The Chinese University of Hong Kong (DOVS, CUHK)
Hong Kong Eye Hospital
Hong Kong

Senmiao Zhan, MD, MS
Resident Physician
Virginia Commonwealth University Health System
Department of Ophthalmology
Richmond, Virginia

Sandy Zhang-Nunes, MD
Director of Oculofacial Plastic Surgery
USC Roski Eye Institute
Kick School of Medicine
Los Angeles, California

Part I

Anatomy and Principles

1 Anatomy of the Eyelids, Orbit, and Lacrimal System

Lora R. Dagi Glass

Summary

This chapter reviews anatomy of the eyelids, lacrimal system, and orbit. Anatomic knowledge is the basis of ophthalmic plastic and reconstructive surgery. By thoroughly understanding the relationship between the various layers and structures, a surgeon can often preserve functionality and cosmesis of the orbit and periocular region.

Keywords: anatomy, eyelid, lacrimal system, orbit

1.1 Eyelids

The eyelid structures are herein described in an anterior-to-posterior approach (▶ Fig. 1.1).

1.1.1 Skin

Eyelid skin is extremely thin, and notably lacking in subcutaneous fat. The upper eyelid skin crease, found 8 to 10 mm above the lid margin in non-Asian eyelids, is composed of fine attachments of the levator aponeurosis through overlying orbicularis muscle to the skin.[1] Asian eyelids may not have an upper eyelid crease, or may have a significantly lower crease.

The medial and lateral canthal angles are the angles created by the joining of the medial and lateral upper and lower eyelids, respectively.

1.1.2 Orbicularis Muscle

The orbicularis oculi muscle is a protractor, or muscle of eyelid closure, and is divided into three portions: orbital, overlying the orbital bone; preseptal, overlying the septum; and pretarsal, overlying the tarsus. As it approaches the eyelid margin, orbicularis muscle is termed "the muscle of Riolan," visualized as the gray line. It is innervated by cranial nerve 7, the facial nerve (▶ Fig. 1.2).

Tissue in this plane onwards is considered part of the anterior lamella of the eyelid. Tissue posterior to this plane is considered posterior lamella of the eyelid.

1.1.3 Septum

Orbital septum is a connective tissue layer arising from the bony orbital margin (arcus marginalis) and inserting onto the levator aponeurosis superiorly, and onto the inferior edge of the tarsus inferiorly (▶ Fig. 1.3). It can be relatively thick in children, but is typically thin in adulthood. It is a crucial zone of differentiation between pre- and postseptal anatomy and processes.

1.1.4 Fat Pads

There are two fat pads superiorly, and three pads inferiorly; all are postseptal, or orbital, and are considered contiguous with extraconal fat. Given their location relative to the levator aponeurosis, the central upper fat pads are typically referred to as "preaponeurotic fat." The upper and lower eyelids have medial and central fat pads. The lower eyelid has a lateral fat pad.

1.1.5 Lacrimal Gland

The orbital portion of the lacrimal gland can be found lateral to the central preaponeurotic fat pad (▶ Fig. 1.3). It will be further described in the Orbit section. It is assisted in tear production by the fornix-based accessory lacrimal glands of Krause and Wolfring.[2]

1.1.6 Eyelid Retractors

The levator palpebrae superioris is the major muscle of upper eyelid retraction (▶ Fig. 1.3). It arises from the lesser sphenoid wing and projects anteriorly until Whitnall ligament just posterior to the orbital rim, at which point the vector is changed to a vertical system of retraction.[1] At approximately the same point of change, the muscle transitions to its aponeurosis, which ultimately inserts onto the anterior face of the tarsus. As previously described, various muscle fibers also travel anteriorly, ultimately forming the upper eyelid skin crease. This muscle is striated and innervated by cranial nerve 3, the oculomotor nerve.

Müller muscle arises from the condensation of the levator palpebrae superioris and Whitnall ligament, and inserts upon the upper tarsal border.[1] Unlike the levator muscle, Müller muscle is a smooth, sympathetically innervated muscle.

The capsulopalpebral fascia is the major retractor of the lower eyelid. It is a fibrous sheet extending from Lockwood ligament, traveling parallel to the inferior rectus and around the inferior oblique prior to inserting along the inferior tarsal border.[1]

1.1.7 Tarsus

Tarsus is a dense tissue plate found just underneath the lid margins (▶ Fig. 1.3). It is up to 10 mm in maximal vertical height in the upper lid, and up to 4 mm of maximal vertical height in the lower lid.[1]

The medial and lateral canthal tendons arise from the medial and lateral tarsal plates, and are further strengthened by orbicularis oculi muscle heads.

1.1.8 Margin

The eyelid margin is an epithelialized platform noted along the upper and lower eyelids. Eyelash follicles lie deep to the eyelid margin anterior to the tarsus, and eyelashes exit the margin anteriorly. The gray line demonstrates the location of orbicularis oculi muscle. Meibomian gland orifices are microscopically visualized in line with the deeper tarsus, which envelops them.

The interpalpebral fissure, or space between the eyelid margins, spans approximately 1 cm vertically, and 3 cm horizontally. The upper eyelid usually falls approximately 1 mm below

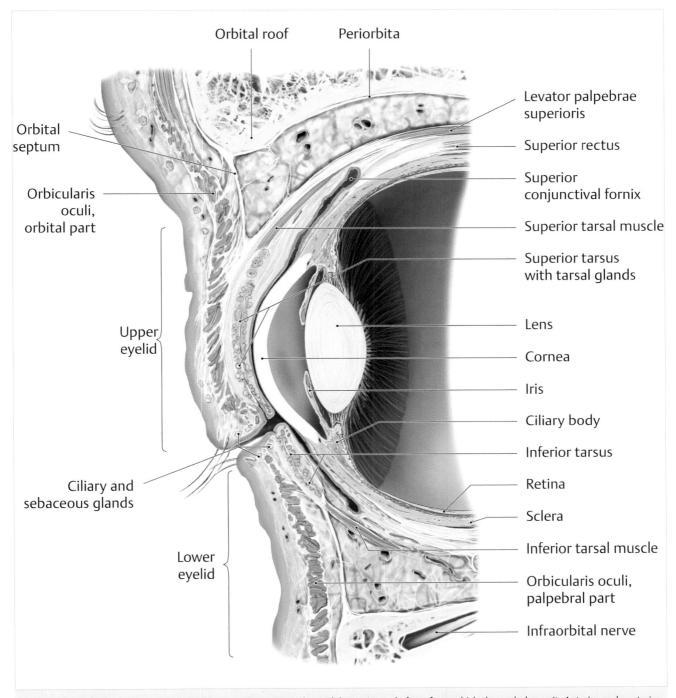

Fig. 1.1 The eyelids are viewed in a sagittal cross-section. Note the eyelid margin, a platform from which the eyelashes exit. Anterior and posterior lamellae are demarcated by the orbicularis oculi muscle. Orbital contents are demarcated by the septum. (From Schuenke M, Schulte E, Schumacher U. Prometheus. Thieme Atlas of Anatomy: Head and Neuroanatomy. Illustrations by M. Voll and K. Wesker. 1st ed. Stuttgart: Thieme; 2010.)

the superior corneal limbus; the lower eyelid usually skirts the inferior limbus.

1.1.9 Conjunctiva

The conjunctival mucous membrane lines the posterior surface of the eyelids, forms the fornices, and is contiguous with the bulbar conjunctiva.

1.1.10 Vascularization

The eyelids are heavily vascularized, with multiple anastomoses passing between the anterior and posterior lamellar vascular supply. In general, the transverse facial, superficial temporal and angular artery branches of the external carotid artery supply the anterior lamellae. The nasal and lacrimal branches of the ophthalmic artery supply the majority of the posterior

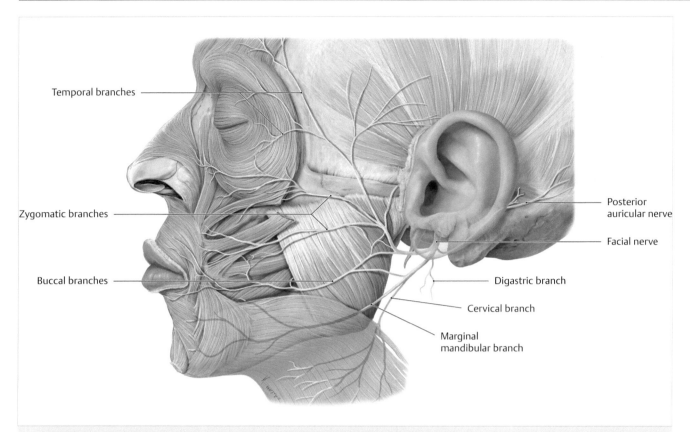

Fig. 1.2 The facial nerve and its branches are delineated, demonstrating innervation of the orbicularis oculi muscle among other muscles of facial animation. (From Schuenke M, Schulte E, Schumacher U. Prometheus. Thieme Atlas of Anatomy: Head and Neuroanatomy. Illustrations by M. Voll and K. Wesker. 1st ed. Stuttgart: Thieme; 2010.)

lamellae. A marginal arcade supplies the upper and lower eyelid margins. A peripheral arcade is found in the upper eyelid just superior to the tarsal plate. Vascular drainage is both orbital and facial.[1]

1.2 Lacrimal Drainage System

Tear drainage begins at the puncta (▶ Fig. 1.3). The upper and lower lids each contain a punctum medially; the punctum is 5 mm from the canthal angle superiorly, and 6 mm from the canthal angle inferiorly. Each punctum drains into a canaliculus. The canaliculi travel vertically for 2 mm, then horizontally for an additional 8 mm. The superior and inferior canaliculi fuse to create a common canaliculus 90% of the time. Then, either in the form of a common canaliculus or as two separate canaliculi, the canalicular structure empties into the lacrimal sac. The valve of Rosenmüller is a fold of tissue that serves as a one-way valve, helping prevent tear reflux from the lacrimal sac into the canalicular apparatus. The lacrimal sac, 1.2 to 1.5 cm in length, sits in the lacrimal sac fossa, cradled by the anterior and posterior lacrimal crests. The anterior lacrimal crest is part of the maxillary bone, whereas the posterior lacrimal crest is part of the lacrimal bone, with a suture line in the fossa. Periorbital tissue spans the lacrimal sac from the anterior to the posterior lacrimal crest. In addition, the medial canthal ligament and orbicularis oculi muscle fibers split, hugging the lacrimal sac and inserting

onto the anterior and posterior lacrimal crests, thereby allowing the orbicularis-derived Horner muscle and muscle of Riolan to contribute to the lacrimal sac pump function.[3]

Inferiorly, the lacrimal sac transitions into the nasolacrimal duct, which travels approximately 1.2 cm through the lacrimal canal.[3] The nasolacrimal canal is surrounded by maxillary bone, with the exception of the superomedial portion, which is ethmoidal. The canal comprises the lacrimal ridge intranasally, which is found anterior to the middle turbinate. The nasolacrimal duct empties into the nasal cavity via the inferior meatus. The valve of Hasner sits just at the opening of the meatus, helping to prevent reflux.[3]

1.3 Orbit

The orbital volume is 30 mL. The orbit serves to house the globe, an essentially spherical, complex structure of visual function approximately 2.4 cm in diameter. Fat envelops all structures of the orbit.[4] This section will focus on the bony structures and soft tissue elements that protect, move, and innervate the globe.

1.3.1 Bone

The orbital bony complex is typically simplified into a floor, roof, and two "walls"—medial and lateral (▶ Fig. 1.4, ▶ Fig. 1.5).

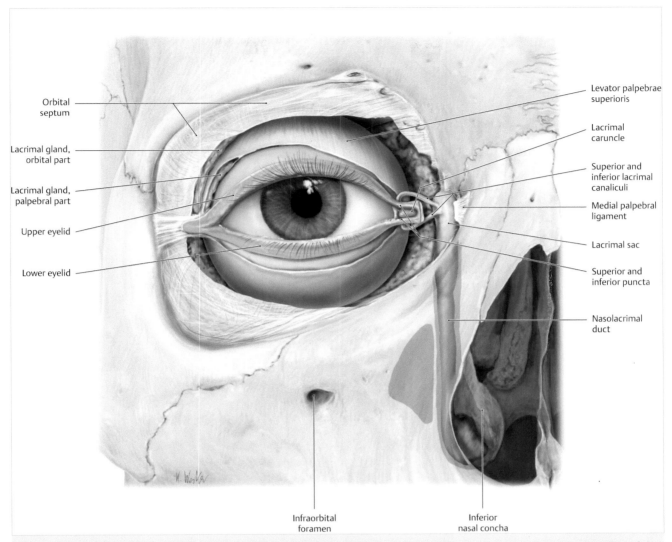

Fig. 1.3 The orbital septum has been partially stripped to demonstrate levator palpebral superioris aponeurosis insertion on the anterior face of the tarsus, and division of the lacrimal gland into its orbital and palpebral lobes by the same. The fat pads lie between the septum and the retractor musculature. This figure also demonstrates the anatomy of nasolacrimal drainage from the puncti, through the canaliculi, into the lacrimal sac, and down through the nasolacrimal duct, emptying through the inferior meatus. (From Schuenke M, Schulte E, Schumacher U. Prometheus. Thieme Atlas of Anatomy: Head and Neuroanatomy. Illustrations by M. Voll and K. Wesker. 1st ed. Stuttgart: Thieme; 2010.)

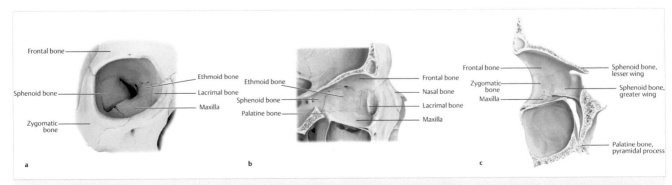

Fig. 1.4 (a) The bones comprising the orbital roof, floor, and walls. The medial wall appears in **(b)**, whereas the lateral wall appears in **(c)**. In both these cases, the surrounding bones are labeled to provide anatomic context. (From Schuenke M, Schulte E, Schumacher U. Prometheus. Thieme Atlas of Anatomy: Head and Neuroanatomy. Illustrations by M. Voll and K. Wesker. 1st ed. Stuttgart: Thieme; 2010.)

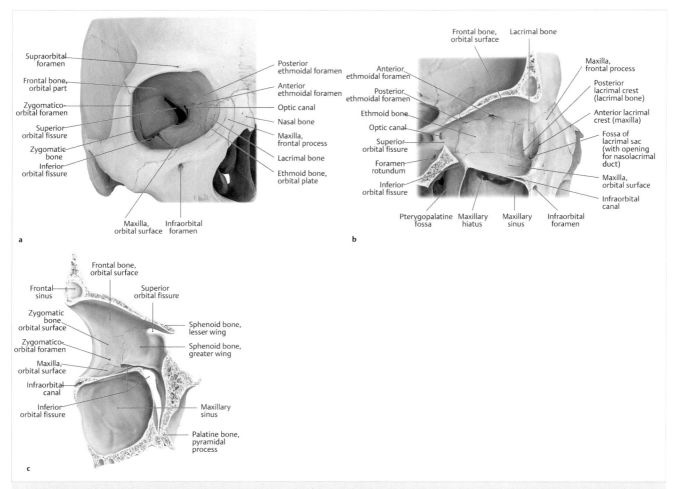

Fig. 1.5 **(a)** Bones, foramina, and fissures. **(b,c)** Note the boomerang shape of the superior and inferior orbital fissures, as well as the optic foramen superior to the boomerang apex. (From Schuenke M, Schulte E, Schumacher U. Prometheus. Thieme Atlas of Anatomy: Head and Neuroanatomy. Illustrations by M. Voll and K. Wesker. 1st ed. Stuttgart: Thieme; 2010.)

Despite this structural description, the orbit is actually rather pear-shaped, with the entrance being approximately 3.5 cm in height and 4 cm in width.[2] It widens approximately 1 cm posterior to the rim.[2] The medial walls are parallel and 2.5 cm apart; the lateral walls track at 45-degree angles to the medial walls. The periorbita is the equivalent of periosteum, and lines the orbital bones and encases the orbital soft tissue. It is strongly adherent at the arcus marginalis of the orbital rim, the lateral orbital tubercle, the optic foramen, and the orbital fissures. It fuses with dura at the optic canal and superior orbital fissure, and with the septum at the arcus marginalis.[4]

The orbital floor is comprised of the maxillary, zygomatic, and palatine bones. The orbital floor does not meet the orbital apex, unlike the other orbital walls, being bounded by the inferior orbital fissure approximately 1.5 cm from the orbital rim.[2] The pterygopalatine fossa sits under the inferior orbital fissure. The infraorbital groove and canal sit in the medial aspect of the orbital floor.

The medial wall is comprised of the maxillary, lacrimal, ethmoid, and sphenoid bones. The ethmoidal portion of the medial wall is called the lamina papyracea and is the thinnest of the orbital walls. Two foramina in the frontoethmoidal suture help delineate the distance traveled from the anterior lacrimal crest, as well as the general level of the anterior cranial fossa floor. The anterior ethmoidal foramen is approximately 2.4 cm, and the posterior ethmoidal foramen is approximately 3.5 cm, from the anterior lacrimal crest. The posterior foramen is approximately 0.2 to 1 cm anterior to the optic canal.[2,4]

The orbital roof is comprised of frontal bone and the lesser wing of the sphenoid bone. It is home to the lacrimal gland fossa laterally, the trochlear fossa medially, and the supraorbital notch or foramen. At the orbital apex, the roof ends at the optic foramen through which the optic nerve travels, and the superior orbital fissure, which will be addressed in greater detail later.

The lateral wall is comprised of the greater wing of the sphenoid bone, frontal bone, and zygomatic bone. It is the strongest bone of the orbit, and measures 4 cm from the rim to the superior orbital fissure.[2] It is home to the zygomaticofacial and zygomaticotemporal canals, as well as the lateral orbital tubercle, upon which coalesce the lateral canthal tendon, the lateral

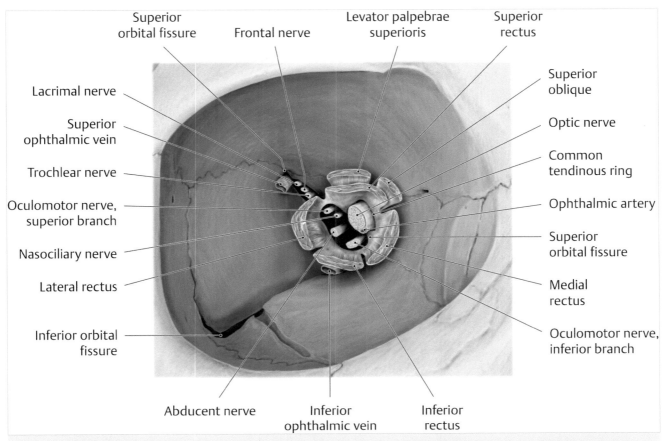

Fig. 1.6 The annulus of Zinn, derived from the rectus muscles, encapsulates the optic foramen and part of the superior orbital fissure. The lacrimal, frontal, and trochlear nerves, as well as the superior ophthalmic vein, pass via the superior orbital fissure outside of the annulus of Zinn. Cranial nerves 2–3, the nasociliary branch of 5_1, cranial nerve 6, and the sympathetic nerves pass through the annulus. The inferior ophthalmic vein passes through the inferior orbital fissure. (From Schuenke M, Schulte E, Schumacher U. Prometheus. Thieme Atlas of Anatomy: Head and Neuroanatomy. Illustrations by M. Voll and K. Wesker. 1st ed. Stuttgart: Thieme; 2010.)

levator aponeurosis, the check ligament of the lateral rectus, Lockwood ligament, and Whitnall ligament. The tubercle is found 9 mm below the frontozygomatic suture line and 4 mm posterior to the lateral orbital rim.[4]

1.3.2 The Superior and Inferior Orbital Fissure and the Optic Foramen

The superior orbital fissure sits between the greater and lesser sphenoid wings (► Fig. 1.5). The sympathetic nerves and cranial nerves 3, 4, 5_1, and 6 enter the orbit via the superior orbital fissure; the superior ophthalmic vein drains the orbit via the same (► Fig. 1.6).

The inferior orbital fissure is bounded by the orbital floor and the lateral wall. It carries the inferior ophthalmic vein and cranial nerve 5[2].

The optic foramen leads to the optic canal, a 0.8 to 1 cm long and 0.6 cm wide structure that sits in the lesser wing of the sphenoid bone separated from the superior orbital fissure by the optic strut.[2,4] It carries cranial nerve 2—the optic nerve—as well as the ophthalmic artery and sympathetic nerves.

1.3.3 Extraocular Muscles and Septa

There are six muscles of extraocular movement, all of which insert upon the globe: the superior and inferior oblique muscles and the superior, inferior, medial, and lateral rectus muscles (► Fig. 1.7). Each of the muscles is enveloped in a sheath and connected to a weblike network of connective tissue septa.

The superior oblique muscle originates superomedial to the optic foramen and travels anteriorly to the trochlea, a cartilaginous ring through which the superior oblique muscle ligament passes; at that point, the ligament runs laterally prior to inserting on the globe.[4]

The inferior oblique originates inferolateral to the lacrimal sac fossa, traveling laterally prior to insertion on the globe. Of note, the inferior oblique muscle sheath combines with that of the inferior rectus, helping to create the globe-suspending Lockwood ligament.[4]

The four rectus muscles originate from the annulus of Zinn (► Fig. 1.6), a fibrous band that arises from the optic foramen and surrounds both the optic foramen and a portion of the superior orbital fissure. Orbital contents within the four rectus muscles are considered intraconal; those outside are extraconal.

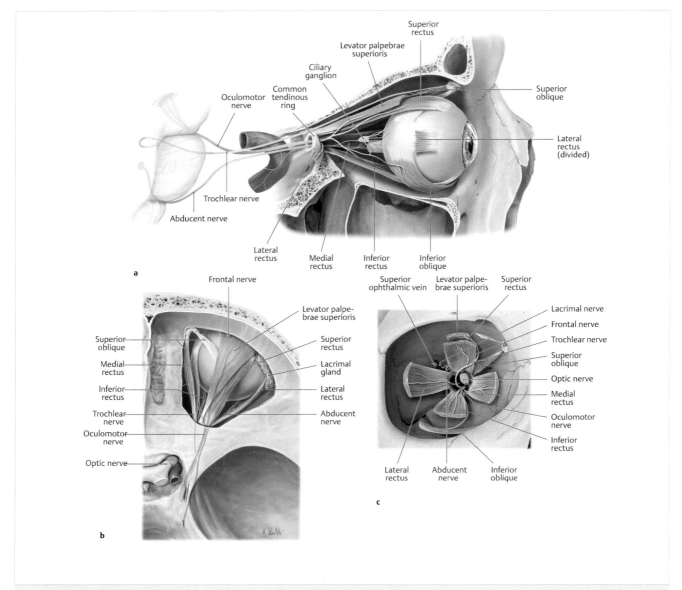

Fig. 1.7 Path of the six muscles of extraocular movement, from their point of origins to their insertion on the globes. In addition, the innervation of the extraocular muscles is highlighted. Images demonstrate extraocular muscles and routes of innervation from the lateral **(a)**, sagittal, **(b)** intracranial/supraorbital, and **(c)** orbital apex views. Note the ciliary ganglion is found between the optic nerve and the lateral rectus muscle. (From Schuenke M, Schulte E, Schumacher U. Prometheus. Thieme Atlas of Anatomy: Head and Neuroanatomy. Illustrations by M. Voll and K. Wesker. 1st ed. Stuttgart: Thieme; 2010.)

1.3.4 Lacrimal Gland

The lacrimal gland is a bilobed orbital structure of tear production measuring approximately $2\,cm \times 1.2\,cm \times 0.5\,cm$.[2] The palpebral lobe sits anteriorly in a postseptal location. The larger orbital lobe is seated in the lacrimal gland fossa of the orbital roof. The two lobes are divided by the lateral horn of the levator aponeurosis. Ducts from the orbital lobe travel unidirectionally to the palpebral lobe, prior to tear exit into the superolateral fornix approximately $0.5\,cm$ above the superior tarsal border.[2]

The lacrimal gland receives afferent innervation from cranial nerve 5_1, and parasympathetic efferent innervation.

1.3.5 Nerves

Cranial nerve 2, the optic nerve, arises from the retinal ganglion cells found in the globe (▶ Fig. 1.8). The orbital component of the optic nerve is 4 mm in diameter and approximately 3 cm in length; of note, it travels 1.8 to 2 cm from the globe to the optic

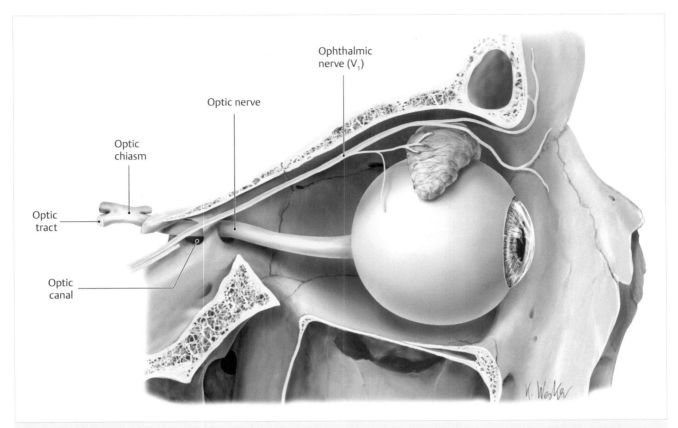

Fig. 1.8 Sinusoidal path of the optic nerve from the globe to the optic canal. (From Schuenke M, Schulte E, Schumacher U. Prometheus. Thieme Atlas of Anatomy: Head and Neuroanatomy. Illustrations by M. Voll and K. Wesker. 1st ed. Stuttgart: Thieme; 2010.)

foramen.[2,4] The excess length allows for ease of globe movement. The nerve dips downward before rising to the optic foramen, thus taking a "sinusoidal path."

Cranial nerves 3, 4, and 6 supply the extraocular muscles (▶ Fig. 1.7). Cranial nerve 3, the oculomotor nerve, enters the orbit through the superior orbital fissure within the annulus of Zinn. It has two orbital branches whose fibers penetrate the underbellies of the innervated muscles. The superior branch innervates the levator palpebrae superioris and superior rectus muscles. The inferior branch innervates the inferior oblique, inferior rectus, and medial rectus muscles. Cranial nerve 4, the trochlear nerve, enters the orbit through the superior orbital fissure above the annulus of Zinn; it travels along the orbital roof prior to entering the superior oblique muscle. Cranial nerve 6, the abducens nerve, enters the orbit through the superior orbital fissure, in the annulus of Zinn; it travels laterally to innervate the lateral rectus muscle.[4]

Cranial nerve 5, the trigeminal nerve, is divided into three branches and provides sensory innervation (▶ Fig. 1.9). The first division, or ophthalmic division (▶ Fig. 1.10, ▶ Fig. 1.11), branches into the lacrimal, frontal, and nasociliary nerves. The lacrimal nerve enters the superior orbital fissure above the annulus of Zinn, ultimately innervating the lacrimal gland and upper eyelid. The frontal nerve gives rise to the supraorbital nerve, which exits the orbit at the supraorbital notch (or supraorbital foramen), and the supratrochlear nerve, which exits the orbit superomedially. Both the supraorbital and supratrochlear branches innervate the conjunctiva, upper eyelid, and forehead. The nasociliary nerve enters through the annulus of Zinn, passing off short ciliary nerve branches to the globe, long posterior ciliary nerve branches to the globe, the anterior and posterior ethmoidal nerves, and ultimately exiting superomedially as the infratrochlear nerve innervating the medial canthal region and lacrimal sac.[4] The second division of the trigeminal nerve, or the maxillary division, provides infraorbital nerve fibers. It travels through the foramen rotundum, across the pterygopalatine fossa, to enter the orbit at the inferior orbital groove, continues along the infraorbital canal, and exits via the infraorbital foramen onto the maxilla.[2]

Parasympathetic fibers follow the inferior branch of the oculomotor nerve and then synapse in the ciliary ganglion inferolateral to the optic nerve (▶ Fig. 1.11). Postsynaptic short ciliary nerves then travel to the globe to innervate the ciliary body and iris sphincter, allowing for accommodation and pupil constriction. Fibers also stimulate the lacrimal gland.[4]

Sympathetic fibers follow the arterial supply through the optic canal and the superior orbital fissure. They allow for pupil dilation and smooth muscle control, including Müller muscle in the eyelid.

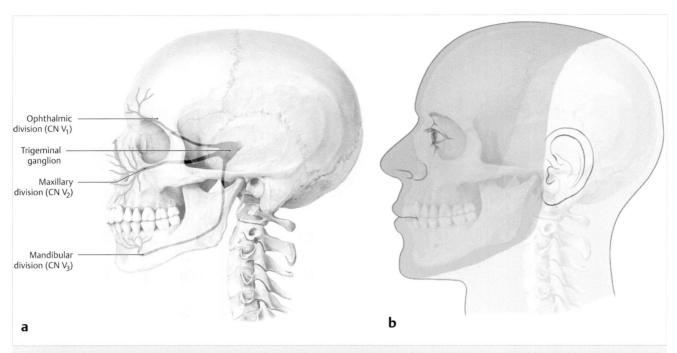

Fig. 1.9 **(a)** Cranial nerve 5 is divided into three main branches: ophthalmic (5_1), maxillary (5_2), and mandibular (5_3). **(b)** Cutaneous sensory innervation of the face according to branch number. (From Schuenke M, Schulte E, Schumacher U. Prometheus. Thieme Atlas of Anatomy: Head and Neuroanatomy. Illustrations by M. Voll and K. Wesker. 1st edn. Stuttgart: Thieme; 2010.)

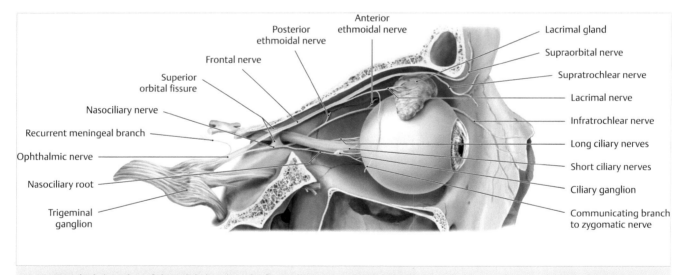

Fig. 1.10 Multiple branches of the ophthalmic branch of cranial nerve 5, or 5_1. In particular, note the course of the lacrimal, frontal, and nasociliary nerves. The frontal nerve ultimately gives rise to the supraorbital and supratrochlear nerves. The nasociliary nerve gives rise to the infratrochlear nerve. (From Schuenke M, Schulte E, Schumacher U. Prometheus. Thieme Atlas of Anatomy: Head and Neuroanatomy. Illustrations by M. Voll and K. Wesker. 1st ed. Stuttgart: Thieme; 2010.)

1.3.6 Vascularization

Branches of both the internal and external carotid arteries serve to supply the orbit, with ample anastomoses between the two (▶ Fig. 1.12). The ophthalmic artery derives from the internal carotid system. It travels with the optic nerve through the optic canal, and soon after releasing multiple branches.

Centrally, the ophthalmic artery branches into the central retinal and the lateral and medial long posterior ciliary arteries. The central retinal artery pierces the underside of the optic nerve 0.8 to 1.5 cm behind the globe.[2] The medial and lateral long posterior ciliary arteries parallel the optic nerve, and branch into multiple short posterior ciliary arteries; these short

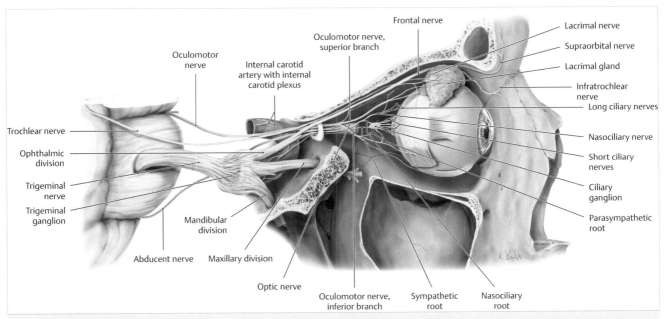

Fig. 1.11 Orbital innervation from cranial nerves 3–6. In addition, parasympathetic fibers following the inferior branch of the oculomotor nerve synapse in the ciliary ganglion inferolateral to the optic nerve are resected in this image. (From Schuenke M, Schulte E, Schumacher U. Prometheus. Thieme Atlas of Anatomy: Head and Neuroanatomy. Illustrations by M. Voll and K. Wesker. 1st ed. Stuttgart: Thieme; 2010.)

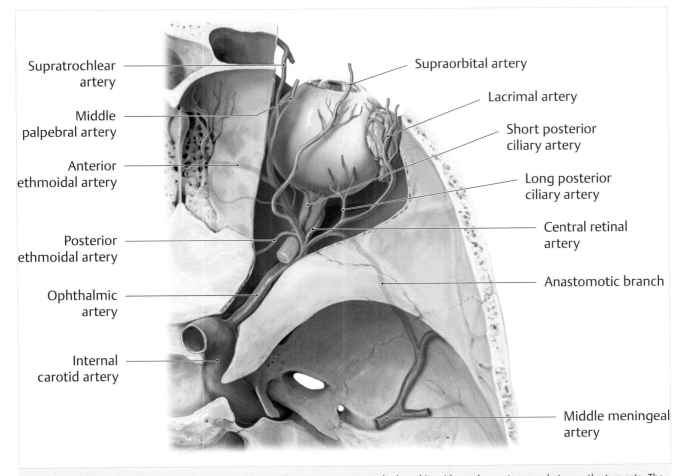

Fig. 1.12 Branches of both the internal and external carotid arteries serve to supply the orbit, with ample anastomoses between the two sets. The ophthalmic artery is of particular import, as it is a branch of the internal carotid artery, and gives rise to multiple crucial branches medially, centrally, and laterally. (From Schuenke M, Schulte E, Schumacher U. Prometheus. Thieme Atlas of Anatomy: Head and Neuroanatomy. Illustrations by M. Voll and K. Wesker. 1st ed. Stuttgart: Thieme; 2010.)

posterior arteries enter the sclera encircling the optic nerve and generally supply the extraocular muscles.[4]

Laterally, the ophthalmic artery branches into the lacrimal artery, which in turn gives rise to the zygomaticotemporal and zygomaticofacial arteries. The lacrimal artery rises superolaterally to pierce the lacrimal gland. The zygomaticotemporal and zygomaticofacial arteries enter their respective foramina, and ultimately anastomose with the transverse facial and superficial temporal arteries.[4]

Medially, the ophthalmic artery branches into the supraorbital, posterior ethmoidal and anterior ethmoidal, and nasofrontal arteries. The supraorbital branch tracks with the frontal nerve to exit through the supraorbital notch. The ethmoidal arteries enter their respective foramina. The nasofrontal artery exits above the medial canthus, giving arterial supply to the eyelids, and coursing on as the supratrochlear and dorsal nasal arteries. It anastomoses with the angular arterial supply.[4]

The superior and inferior ophthalmic veins drain the orbit (▶ Fig. 1.13). Collateral venous drainage runs between the superior and inferior ophthalmic veins.

The superior ophthalmic vein drains venous blood from the angular vein, supratrochlear, supraorbital, medial, and superior rectus muscles, levator palpebrae superioris muscle, superior vortex, anterior ethmoidal and lacrimal veins. Its course begins in the superomedial orbit; it crosses laterally and travels below the superior rectus muscle at mid-orbit, taking an intraconal path to the superior orbital fissure and ultimately emptying into the cavernous sinus.[4]

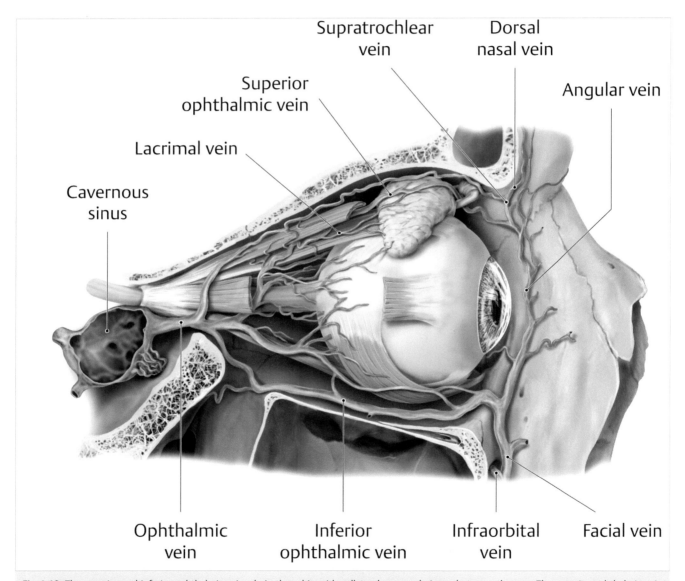

Fig. 1.13 The superior and inferior ophthalmic veins drain the orbit, with collateral venous drainage between the two. The superior ophthalmic vein drains into the cavernous sinus; one branch of the inferior ophthalmic vein joins the superior ophthalmic vein, whereas another branch drains into the pterygoid plexus. (From Schuenke M, Schulte E, Schumacher U. Prometheus. Thieme Atlas of Anatomy: Head and Neuroanatomy. Illustrations by M. Voll and K. Wesker. 1st ed. Stuttgart: Thieme; 2010.)

The inferior ophthalmic vein drains the inferior rectus muscle, lateral rectus, inferior oblique muscle, and inferior vortex veins. After traveling along the inferior rectus, it ultimately joins with the superior ophthalmic vein. Another branch travels through the inferior orbital fissure to drain into the pterygoid plexus.[4]

References

[1] Dutton JJ. Eyelid anatomy. In: Atlas of Oculoplastic and Orbital Surgery. Philadelphia, PA: Lippincott Williams & Wilkins; 2013:7–9

[2] Rootman J. Orbital anatomy. In: Orbital Surgery: A Conceptual Approach. 2nd ed. China: Lippincott Williams & Wilkins; 2014:51–116

[3] Dutton JJ. Surgical anatomy of the lacrimal drainage system. In: Atlas of Oculoplastic and Orbital Surgery. Philadelphia, PA: Lippincott Williams & Wilkins; 2013:216–217

[4] Dutton JJ. Surgical anatomy of the orbit. In: Atlas of Oculoplastic and Orbital Surgery. Philadelphia, PA: Lippincott Williams & Wilkins; 2013:252–255

2 Fundamental Principles and Techniques of Ophthalmic Plastic Surgery

Victoria Starks and Suzanne K. Freitag

Summary

Surgical outcomes are impacted by the combined effects of preoperative assessment, surgical planning, surgical technique, and patient-specific factors that influence healing. The first three components are modifiable. Careful preoperative evaluation and comprehensive patient counseling allows the surgeon to optimally plan and appropriately set patient expectations. Attention to anatomy, technical knowledge, and experience minimize intraoperative complications. Good tissue handling affects tissue healing and the quality of histopathology specimens. Attention to detail in each step of this process will promote good outcomes and patient satisfaction.

Keywords: periorbital surgery, surgical technique, surgical principles, periorbital surgical instruments, perioperative management

2.1 Preoperative Assessment and Discussion

A comprehensive preoperative examination and assessment is essential for surgical planning. In addition, the surgeon should counsel the patient about the proposed procedure, address the patient's concerns, and set reasonable expectations. The patient's other medical comorbidities should be optimized. Elective procedures are often best delayed in the setting of urgent health issues.

2.1.1 Essential Components of Preoperative Assessment

- Periorbital and complete ophthalmic examination.
- For trauma cases:
  - Careful ophthalmic examination to rule out an open globe or foreign body.
  - Consider CT imaging of orbits if indicated as well as B-scan ultrasound of the globe if poor view of the posterior pole.
  - Tetanus booster and/or tetanus immune globulin as indicated.
- Documentation via medical record and photography.
- Discussion of goals and expectations.

2.1.2 Anticoagulation

Stopping anticoagulation is important for patient safety. The primary concern is development of a retrobulbar hemorrhage with the possibility of subsequent optic neuropathy due to orbital compartment syndrome. Exceptions to this policy include obtaining biopsies of potentially malignant neoplasms or other small preseptal lesions, which should not be delayed. Patients are prescribed anticoagulation for a myriad of reasons and durations; thus, communication with the prescribing physician is important to ensure patient safety on stopping these medications. Anticoagulation is typically resumed on the first postoperative day. Suggested cessation schedules are as follows: warfarin for 3 to 5 days (preoperative international normalized ratio goal < 1.5), aspirin for a minimum of 5 to 7 days, platelet $P2Y_{12}$ inhibitors for a minimum of 7 days, direct thrombin or factor Xa inhibitors for 2 to 3 days, and nonsteroidal anti-inflammatory drugs for a minimum of 7 days. Other supplements with anticoagulative properties are held for 1 to 2 weeks.

2.2 Perioperative Antibiotics

The infection rate for routine eyelid surgery is very low, likely due to the abundant vascular supply to the ocular adnexa.[1] As a result, systemic antibiotics intraoperatively or postoperatively are not routinely used by all surgeons. However, many surgeons prescribe antibiotic prophylaxis for their patients, and perioperative antibiotics are strongly recommended in cases of trauma, foreign body implantation, or tissue grafting. When using systemic antibiotics for prophylaxis, intraoperative cefazolin is often adequate with an appropriate postoperative oral antibiotic for 5 to 7 days. Topical ophthalmic antibiotic ointment is routinely prescribed for 1 to 2 weeks postoperatively for both infection prevention and wound and ocular surface lubrication.

2.3 Local Anesthesia and Surgical Site Preparation

Local anesthesia is used for both its anesthetic and vasoconstrictive effects. Thus, even for cases under general anesthesia, lidocaine with 1:100,000 epinephrine is infiltrated into the surgical site, allowing 10 to 15 minutes for vasoconstriction prior to making the incision. Bupivacaine can be included to extend the duration of anesthesia. The addition of hyaluronidase allows the local anesthetic effect to diffuse more widely through tissue, therefore requiring less anesthesia. Surgical markings are best performed before infiltrating and distorting the tissue with local anesthesia.

Standard preoperative site preparation includes cleaning the skin with an iodine-based solution or another antiseptic. Care should be taken to avoid the use of flammable prep solutions such as alcohol because of the risk of intraoperative fire if the surrounding drapes remain saturated. Sterile drapes are then used to define the surgical field. Many surgeons leave the full face in the sterile field. Placement of corneoscleral shells is important to protect the eye from inadvertent damage. In cases of trauma, contaminated wounds are irrigated and foreign bodies removed.

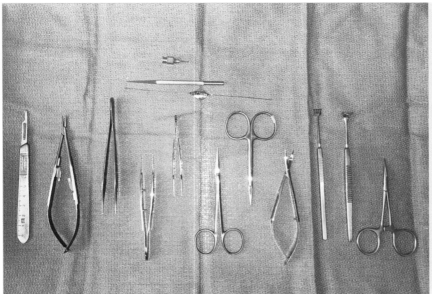

Fig. 2.1 Standard periorbital surgery instruments. From left to right: Number 15 Bard-Parker blade on blade handle, Castroviejo needle holder, Adson forceps, 0.5 mm Castroviejo forceps, Bishop-Harmon forceps, straight iris scissors, curved Stevens tenotomy scissors, Westcott scissors, skin retractor, Desmarres retractor, fine hemostat. Superiorly: lacrimal irrigation cannula, punctal dilator, lacrimal probe.

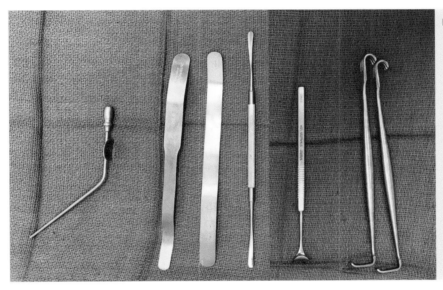

Fig. 2.2 Specialized instruments for orbitotomy.

2.4 Instruments

The thin skin of the periorbita requires the use of fine suture and precision instruments (▶ Fig. 2.1). The basic periorbital instruments include the following:

- Precision blades (#15 and #11 Bard-Parker blades) and blade handles.
- Locking, fine-tipped needle holders (Castroviejo).
- Fine-tipped toothed forceps (Bishop-Harmon or Castroviejo).
- Fine spring handle scissors (Westcott).
- Dissection instruments (Stevens tenotomy scissors, hemostat).
- Eyelid eversion instruments (Desmarres retractor).
- Fine skin hooks.

Orbit and lacrimal surgery require the addition of a variety of tools including a fine suction tip, malleable orbital retractors of various sizes, a periosteal elevator, curved retractors, and orbital retractors (▶ Fig. 2.2). The set for lacrimal surgery, such as dacryocystorhinostomy, includes lacrimal stents, lacrimal probe, punctal dilator, nasal speculum, and bone rongeurs (▶ Fig. 2.3).

There are numerous options for cautery. Disposable battery-operated hot-wire cautery units are simple, inexpensive, and do not require grounding the patient. High-frequency monopolar (Bovie) electrocautery requires that the patient be grounded and cannot be used if the patient has metal implants or a pacemaker. Bipolar electrocautery transmits current only between the tips of the instrument; thus, it may be used when

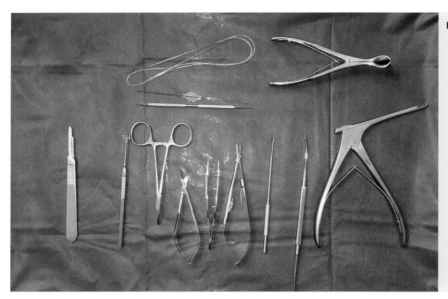

Fig. 2.3 Lacrimal instruments.

Table 2.1 Dissolvable suture

Suture material	Duration of tensile strength	Filament type	Tissue reaction	Uses
Plain gut	7–10 d	Monofilament	Mild	Skin
Fast absorbing plain gut	5–7 d	Monofilament	Mild	Skin
Chromic gut	10–14 d	Monofilament	Mild	Skin
Polyglycolic acid (Vicryl, Dexon, Polysorb)	14 d	Braided	Mild	Buried, skin
Polydioxanone (PDS)	14 d	Monofilament	Minimal	Buried
Polytrimethylene (Maxon)	14 d	Monofilament	Minimal	Buried

monopolar is unsafe. Fine jeweler-tipped handpieces are available for bipolar electrocautery. Fire risk exists for all forms of cautery, especially for monopolar cautery or battery-operated cautery; hence, supplemental oxygen must be turned off and flammable materials held at a distance.

2.5 Suture and Needles

The first component of suture selection is the suture material. One must consider the desired duration, and risk for inflammatory reaction and microbial infection. Absorbable suture is degraded more rapidly by the body, while nonabsorbable suture remains in place and holds tension for longer. With absorbable suture use, there is no need for suture removal, which is a benefit in children and patients who may be lost to follow-up. These sutures support the wound during initial tissue remodeling and then are broken down by enzymatic degradation. The suture's tensile strength is gone before the suture material is completely degraded. Commonly used absorbable sutures are listed in ▶ Table 2.1.

Nonabsorbable or "permanent" sutures are more resistant to degradation and are often less inflammatory. This may be advantageous in certain patients to prevent hypertrophic scarring. In such patients, permanent suture can be used to close skin and removed at 5 to 7 days postoperatively. Sutures in the eyelid margin are left in place for 10 to 14 days to ensure full healing. Commonly used nonabsorbable sutures are listed in ▶ Table 2.2.

2.5.1 Suture Size

The diameter of the selected suture material should increase as the skin thickness increases.
- Thin eyelid skin is closed with 6–0 suture.
- Larger suture such as 4–0 or 5–0 suture is used for thicker glabellar, brow, or cheek skin.
- Finer 7–0 suture may be used in the eyelid margin or at the lash line.

2.5.2 Needle Selection

The choice of needle type depends on the tissue in which it will be used (▶ Fig. 2.4).
- Cutting or reverse cutting needles: pass easily and atraumatically through tissue. Excellent for closing skin or buried sutures.
- Spatulated needles: allow partial thickness passes through dense tissue such as the tarsus or sclera. The flat bottom surface of the needle reduces the risk of perforating the structure below the needle path.
- Tapered needles: only cut at the point and displace but do not cut with the rounded body. Hence, they cause minimal

Table 2.2 Permanent suture

Suture material	Filament type	Tissue reaction	Elasticity	Uses
Silk	Braided	Minimal reaction	None	Lid margin, vascular ties
Polyamide (Nylon)	Monofilament	Nonreactive	Minimal stretch	Skin
Polypropylene (Prolene)	Monofilament	Nonreactive	Moderate stretch	Skin, tarsal strip
Polyester (Dacron, Mersilene)	Braided or monofilament	Minimal reaction, encapsulated	Minimal stretch	Tarsal strip
Steel	Monofilament	Nonreactive	None	Transnasal wiring

trauma as they pass through tissue; however, there is significant drag on the tissue being sutured, making passage more difficult than with a cutting needle.

- Moderately curved needles (1/4 circle or 3/8 circle curvature): commonly used to suture skin or tarsus.
- Highly curved (1/2 circle): useful for small, difficult to access spaces or for buried sutures.

2.6 Periorbital Surgical Technique

Planned incisions are best marked prior to injecting local anesthetic because this can distort anatomy. Skin incisions are best created with a scalpel. When using a scalpel, the blade handle is held like a pencil with the blade perpendicular to the skin. Occasionally, the incision is intentionally beveled, for instance, to preserve hair follicles. Prior to incising, the skin is held tautly. The tip of the blade begins the incision, the belly of the blade is used to create the incision, and the blade tip is used to precisely complete the incision. The incision should be one smooth movement and incise through the dermis, allowing the wound edges to separate.

Delicate handling of tissue is very important in the periorbital area. This is accomplished by efficient, precise surgery. Iatrogenic tissue trauma can affect healing, cosmesis, the condition of specimens, and cause tissue edema and distortion.[2] Tissue should be grasped with the minimum force necessary to prevent crush injury and ideally not regrasped. Grasping across the eyelid margin may cause notching of the margin. Cautery should be used conservatively to maintain hemostasis but not cause unnecessary charring or shrinkage of tissue.

Wound closure in the periorbital area is primarily performed with sutures. Simple, shallow, nonmarginal wounds under minimal tension may be closed with cyanoacrylate tissue adhesive. In cases of small, cutaneous defects that are in locations not likely to induce traction on the eyelids, the wound may be allowed to heal by secondary intention. Scarring is minimized if the skin edges of a wound are apposed with no intervening foreign bodies or granulation tissue. Granulation tissue can be debrided or excised with fine scissors or scraping the wound edges with a scalpel.

2.6.1 Suturing

Precise placement of cutaneous sutures is important for wound healing and cosmesis and is important to the patient because it is the part of the surgery that they will scrutinize. Forceps are used to stabilize tissue immediately adjacent to the point of suture entry. The needle enters perpendicular to the skin.

Delicate movements of the fingers and wrist allow the needle to remain perpendicular as it passes through tissue. Minimal force is required if the surgeon follows the curvature of the needle. Skin sutures should result in slight eversion of the wound edges, which will flatten as the wound contracts. In addition, skin sutures are tightened enough to bring the wound edges together but not so much that the skin is compressed into irregular waves or strangulated.

- Interrupted suture: a simple, looped trapezoid. Tightening the suture causes mild skin eversion. Useful for skin closure with minimal or no tension. Good for irregular wounds (▶ Fig. 2.5a).
- Vertical mattress suture: Induces more eversion than simple interrupted sutures. Two layers of sutures evert the deeper and more superficial tissue (▶ Fig. 2.5b).
- Horizontal mattress suture: May be buried to close deep tissue planes. A partially buried horizontal mattress suture can be used for corners, and is useful to secure tarsus to the periosteum of the lateral orbital rim (▶ Fig. 2.5c).
- Continuous (running) sutures: Used to efficiently close regularly shaped wounds under minimal or no tension (▶ Fig. 2.5d).
- Continuous locking suture: Efficient method of closure for minimal wound tension (▶ Fig. 2.5e).

2.6.2 Principles of Skin Closure

The approach to closing skin incisions, wounds, or skin defects of the periorbita may be thought of as a hierarchy of techniques with not only increasing defect coverage but also increasing morbidity.

- Healing by secondary intention: Acceptable for small periorbital skin defects that are unlikely to induce retraction of the eyelids, such as those located in the medial canthus.
- Primary closure of a skin defect: Useful for incisions or skin defects with minimal tension and without vertical tension on the eyelid. Tension must be oriented horizontal to the eyelid, along the relaxed skin tension lines (a vertical line of closure) to prevent eyelid retraction.[3] Elliptical incisions with a ratio of 1:3 or 1:4 are optimal for closure.[2] Skin defects may be converted to an ellipse for primary closure by various methods. Undermining of the tissue edges facilitates direct closure.
- Skin flaps: Useful for closing larger skin defects or to control the orientation of the resulting scar. Descriptions of various flaps used in the periorbital area are discussed in subsequent chapters.
- Full-thickness skin grafting is useful in a variety of ocular adnexal procedures, including eyelid reconstruction, repair of

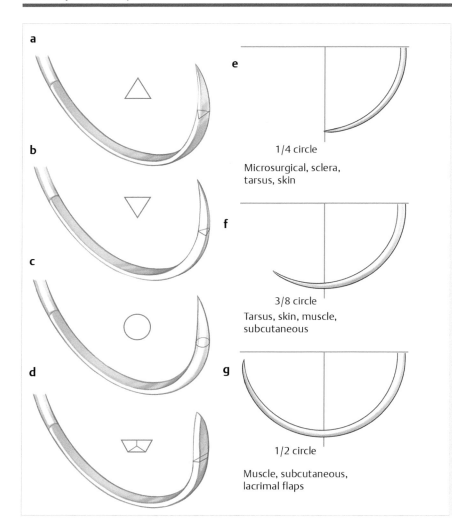

Fig. 2.4 (a–g) Needle styles used in ophthalmic plastic surgery.

1/4 circle

Microsurgical, sclera, tarsus, skin

3/8 circle

Tarsus, skin, muscle, subcutaneous

1/2 circle

Muscle, subcutaneous, lacrimal flaps

cicatricial lower eyelid retraction, and scar revision. A donor site is chosen that is similar in appearance to the recipient area. For eyelid skin, common donor sites include ipsilateral or contralateral upper eyelid skin, preauricular and retro-auricular skin, or supra-clavicular skin.

- Partial-thickness skin grafting is sometimes used in the periocular area in the treatment of burns or to line the exenterated socket. This procedure involves using a dermatome to harvest a split-thickness skin graft.

2.6.3 Tips and Pearls

- Excising dog ears: When there is a mismatch of skin length on either side of an incision, the result is an unsightly standing cone deformity or dog ear. To excise the skin, the redundant skin is held tautly above the incision and the line

of the incision is extended, then the remaining skin is folded over the incision and truncated (▶ Fig. 2.6).
- Relaxed skin tension lines: Understanding the natural skin lines created by the muscles of facial expression allows the surgeon to maximize concealment of scars. For example, the eyelid crease is often utilized to place an incision for access to the deeper structures or to harvest a flap (▶ Fig. 2.7).
- Full-thickness skin grafts are measured and marked based on the skin defect prior to harvesting. Suturing into the recipient bed is best initiated with cardinal interrupted sutures to align the graft correctly in the bed and distribute tension equally. Interrupted sutures are then placed to close the skin. A bolster or pressure dressing is used to maintain good contact between the graft and donor bed for several days to allow for diffusion of oxygen.

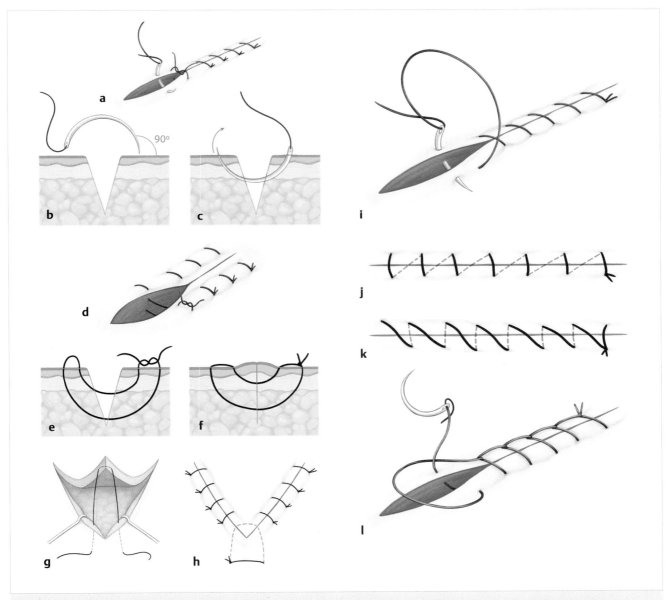

Fig. 2.5 (a–c) Simple interrupted suture, (d–f) vertical mattress suture, (g,h) partially buried horizontal mattress, (i–k) continuous suture, (l) continuous locking suture.

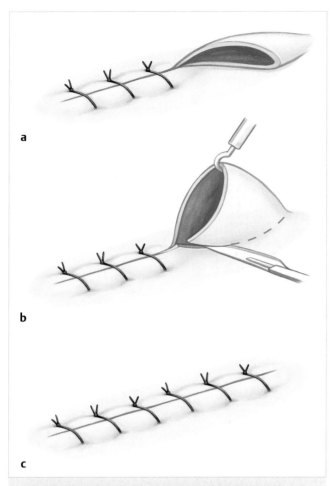

Fig. 2.6 (a–c) Excision of a standing cone deformity (dog ear).

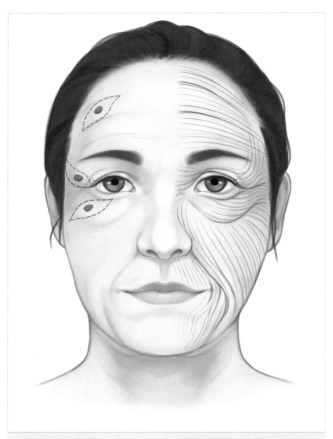

Fig. 2.7 Taking advantage of relaxed skin tension lines allows concealment of incisions.

References

[1] Lee EW, Holtebeck AC, Harrison AR. Infection rates in outpatient eyelid surgery. Ophthal Plast Reconstr Surg. 2009; 25(2):109–110

[2] McCord C, Tanenbaum M, Nunery W, eds. Oculoplastic Surgery. 3rd ed. New York, NY: Raven Press; 1995

[3] Lelli GJ, Zoumalan C, Nesi F. Basic principles of ophthalmic plastic surgery. In: Black E, Nesi F, Calvano C, Gladstone G, Levine M, eds. Smith and Nesi's Ophthalmic Plastic and Reconstructive Surgery. New York, NY: Springer; 2012:61–79

Part II

Eyelid Trauma

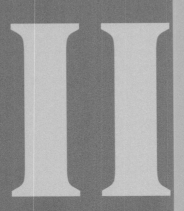

II

3 Traumatic Eyelid Laceration

Pete Setabutr and Chau Pham

Summary

Traumatic eyelid lacerations are a common condition seen by just about every ophthalmologist, plastic surgeon, and emergency room physician. Despite the fact that each case is unique and the severity of injury is varied, a thorough understanding of anatomy and consideration of a few basic principles can help maximize outcomes. This chapter will review some essential steps in the evaluation and treatment of eyelid lacerations.

Keywords: trauma, eyelid laceration, eyelid repair, ocular trauma, periocular trauma, foreign bodies

3.1 Goals

- Anatomical repair resulting in maximum aesthetic and functional outcome.[1]
- Eyelids that adequately protect the eye, lubricate the cornea, and allow for optimal vision.
- Creation of a stable eyelid margin, adequate vertical eyelid height, adequate eyelid closure, and development of an epithelized internal surface.
- Cosmesis and symmetry.

3.2 Advantages

Primary repair of traumatic eyelid lacerations as close to the time of initial injury as possible can optimize results. Increased blood flow, release of cytokines, and interruption of normal lymphatic drainage channels lead to post-traumatic edema that makes tissue planes difficult to identify and closure more challenging. Delay of repair until after formation of scar and granulation tissue has begun can likewise result in unsatisfactory closure. Should other circumstances preclude immediate intervention however, delayed repair may result in increased complications.[2] In such instances, the area should be cleaned, kept lubricated with ointment, and covered with a loose non-stick dressing.

3.3 Expectations

- Eyelids that protect the globe, lubricate the cornea, and do not obstruct vision.
- An aesthetically favorable result.

3.4 Key Principles

No two traumatic eyelid lacerations are the same and the severity can vary widely. Several key principles in the approach to all traumatic eyelid lacerations can be utilized, and adherence to these principles can go a long way to maximizing outcomes. Life-threatening injuries should be ruled out and the patient should be stabilized prior to addressing ocular and adnexal injuries. Ocular injuries should be assessed and eyelid repair should be deferred in the setting of open globe injuries. Fractures, if operative, should be repaired prior to soft tissue repair. To avoid complications related to cicatricial lagophthalmos, the tension of closure should be horizontal and vertical traction should be minimized. Anatomical canthal fixation should be maintained when possible. When used, free grafts cannot be utilized for both anterior and posterior lamella. Canalicular repair should be attempted when it is reasonable to avoid epiphora in the future. Traumatic canalicular lacerations are often associated with medial canthal tendon injury, and bicanalicular silastic intubation in this setting can reinforce anatomical canthal fixation. A consideration in the pediatric population is the potential for amblyopia—young children with damage to the levator and resultant ptosis should be monitored for development of amblyopia.

3.5 Indications

- Eyelid lacerations in a systemically stable patient.

3.6 Contraindications

- Intraocular injury.
- Cardiopulmonary or neurologic instability.
- Other grave bodily injuries requiring more urgent repair.
- Lack of equipment or facilities to properly carry out the repair.

3.7 Preoperative Preparation

Prior to surgical repair of an eyelid laceration, a thorough systemic and ocular exam should be performed. Grave cardiopulmonary and neurologic injuries should be stabilized prior to repair of ocular and adnexal tissues. An accurate history including timing and nature of the injury should be obtained. Care should be taken to illicit information that may suggest foreign bodies, chemicals, or animal bites. If there is an animal bite, the rabies vaccination status of the animal should be determined.[3,4] If a foreign body is suspected, radiographic imaging with plain films, CT, or MRI should be obtained. Suspicion for an intraorbital or intraocular foreign body should be suspected by the presence of free air.[5] Questions aimed at differentiating between blunt and penetrating injuries should be asked.

Next, evaluation of the face looking for evidence of foreign bodies, missing tissue, or penetrating wounds is performed. Proper visualization of the full extent of wounds is often difficult due to obscuration by blood, debris, or hair as well as patient tolerance.[3] Gentle cleaning with sterile saline should be carried out and patient tolerance can be aided by light sedation or local infiltrative anesthesia.

A complete ocular exam, including a dilated fundus exam is required. Ruptured globes, hyphema, angle recession, and retinal detachments have all been associated with eyelid trauma. If a ruptured globe is present, all repairs of the eyelids should be

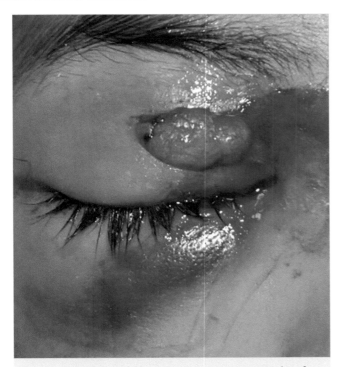

Fig. 3.1 Right upper eyelid laceration in a young patient resulting from a sharp penetrating injury. The prolapsed orbital fat signals that the orbital septum has been breached and there should be concern for deeper orbital or globe injury or possible orbital foreign body. Courtesy of Michael K Yoon, MD.

anticipated length of time needed, whether cardiopulmonary monitoring would be required, what sort of anesthesia might be required, and will there be adequate space, lighting, tools, and instrumentation available to accomplish the repair. Understanding and anticipating these factors can aid in the choice to perform the repair at bedside in the Emergency Department or inpatient floor, the procedure room, or in the operating room.

Once the decision on the timing and location of repair is made, consent should be obtained from the patient, next of kin, or individual with power of attorney, and communication and coordination with any other medical team should proceed.

3.8 Operative Technique

The general approach to eyelid laceration repair is to ensure good approximation of wound edges (without step-off of the two edges of the wound) and minimize tension on the wound to limit wound contractures that can lead to eyelid malposition. Contaminated wounds should be irrigated and sterile technique should be employed when possible to minimize risks of postoperative infection. If wounds are deep and they are located away from the thin layers of the upper and lower eyelid (e.g., above the brow or lateral to the lateral canthus), deep buried sutures can eliminate dead-space and reduce tension on superficial closures. When needed, undermining of the dermal layer can relieve wound tension and aid in skin closure.[4] Wound edge eversion and use of atraumatic tissue handling technique can minimize scar formation. If good follow-up is ensured, use of non-absorbable sutures may be less inflammatory and can potentially further minimize scar formation and maximize aesthetic results.

Small wounds or abrasions that do not involve exposure of vital structures such as orbicularis or septum, and are not in a location where scar formation may interfere with eyelid function or cosmesis may be left to heal by secondary intention. Application of ophthalmic antibiotic ointment and application of non-stick dressings may be all that is required.[3]

For simple, superficial non-margin involving lacerations of the upper and lower eyelids without missing tissue, simple closure of the superficial tissue using non-absorbable suture is often all that is needed. Simple interrupted sutures may be used (and are preferred in pediatric patients where eye rubbing may result in broken sutures); however, horizontal or vertical mattress sutures may be employed if the wound is under tension. The approach to repairing irregular lacerations can begin with approximation of key anatomical landmarks—brow hair, eyelashes, and natural eyelid creases can be observed and used as key points of initial fixation followed by repair of the remaining wound.[4] Taking care to direct the tension of closure horizontally rather than vertically will prevent cicatricial ectropion in the lower eyelid, and lagophthalmos of the upper eyelid.[1,3,4,8,9] The use of non-absorbable monofilament suture can minimize inflammation and help mitigate scar formation; however, the ability of the patient to follow up for suture removal should be considered in choice of material.

For deep lacerations, thorough exploration with removal and debridement of any foreign materials followed by irrigation with sterile saline is essential. Prolapsed fat is suggestive of

deferred and manipulation of the surrounding periorbital tissue discontinued.[1,3,4]

Thorough evaluation of the eyelids noting lacerations, tissue avulsion, foreign bodies, ecchymosis, and abrasions can be performed once the globe has been identified as stable. The presence of orbital fat may suggest a deep injury with potential trauma to the levator muscle (Fig. 3.1). In such cases, a traumatic ptosis may be present.[4] Medial eyelid injuries and dog-bite injuries (in children in particular) can be associated with injury to the lacrimal system and canalicular probing/irrigation should be performed to ascertain the extent of injury.[6] Though the lower canaliculus is most commonly involved, simultaneous globe injury has been found to be more common with upper canalicular involvement.[7] Rounding of the canthal angles or shortening of the palpebral fissure suggests canthal tendon injury or avulsion.[1] Assessment of the integrity of the medial and/or lateral orbital walls should be carried out and fractures should be repaired, if necessary, prior to canthal reconstruction.[8]

Debridement of all foreign materials should be carried out to maximize wound healing and minimize infection and inflammation. Due to the excellent blood supply of the eyelids, often little to no debridement of eyelid tissue is necessary, and even damaged or avulsed tissue may be viable.[4] Thorough irrigation using sterile saline should be carried out for all contaminated wounds or noncontaminated wounds more than 6 hours old.[3]

Once a complete examination of the injury has been performed, attention should be turned to deciding the optimal timing and setting for the repair. Factors to consider include the violation of the orbital septum and possible injury of the levator muscle.[1,4] If the levator is found to be damaged, repair should proceed at the time of initial surgery. Incorporation of orbital septum into the laceration repair should be avoided and laceration of the septum should not be sutured.[1,3,4,8,9] Fig. 3.2 and Fig. 3.3 demonstrate eylid lacerations pre- and post repair.

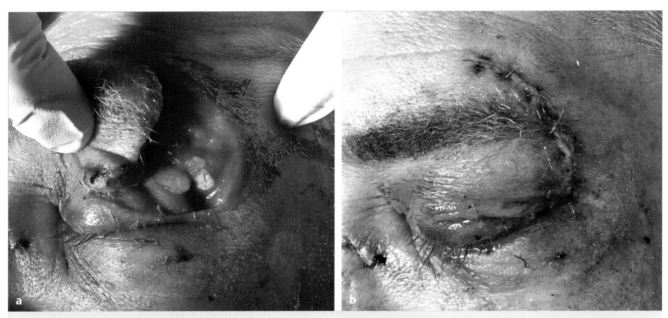

Fig. 3.2 (a) Left upper eyelid crease laceration extends superior to involve the lateral eyebrow and extends deep to bone. (b) After repair, the lid crease has been reformed with careful sutured closure, the eyebrow cilia are properly realigned and the wound edges everted for optimal healing. Courtesy of Natalie Wolkow, MD, PhD.

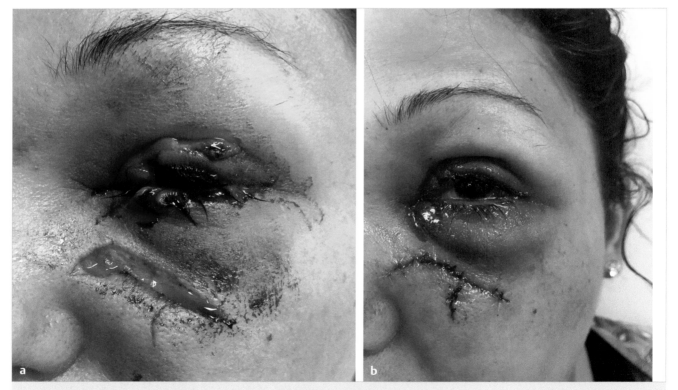

Fig. 3.3 (a) Left eyelid lacerations involving upper and lower lids including margins as well as left lower lid and cheek, where the wound is beveled and involves the skin, subcutaneous tissue and malar fat pad. (b) After repair, the lid margins are well aligned and the lower lid and cheek laceration is closed with a layer of deep followed by cutaneous interrupted sutures. There is excellent apposition of the wound edges and no downward traction on the lower eyelid margin. Courtesy of Victoria Starks, MD.

3.9 Tips and Pearls

- Use of small-caliber sutures with early removal can lower the risk of unnecessary scarring.
- Find and use anatomical landmarks to help ascertain where tissue needs to go. A temporary suture can be placed to aid in repair then removed and replaced as the tissues begin to come together.
- Other than with animal bites, tissue is rarely missing.
- When working in the brow area, noting the direction of hair growth can help identify the correct placement of tissues.
- It's ok to cut out sutures and start over!

3.10 What to Avoid

Common mistakes in the repair of traumatic eyelid laceration often occur due to improper preoperative assessment or due to improper wound closure technique. Failure to recognize grave systemic injury or globe injury can result in significant morbidity and mortality. The failure to recognize and remove foreign bodies, or to recognize and repair specialized adnexal structures can result in significant postoperative complications and increase the likelihood of the need for further surgical intervention.[9] Suturing of the orbital septum may result in lagophthalmos and tethering of the eyelid to the orbital rim. Excessive or inappropriate tissue handling, overutilization of cautery, non-anatomic re-approximation of tissues, suture tension that is too tight or too loose, or improper eversion of wound edges may lead to poor aesthetic and functional outcomes.[1,4,9] Improper timing of suture removal may lead to wound dehiscence if too early and formation of epithelialized suture tracts or inclusion cysts if too late.[8]

3.11 Complications/Bailout/Salvage

- Nonadherence to the principles of wound repair can yield eyelid deformities which maximize risk for ocular irritation, dryness, and ultimately, permanent damage.
- Eyelid retraction and lagophthalmos from fixation of orbital septum may result in exposure keratopathy. Ocular irritation and exposure may be managed medically with topical lubrication; however, more severe cases may need secondary surgical repair to correct.
- Improper fixation of the eyelid margin may cause trichiasis and resultant corneal irritation and injury—epilation, cryotherapy, laser ablation, or eyelid margin repositioning are all options for management of this complication.[1,4,8]
- Preoperative identification of injury to specialized adnexal tissue and subsequent repair of these tissues may avoid eyelid or punctal malposition, palpebral fissure shortening, rounding of the canthal angles, or epiphora.
- Improper repair of posterior lamellae prevents proper re-epithelialization and may result in subsequent symblepharon formation.
- Traumatic ptosis of myogenic origin may be avoided by identification and repair of a damaged levator at the time of initial surgery. Residual ptosis should be observed for 6 to 12 months for spontaneous resolution before secondary repair is undertaken.[1,4]
- Improper adherence to the principles of wound repair may lead to complications such as unacceptable scarring and poor cosmesis. Scarring may resolve spontaneously over time; alternatively, intralesional steroid injection or application of laser may be applied.[4]
- Avoidance of complications is best accomplished by proper preoperative evaluation, planning, and adherence to proper suturing techniques.

3.12 Postoperative Care

Assessment should focus on signs of infection, excessive scar tissue, cicatricial changes, and unwanted eyelid malposition. Furthermore, postoperative care of the traumatic eyelid laceration often occurs simultaneously with other ocular injuries incurred (e.g., lens dislocations, hyphema, traumatic iritis). Therefore, a multidisciplinary approach is often needed.

Tetanus vaccination status should be ascertained and updated. Due to the excellent vascular supply of the eyelid, wounds typically heal very well with low risk of infection. Often a topical broad-spectrum antibiotic formulated for ophthalmic use is adequate to prevent wound infection and ocular surface irritation. Systemic antibiotics should be considered when the patient is immunocompromised, diabetic, or a smoker (owing to poor microvascular supply). Animal bites and deep puncture wounds (particularly those with vegetable matter) are more likely to be contaminated and are at high risk for infection. Systemic antibiotics should be used in these instances.[3,4] Broad-spectrum antibiotics such as amoxicillin-clavulanate are often employed; however, local resistance patterns, the patient's MRSA (methicillin-resistant *Staphylococcus aureus*) risk factors, and the severity of the injury should be considered.

Removal of non-absorbable suture should occur in a timely manner (ideally within 7 days) to prevent epithelialization of the suture tract and possible foreign body reaction, sterile abscess, or scarring.[10]

Hypertrophic scars can form and may take up to a year to mature. Minor scarring often resolves in time without intervention and patients can be instructed to perform massage or use UV-blocking creams to prevent progression. Once scars form, treatments include silicone gel sheeting, intralesional injections of corticosteroids, interferon, 5-fluorouracil, or dermal radiofrequency. Surgical excision is warranted when contractures result in loss of function or ocular compromise.[10]

References

[1] Foster JA, Carter KD, Durairaj VD, et al. Classifications and management of eyelid disorders: Eyelid Trauma. In: Cantor LB, Rapuano CJ, Cioffi GA, eds. Basic and Clinical Science Course (BCSC) Section 7: Orbit, Eyelids, and Lacrimal System. San Francisco, CA: American Academy of Ophthalmology; 2017:187–196

[2] Chiang E, Bee C, Harris GJ, Wells TS. Does delayed repair of eyelid lacerations compromise outcome? Am J Emerg Med. 2017; 35(11):1766–1767

[3] Ko AC, Satterfield KR, Korn BS, Kikkawa DO. Eyelid and periorbital soft tissue trauma. Facial Plast Surg Clin North Am. 2017; 25(4):605–616

[4] Nelson CC. Management of eyelid trauma. Aust N Z J Ophthalmol. 1991; 19 (4):357–363

[5] Lustrin ES, Brown JH, Novelline R, Weber AL. Radiologic assessment of trauma and foreign bodies of the eye and orbit. Neuroimaging Clin N Am. 1996; 6(1): 219–237

[6] Sadiq MA, Corkin F, Mantagos IS. Eyelid lacerations due to dog bite in children. J Pediatr Ophthalmol Strabismus. 2015; 52(6):360–363

[7] Naik MN, Kelapure A, Rath S, Honavar SG. Management of canalicular lacerations: epidemiological aspects and experience with Mini-Monoka monocanalicular stent. Am J Ophthalmol. 2008; 145(2):375–380

[8] Uzcategui N. Eyelid lacerations and acute adnexal trauma. In: Yen MT ed. Surgery of the Eyelids, Lacrimal System, and Orbit. New York, NY: Oxford University Press; 2012:3–14

[9] Kronish JW. Eyelid reconstruction. In: Tse DT, Wright KW, eds. Oculoplastic Surgery. Philadelphia, PA: J.B. Lippincott Company; 1992:245–294

[10] Rabello FB, Souza CD, Farina Júnior JA. Update on hypertrophic scar treatment. Clinics (São Paulo). 2014; 69(8):565–573

4 Eyelid Margin Laceration Repair

Neil Shah and Peter W. MacIntosh

Summary

A margin-involving eyelid laceration requires special attention to prevent postrepair complications such as eyelid notching and trichiasis. In this chapter, we will review the important techniques to successfully repair margin-involving eyelid lacerations.

Keywords: eyelid margin, everting suture, tarsus, cornea

4.1 Goals

- Become comfortable with the basics of repairing an eyelid margin laceration.
- Understand the possible complications of eyelid laceration repair and how to prevent them.

4.2 Advantages

A thoughtful and well-planned approach will provide the patient with the most optimal functional and aesthetic outcome.

4.3 Expectations

- Learn the steps to reapproximate the eyelid margin.
- Learn how to avoid postoperative complications.

4.4 Key Principles

The most important initial step in any eyelid injury is to ensure that any other head and systemic injuries have been addressed. Next, ensure the integrity of the globe, and address any open globe repair before eyelid repair. Under most circumstances, primary eyelid laceration repair is preferable to delayed repair.

Missing tissue is rare after eyelid margin laceration. As a result, tissue rearrangement and skin grafting are typically not needed for most eyelid margin laceration repairs, and these techniques will not be discussed in this chapter.

4.5 Indications

- Full-thickness upper or lower eyelid margin lacerations.

4.6 Contraindications

- Eyelid laceration with tissue missing/excessive tension.

4.7 Preoperative Preparation

Preoperatively, several factors should be taken into consideration in order to achieve an optimal outcome. This includes the size and orientation of the eyelid margin laceration, surrounding vascular supply, age of the patient, prior eyelid repair surgery, age of the wound, and any history of radiation therapy, all of which may affect healing.

When eyelid margin defects are associated with trauma, the first priority is to assess for and stabilize any concomitant life-threatening injuries. Once stabilized, a complete history, with special attention to the mechanism of injury should be taken. Any history of projectile objects, gunshots, and penetrating foreign bodies such as a pencil or tree branch should raise suspicion for a retained foreign body. In cases of severe head trauma, it is also essential to obtain imaging, typically a computed tomography (CT) scan of the head and orbits to assess for intracranial hemorrhage and craniofacial bony fractures.

These evaluations should be followed by a complete eye exam to evaluate for globe perforation, and retinal and optic nerve injuries. Fat prolapse from the wound suggests a deep laceration, and in the upper eyelid, damage to the levator aponeurosis or muscle should be suspected. All wounds should be thoroughly explored and irrigated to evaluate their extent and to ensure no retained foreign body, especially vegetative debris. The edges of traumatic eyelid lacerations are often jagged and irregular, but usually tissue is not missing. Efforts should be made to preserve all eyelid tissue, but if necrosis is present, then cautious debridement is important before reconstruction can begin. Primary repair undertaken within the first 24 hours of injury can usually prevent necrosis and tissue loss.

If a medial upper or lower eyelid laceration is present, the surgeon must rule out canalicular involvement (see section on canalicular repair).

Prophylactic antibiotic use is controversial; however, most surgeons agree that they should be given perioperatively in heavily contaminated wounds, especially in cases of a human or animal bite. First-generation cephalosporins will typically cover against skin originating methicillin-sensitive *Staphylococcus aureus* and other gram-positive species. For animal/human bites, amoxicillin-clavulanate is the first-line antibiotic and for immunosuppressed patient, broader spectrum agents may also be considered.[1]

Tetanus prophylaxis is required if not given in the last 5 years or if it is unknown when last given. It is also important to note time of last meal, as this may affect the timing of surgical repair, especially in a patient who requires general anesthesia (children and uncooperative patients)—for which, usually no oral intake for the prior 8 hours is required. Animal bites should be reported according to local protocol.[2]

Timing of eyelid laceration repair is very important to achieve the best cosmetic outcome. Though there exists some variability among surgeons on the absolute latest an eyelid laceration can be repaired, in general these should be closed as quickly as possible, ideally within 24 hours of injury. Given that many of these lacerations will present in the setting of trauma, management of life-threatening emergencies will always take precedence. In these situations, every attempt should be made to repair the eyelid laceration within 48 to 72 hours. Maintaining the integrity of the tissue with antibiotic ointment and wet dressing is important if there will be a delay in surgical repair.

4.8 Operative Technique

4.8.1 Anesthesia

Apply a drop of topical anesthetic (e.g., tetracaine or proparacaine) in both eyes. Inject local anesthetic with epinephrine subcutaneously and into the wound. Regional nerve blocks may also be employed, as these may minimize the need for local anesthetics that can distort the eyelid structures.

4.8.2 Upper and Lower Eyelid Lacerations, Not Involving the Medial or Lateral Canthi

Place a corneal protective shield. Manually reapproximate the eyelid margin to assess tension and position. Focus on aligning the posterior lamella first. Use 6–0 or 7–0 polyglactin suture. Alternatively, silk sutures may be used; however, these are not dissolvable. Place a vertical mattress suture at the posterior eyelid margin by passing it through the meibomian gland orifices to align and evert the wound edges (▶ Fig. 4.1). Cinch the sutures together to approximate the wound edges and assess for eversion and alignment, but do not tie it yet. Leave the suture tails long. Using up to three interrupted 6–0 polyglactin sutures, reapproximate the non-marginal tarsal plate (▶ Fig. 4.2). If the full height of the central tarsus is lacerated in the upper eyelid, typically three sutures are used to reapproximate and support the full height of tarsus. If the laceration is more medial or temporal or in the lower eyelid, only one or two sutures may be needed, as the tarsus tapers and may be several millimeters shorter than the central, upper eyelid tarsus. These sutures should be partial thickness passes and stay in the anterior layer of tarsus to avoid the sutures abrading the underlying

cornea. Tie the vertical mattress suture previously placed at the posterior eyelid margin. Place a 6–0 or 7–0 polyglactin suture at or just anterior to the gray line to realign the eyelashes and provide further eversion of the lid margin (▶ Fig. 4.3). This may also be placed as a vertical mattress suture. Leave the suture tails long.

Alignment of the eyelid is key regardless of what type of suture you use. If there is any concern about poor approximation, use a third suture at the eyelash line to help line it up, or replace the posterior or gray line sutures. Close the skin with the leftover polyglactin or silk suture in a simple interrupted fashion. Start with the first suture close to the eyelid margin and work away from it by first passing the suture and tying one knot. Fold the tails of the previously placed margin sutures over the knot, and tie two more knots to secure them (▶ Fig. 4.4). This will keep the tails and knots of the margin sutures away from the cornea. If at this point, the wound seems under tension, consider using the leftover polyglactin suture to approximate the deeper orbicularis muscle before closing skin.

Eyelid margin sutures should be left in place for 7 to 10 days, and then removed regardless of the suture type used. However, if you suspect a patient may not or cannot return for suture removal, polyglactin sutures should be used since they are dissolvable and will eventually fall out on their own. Silk sutures must be removed.

4.8.3 Upper and Lower Eyelid Lacerations, Involving the Lateral Canthus

Inject local anesthetic with epinephrine into the lacerated skin and the lateral canthal skin and muscle. If a stump of the lateral canthal tendon can be identified at the lateral orbital rim and

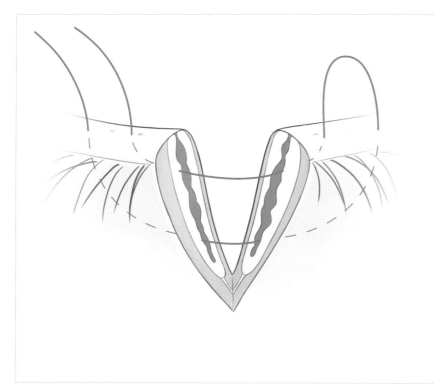

Fig. 4.1 Precise vertical alignment of the edges of the tarsus is key to a successful repair using 6–0/7–0 polyglactin suture through the meibomian gland orifices. Suture tails are left long.

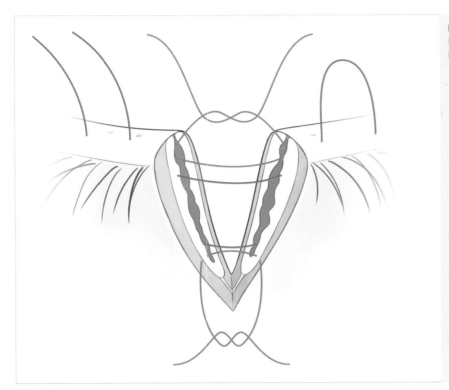

Fig. 4.2 Non-marginal tarsal plate is reapproximated using interrupted 6–0 polyglactin sutures with partial thickness passes.

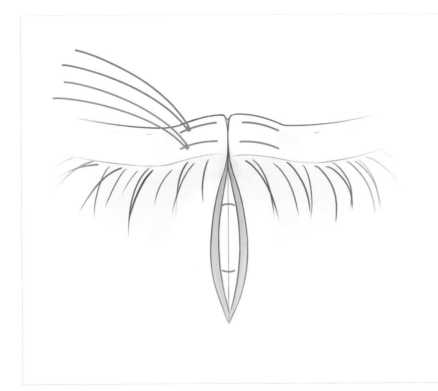

Fig. 4.3 Vertical mattress suture is passed through the anterior lamella along the eyelid margin to realign the eyelashes. Suture tails are left long.

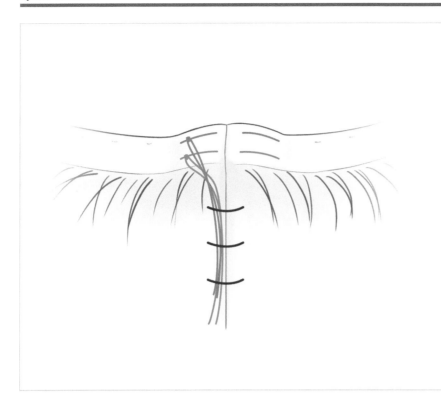

Fig. 4.4 Skin is closed in a simple interrupted fashion incorporating margin suture tails.

grasped, it can be sutured to the lateral edge of the avulsed eyelid tarsus with two or three simple interrupted 4–0 or 5–0 polyglactin sutures. Since this location is distant from the cornea, special wound everting sutures may not be required. The skin can then be closed with fast absorbing gut suture.

If the lateral canthal tendon has been completely avulsed from the lateral orbital rim, it can be sutured to the periosteum at Whitnall's tubercle with mattress 4–0 or 5–0 polyglactin or polypropylene suture. If the lateral canthal tendon cannot be identified, a lateral tarsal strip may need to be fashioned from the remaining tarsus and sutured to the periosteum overlying Whitnall tubercle. See descriptions for lateral tarsal strip in separate section. If the lateral canthal angle skin has been lacerated, place a cerclage 6–0 polyglactin suture to reestablish the sharp canthal angle. Close the skin over the tarsus with interrupted fast-absorbing gut sutures.

4.9 Tips and Pearls

1. The architecture of the medial eyelid makes it very susceptible to traumatic laceration and avulsion. In any eyelid laceration, even if there is no obvious injury to the medial eyelid, be sure to formally check this area for laceration and avulsion.
2. When placing the posterior marginal vertical mattress suture, try to position the knot on the side of the wound farthest from the cornea to reduce the risk of abrasion, should the knot rotate posteriorly. This may be a moot point if the eyelid laceration lines up with the center of the cornea.
3. When reapproximating the nonmarginal tarsus, use a spatulated needle. As described earlier, the tarsus is only

1 mm thick, so a spatulated needle will make passing the suture through this thin structure much easier. You can use a spatulated needle for the eyelid margin as well, reusing the same needle and suture.
4. Close the eyelid skin with the same suture used to close the eyelid margin. This saves expense since you are not using additional sutures, and will ensure that the sutures hold the tails of the eyelid margin sutures for as long as you need them to. Catgut or plain gut sutures may dissolve or break before you want them to.

4.10 What to Avoid

1. **Missing a full-thickness laceration:** When an eyelid laceration appears small, or to just involve the skin, be sure to evert the eyelid to fully evaluate for a full thickness laceration.
2. **Damaging tarsus:** Be careful when holding and manipulating the tarsus. Avoid holding the tarsus with fine forceps that can lacerate it if too much pressure is applied. Instead, hold the eyelid by the skin, or use the Adson forceps with teeth or Von Graefe lid fixation forceps.
3. **Polypropylene sutures:** This suture material is more rigid than polyglactin or silk and has internal "memory." These characteristics prevent it from folding flat and away from the cornea as easily as polyglactin and silk sutures do. Using polypropylene suture would increase the risk of corneal abrasion. An exception to this rule is use to reapproximate an avulsed lateral canthal tendon, where the suture will not be used at the eyelid margin.

4. **Removing the sutures too early:** Sutures in many other parts of the face are often removed after as little as 3 to 5 days due to its excellent vascularity and healing properties. However, the eyelid margin requires more time due to the tension on the eyelid that may pull the wound apart or result in eyelid notching if the suture is removed too early.

4.11 Complications/Bailout/Salvage

1. **Corneal abrasion:** If the posterior eyelid margin or tarsal sutures are not tied anteriorly, they may abrade the cornea. The placement of each suture must be diligently checked at the time of suture placement, and it should be replaced if it appears to be too posterior.
   Management: If an abrasion from the suture is noticed at a postoperative visit, a bandage contact lens may be placed with antibiotic eye drops to protect the cornea until the sutures are removed. If a contact lens is not appropriate, the suture may have to be removed, with the risk of eyelid notching if it cannot be replaced.

2. **Eyelid notching:** If the posterior eyelid margin is not adequately approximated and everted, a notch may develop.
   Management: Small notches that do not result in exposure keratitis, and are cosmetically acceptable, may be observed. Large eyelid notches that result in corneal exposure or that are cosmetically unappealing will require revision by a full thickness wedge resection.

3. **Trichiasis:** If the eyelid margin alignment was not adequate, the eyelashes may rotate against the globe.
   Management: One or a few lashes may be mechanically epilated, but it will require repeat treatment every few weeks. Alternatively, the trichiatic lashes may be hyfrecated for a more permanent solution. Severe trichiasis with entropion will require revision surgery with a full-thickness wedge resection and reapproximation of the wound edges.

4. **Ptosis:** The eyelid may be tight and slightly edematous immediately postoperatively. There may also be mild conjunctival injection.
   Management: Ptosis due to eyelid edema will typically resolve over weeks and the patient should be educated about this process. Residual ptosis lasting greater than 6 to 12 months may require secondary ptosis surgery.

4.12 Postoperative Care

Patient should place antibiotic ointment to the sutures four times a day for 1 week. Patching is usually not necessary.

References

[1] Stevens DL, Bisno AL, Chambers HF, et al. Infectious Diseases Society of America. Practice guidelines for the diagnosis and management of skin and soft tissue infections: 2014 update by the Infectious Diseases Society of America. Clin Infect Dis. 2014; 59(2):e10–e52

[2] Kaufman SC, Lazzaro DR, Eds. Textbook of Ocular Trauma: Evaluation and Treatment. New York, NY: Thieme; 2012

Suggested Readings

[1] McCord CD, Nunery WR, Tanenbaum M. Reconstruction of the lower eyelid and outer canthus. In: McCord CD, Tanenbaum M, Nunery W, eds. Oculoplastic Surgery, 3rd ed. New York: Raven Press, 1995. Pp 119-144

[2] Dutton JJ, Waldrop TG. Atlas of Oculoplastic and Orbital Surgery. Philadelphia, PA: Wolters Kluwer/Lippincott Williams & Wilkins Health; 2013

[3] McCord CD, Nunery WR. Reconstruction of the lower eyelid and outer canthus. Oculoplastic Surgery. 1995:119–144

[4] Nerad JA, Ed. Techniques in Ophthalmic Plastic Surgery: A Personal Tutorial. Philadelphia, PA: Saunders; 2010

[5] Tse DT, Ed. Color Atlas of Oculoplastic Surgery. Philadelphia, PA: Wolters Kluwer Health/Lippincott Williams & Wilkins; 2011

5 Canalicular Laceration and Medial Canthal Tendon Avulsion Repair

Kyle J. Godfrey, Kristen E. Dunbar, and Gary J. Lelli, Jr.

Summary

Early identification and repair of canalicular and medial canthal tendon trauma is essential to restoring the anatomical structure–function relationships that maintain adequate tear drainage and eyelid function. High levels of surgical success can be obtained irrespective of stent selection, provided the key principles of surgical repair are maintained: identification of both ends of the canaliculi, reapproximation, intubation, and anatomic restoration of the eyelid margin position with adequate posterior vector of the medial eyelid and adequate medial canthal tendon support. It is our preference to perform bicanalicular intubation whenever possible. To this end, in the appropriate context, we perform surgical repair in the operating room under general anesthesia. Several techniques may assist the surgeon in locating the lacerated end of the proximal canaliculus, such as the use of phenylephrine, viscoelastic, fluorescein dye, or a pigtail catheter. Stents should be left in place for approximately 4 to 6 months following surgical repair, if they are properly positioned. Medial canthal tendon avulsions should be addressed at the time of canalicular laceration repair, and will help maintain adequate tone and marginal position of the eyelids. With adequate primary repair, the success of canalicular repair may approach 100%.

Keywords: canaliculus, medial canthal tendon, laceration, trauma, injury epiphora, ectropion

5.1 Goals

- To review medial canthal and nasolacrimal anatomy relevant to the treatment of canalicular lacerations and medial canthal tendon avulsions.
- To describe indications and contraindications for repair of medial canthal trauma.
- To review key principles, surgical options, and stenting options in canalicular laceration repair, including pre- and postoperative considerations.
- To review rescue maneuvers that can be employed if the lacerated ends of the canaliculus cannot be easily located.
- To review tips and pearls relevant to the repair of medial canthal tendon trauma.

5.2 Advantages

The goal of oculoplastic repair of the medial canthal area is to restore the anatomic relationships of the eyelids, puncta, and canaliculi to the globe and nasolacrimal system. Surgical failure can be defined broadly as either failure of reapproximation of the lacerated canaliculi, or poor apposition of the eyelid and puncta to the globe in the form of medial ectropion. Accordingly, it is our preference to perform bicanalicular intubation of the nasolacrimal system whenever possible. To this end, we prefer to perform surgical repair in the operating room under general anesthesia. This approach provides the highest certainty of anatomic reapproximation of the canaliculi at the time of primary repair, allows adequate exploration of the medial canthal tendon complex and complete anatomic repair, and provides greatest patient comfort and cooperation during the procedure.

5.3 Expectations

- Patients can expect minimal-to-moderate postoperative pain, bruising, swelling similar to other oculoplastic surgical procedures, depending on the extent of repair required.
- Patients may experience postoperative tearing until the silicone stent is removed.

5.4 Key Principles

Essential to their function of modulating the healthy ocular surface environment by distributing the precorneal tear film, the eyelids must maintain proper position relative to the ocular surface and provide adequate lacrimal outflow. The components of a properly functioning lacrimal outflow system include patency and apposition of the marginal punctum to the ocular surface and tear lake, intact orbicularis oculi pump function, and patency of both the upper and lower segments of the nasolacrimal excretory system. In the context of trauma, care must be taken to ensure that these anatomic structure–function relationships are preserved, and when necessary, appropriately repaired.

Although in cases of monocanalicular trauma there is evidence that compensatory drainage through the contralateral canaliculus may be sufficient in draining basal tear flow, it has also been reported that over half of patients with monocanalicular obstruction will experience symptoms of watery eyes, blurred vision, redness, and crusting in situations of reflex tearing.[1,2,3] Furthermore, while there is a disagreement in the literature on the relative contributions of the upper and lower canaliculi to tear outflow, it can be concluded that there is variation between individuals and eyes, further advocating for repair of monocanalicular lacerations of either the upper or lower canalicular system.[2,4,5] Given the high success rates of monocanalicular repair of greater than 90%, it is our opinion that all monocanalicular lacerations should be repaired when possible.[6,7]

As a concise review of the relevant anatomy, the upper and lower eyelid puncta are medial and lateral to the plica semilunaris, respectively, and have a diameter of approximately 0.3 mm at the mucocutaneous junction directed posteriorly into the tear lake. The puncta overlie the canaliculi, which travel approximately 2 mm vertically, turn medially at 90 degree angles, and travel 8 to 10 mm within the orbicularis oculi muscle (► Fig. 5.1). In the vast majority of individuals, the upper

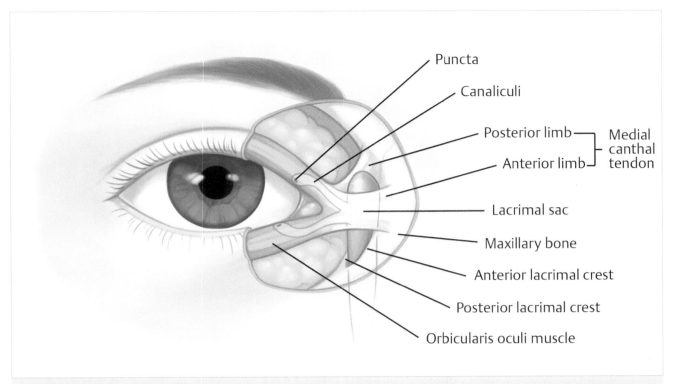

Fig. 5.1 Normal medial canthal anatomy, demonstrating the relationship between the puncta, canaliculi, anterior, and posterior limbs of the medial canthal tendon, lacrimal sac, and bony lacrimal fossa.

and lower canaliculi converge to form a common canaliculus before entering the posterolateral nasolacrimal sac deep and slightly superior to the anterior crus of the medial canthal tendon.[8,9] Without support from the tarsus, which terminates near the punctum, the medial eyelid has only soft tissue support and is vulnerable to injury.

The medial canthal tendon has a close relationship with the lacrimal drainage apparatus. The preseptal and pretarsal orbicularis oculi fibers extend nasally to form the medial canthal tendon, which subsequently divides into anterior and posterior limbs. The anterior limb passes in front of the lacrimal sac and inserts on the anterior lacrimal crest of the maxillary bone. The posterior limb passes behind the lacrimal sac and inserts on the posterior lacrimal crest of the lacrimal bone. Stability of the posterior limb is disproportionately critical in maintaining the horizontal tone and posterior vector of the medial eyelid that keeps the eyelid punctum well apposed to the ocular surface and directed toward the tear lake.

Due to their relative proximity, concurrent injury to both the canaliculi and medial canthal tendon is common. A high index of suspicion for canalicular laceration or medial canthal tendon avulsion should be maintained in all cases of eyelid trauma, particularly when there is evidence of trauma medial to the punctum. As in all cases of trauma, history regarding the circumstances of the trauma should be collected whenever possible. Canthal avulsions and canalicular lacerations most commonly occur secondary to blunt trauma, animal bites, motor vehicle collisions, falls, and assault with lateral traction to the eyelid. They are often associated with avulsion of the medial canthal tendon.[10,11,12] Lacerations of the inferior system are more common than the superior.[6,13] If injury is not identified and repaired in a timely fashion, insufficient lacrimal outflow with resultant epiphora and its associated ocular and visual symptoms may occur. Optimally, canalicular lacerations should be repaired within 24 to 48 hours, although there is evidence that acceptable outcomes may be obtained with delayed repair beyond 48 hours.[14] Adequate primary repair is crucial, as delayed repair to the canalicular system in symptomatic individuals may necessitate conjunctivodacryocystorhinostomy.

The key principles of successful canalicular laceration repair are identification of both ends of the lacerated canaliculus, canalicular reapproximation, canalicular intubation, and anatomic restoration of the eyelid margin position with adequate posterior vector of the medial canthus and posteriorly directed puncta into the tear lake. Practically speaking, surgical magnification is helpful, either through surgical loupes or an operating room microscope. In the case of concomitant medial canthal avulsion and canalicular laceration, intubation of the canaliculus should be performed first, followed by tendon repair.

In addressing the canalicular laceration, identification and location of the cut ends of the canaliculi must be performed preeminently. These cut ends appear as white or pink rings of mucosal tissue. Given the direction of the canalicular pathway, the more medial the laceration, the more posterior or deep the cut end of the canaliculus will be found. This is particularly true in the case of medial canthal avulsions, where the canaliculus may be avulsed at the level of the lacrimal sac. Copious irrigation, and gentle cleaning and debridement of the laceration

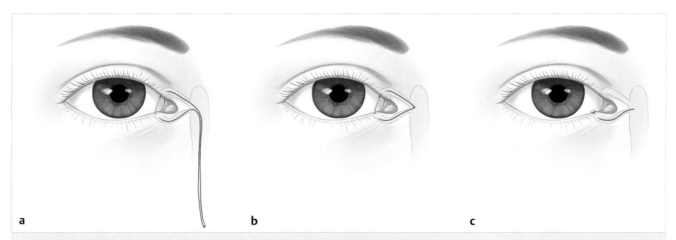

Fig. 5.2 Lacrimal stent variations: **(a)** Bicanalicular, Crawford-type stent through the upper and lower canaliculi and the nasolacrimal duct into the nose; **(b)** bicanalicular, stent of the upper and lower canaliculi placed using a pigtail probe; **(c)** monocanalicular stent of the lower canaliculus.

using moist cotton tipped applicators, is useful. When performing the repair under general anesthesia, we prefer to avoid use of local anesthetic to evade distortion of the normal anatomy. Once both ends have been identified, the stent may be passed through the proximal and distal ends.

Regarding stent selection and canalicular intubation, several options exist, which may be broadly grouped into three categories: (1) bicanalicular intubation of the upper and lower canaliculi and nasolacrimal duct, (2) bicanalicular intubation of the upper and lower canaliculi alone, (3) monocanalicular intubation (▶ Fig. 5.2). It should be noted that excellent functional results can be obtained with a variety of the stents and surgical techniques.[6,15,16,17,18,19,20,21,22,23] However, it is our preference, when possible, to perform bicanalicular intubation with a Crawford-type stent for both monocanalicular lacerations and bicanalicular lacerations as this may increase the likelihood of surgical success.[12] Advantages include the strength of a closed loop stent, assurance of reapproximation of the lacerated ends, and a posteromedial directed vector of force that minimizes the risk of postoperative eyelid margin and punctum malposition.

5.5 Indications

- Given the high success rates of canalicular repair, it is our opinion that all canalicular lacerations should be repaired when possible, irrespective of location in the upper or lower eyelid.
- To prevent the development of ectropion and epiphora, surgical repair of an avulsed medial canthal tendon is indicated whenever proceeding with repair is possible.

5.6 Contraindications

- Contraindication to repair of canalicular lacerations or medial canthal tendon avulsions are generally limited to situations in which the patient is medically unstable to undergo surgical repair in the operating room or at the bedside, or demonstrates appropriate decision-making capacity and declines repair.

- Ruptured globe and other vision- or life-threatening injuries should be addressed prior to exploration and repair of the canalicular system and medial canthal tendon.
- The most common reasons for postponing repair are traumatic brain injury, facial fractures, long bone fractures, chest injury, lung disease, and delay in seeking care.[14,24]

5.7 Preoperative Preparation

After life-threatening injuries and any globe injuries have been addressed, a careful examination of the eyelids and lacrimal system should be performed, including dilation and probing when canalicular injury is suspected due to evidence of trauma medial to the puncta. Punctal dilation allows for the introduction of a #0 Bowman probe. If the probe cannot be passed into the nasolacrimal sac, as indicated by a hard stop, canalicular injury must be suspected. Often the probe will become visible through the lacerated end of the canaliculus confirming the diagnosis (▶ Fig. 5.3). Alternatively, a lacrimal irrigation cannula on a saline-filled syringe can be used to irrigate the nasolacrimal system to evaluate patency. Similar to the Bowman probe, if there is difficulty advancing the cannula, or if there is dynamic reflux of saline, laceration should be suspected and further explored. Medial canthal avulsion is suggested by laxity of the medial canthal complex with increased distractibility of the lower eyelid laterally and anteriorly.

Once canalicular or medial canthal injury is diagnosed or suspected, the decision can be made to proceed with repair at the bedside or in the operating room. In most situations, the controlled environment of the operating room provides the optimal conditions for successful primary repair and greatest patient comfort. Additionally, some reports demonstrate higher success rates for repairs performed in the operating room.[12] General anesthesia is preferred in most situations as it allows placement of bicanalicular, Crawford-type stents and the required nasal manipulation, which may be intolerable for some patients in an office setting or under monitored anesthesia care. As in all cases of ocular adnexal trauma, if the associated lacerations and adnexal trauma are substantial, or if there

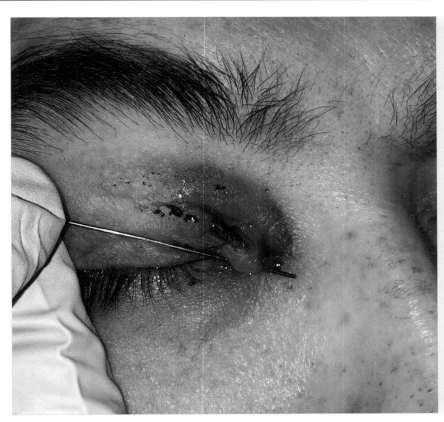

Fig. 5.3 A medial right upper eyelid laceration involving the canaliculus, as demonstrated with a Bowman probe. Note the distal end of the Bowman probe is visible through the end of the lacerated canaliculus.

is contamination of the wound, copious irrigation and cleaning should be performed, and antibiotics should be considered. If the patient has not received a tetanus immunization within 5 years, tetanus toxoid should be given. If they have never received a tetanus immunization, human tetanus immune globulin should be given. If an animal bite occurred, the animal should be investigated and rabies prophylaxis should be considered.[25,26] Preoperative surgical preparation and draping should be performed with betadine in the standard fashion for ophthalmic plastic surgery.

5.8 Operative Technique

First, attention is directed to identification and intubation of the proximal and distal cut ends of the canaliculi. Both upper and lower canaliculi are inspected to ensure that occult injury is not missed. Cotton tipped applicators are used to debride the wound and identify the lacerated canaliculi. The bicanalicular, Crawford-style lacrimal stent is passed first through the punctum (after punctal dilation when necessary) and proximal canaliculus, then through the distal ends beyond the laceration. Once a hard stop is felt in nasolacrimal sac, the stent is rotated vertically and directed slightly posteriorly and laterally and advanced through the nasolacrimal duct and into the nose. It can then be retrieved using a Crawford hook, or similar instrument, beneath the inferior turbinate. This is then repeated through the opposite canaliculus.

The pericanalicular tissues should then be repaired. We use 7–0 polyglactin suture to reapproximate the mucosal edges of

the lacerated canaliculi or at least reapproximate the pericanalicular tissues (▶ Fig. 5.4). When possible, several sutures are placed in an interrupted fashion through these tissues. The orbicularis and skin can then be closed according to the surgeon's preference. It is our practice to use 6–0 polyglactin suture to reapproximate the orbicularis and 6–0 nylon, polypropylene, or fast-absorbing gut suture to close the skin in an interrupted or running fashion. The ends of the stent are then collected, gentle traction is placed, and an empty needle driver is placed on the stent at the level of the nostril and it is tied in a 1-1-1 fashion. This smaller knot allows for the stent to be rotated and retrieved through the palpebral aperture if necessary. In adults, a single permanent suture, such as 6–0 polypropylene, can be placed through the lateral nasal mucosa and loosely tied around the looped stent to facilitate retrieval through the nose and prevent migration or extrusion of the stent from the palpebral aperture. In this instance, care should be taken to ensure there is not excess tension from the stent on the eyelids and puncta. In children, we avoid this lateral nasal wall suture to allow the stent to be removed in the office through the palpebral aperture without additional anesthesia.

If bicanalicular intubation is not possible, monocanalicular intubation can be performed using a mono-Crawford, Mini-Monoka, or similar stent. In this situation, it is especially important to get excellent reapproximation of the pericanalicular tissues to give the patient the best chance of postoperative canalicular patency. Some monocanalicular stents (e.g., Mini-Monoka) may not reach all the way to the nasolacrimal sac, and, as such, are not well suited for the deepest lacerations or canalicular avulsions at the level of the sac. However, excellent

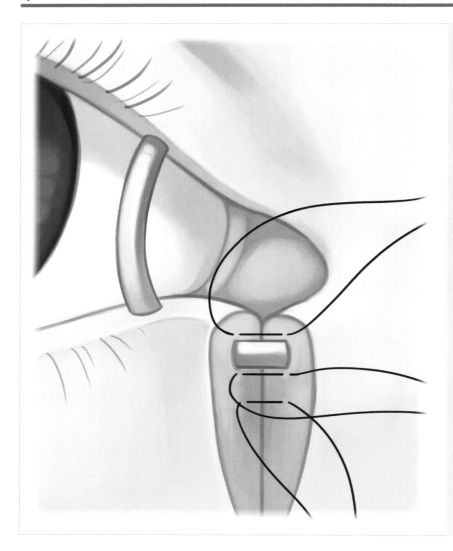

Fig. 5.4 Reapproximation of the pericanalicular tissues following canalicular intubation. Our preference is to use 7–0 polyglactin suture.

success rates have been reported with this approach in appropriately chosen cases where tendon reconstruction is not needed.[12,18,27] We note good success in smaller lacerations, proximal to the lacrimal sac without extensive tendon damage.

If bicanalicular and nasolacrimal intubation is not possible, or the proximal end of the lacerated canaliculus cannot be located, bicanalicular intubation using a pigtail probe can be attempted. Although this requires the presence of a common canaliculus, it does not require nasolacrimal stimulation, making it an option for bedside repair in which bicanalicular intubation is desired, despite a small risk of iatrogenic damage to the intact canaliculus. This technique is more difficult in situations where both canaliculi have been damaged, although it is still possible. In situations of monocanalicular trauma, the pigtail probe is passed first through the intact punctum and rotated through the intact canaliculus and posterior to the medial canthal tendon through the common canaliculus, exiting out the cut end of the damaged canaliculus. Alternatively, the probe can be passed in a reverse fashion, first through the lacerated end and exiting the intact punctum. In either case, once the probe has been rotated through the upper canalicular system, a suture (typically a 6–0 nylon with the needle removed) is threaded through the eyelet

of the probe (▶ Fig. 5.5). The probe is then rotated back out of the canalicular system, pulling the suture with it, allowing the suture to act as a guide wire through the canalicular system over which the stent can be passed. Silicone tubing (0.25 mm external diameter) is threaded over the suture and pulled through the canaliculus. Smooth forceps can help introduce and guide the stent through the canalicular system. Once the canaliculi are intubated, the pericanalicular tissues can be repaired as previously described. The nylon suture is then tied so as to pull the knot into the stent while avoiding kinking or buckling it. When the tails of the knot are cut, they should retract into the tubing. Finally, the stent should be rotated so the knot and ends of the stent are not exposed in the palpebral aperture.

Once intubation of the canalicular system has been performed, repair of the medial canthal complex should proceed if indicated. First, careful examination should be performed to determine whether both the anterior and posterior horns of the medial canthal tendon have been damaged. As mentioned previously, the posterior limb is critical to proper eyelid position and function and should always be repaired. Additionally, careful examination should be performed to evaluate for bony fracture, as proper repair of the medial canthal complex is

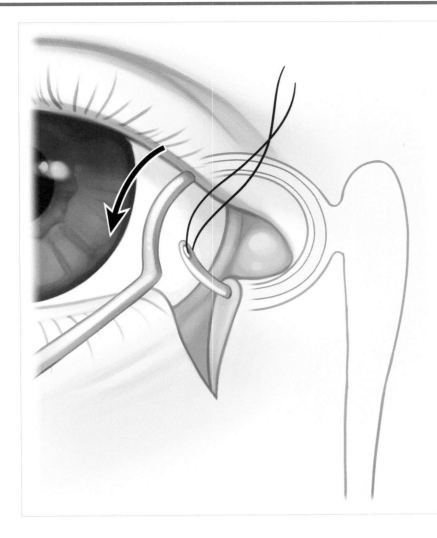

Fig. 5.5 A pigtail probe being passed through the intact upper eyelid canaliculus, exiting through the cut end of the lower eyelid canaliculus. A suture can be passed through the eyelet of the probe and rotated back through the canalicular system to act as a guidewire over which the silicone stent can be passed through the upper and lower eyelid canaliculus. The pigtail probe can also be used to help locate the nasal end of the lacerated canaliculus.

dependent on stable bony anatomy. Of note, if the medial canthal tendon has been avulsed, the bicanalicular stent is particularly useful for providing posteromedial traction and anatomic reapproximation of the medial canthal complex.

In the case of medial canthal trauma, three conditions exist relative to the soft tissues: (1) a severed medial canthal tendon where both ends of the tendon can be located, (2) an avulsed medial canthal tendon where the distal portion of the tendon cannot be identified, but intact periosteum is present, (3) an avulsed medial canthal tendon and periosteum with complete avulsion of the soft tissue from the bone. In situations where both ends of the lacerated canthal tendon can be located, it can be repaired using a non-absorbable suture such as 4–0 polyester suture on a P2 needle passed in a horizontal mattress fashion, first through the distal end then anteriorly through the proximal portion. If the distal end cannot be identified, but periosteum is intact, the tendon can then be repaired by passing a 5–0 braided multifilament absorbable suture through the periosteum of the medial wall and the canthal tendon. In the case of complete soft tissue avulsion, a microplate can be used to fixate the medial canthal tendon to bone. The screws should be placed through the thicker maxillary bone of the anterior lacrimal crest and the posterior portion used to anchor the tendon. If any previously identified bony nasolacrimal fractures cannot be stabilized, transnasal wiring should be performed to stabilize the medial canthal complex.

5.9 Tips and Pearls

- Whenever possible, bicanalicular intubation through the canaliculi and nasolacrimal system using Crawford-type stents should be attempted. The advantages of this include increased certainty of canalicular reapproximation, and, importantly, the added posteromedial vector of force that helps support the medial canthal complex and promotes lid apposition to the globe.
- Another technique for ensuring an adequate superior and posteromedial vector during primary repair is placing a temporary supporting suture through the lower eyelid. A 4–0 double armed silk or polypropylene suture can be passed through a bolster then in a horizontal mattress fashion through the lower eyelid skin and orbicularis muscle proximally, down to the periosteum of the nasal bone, then up through the skin over the origin of the anterior medial canthal tendon. These can then be tied over two bolsters (one along the lower lid and one directly over the tendon) such as

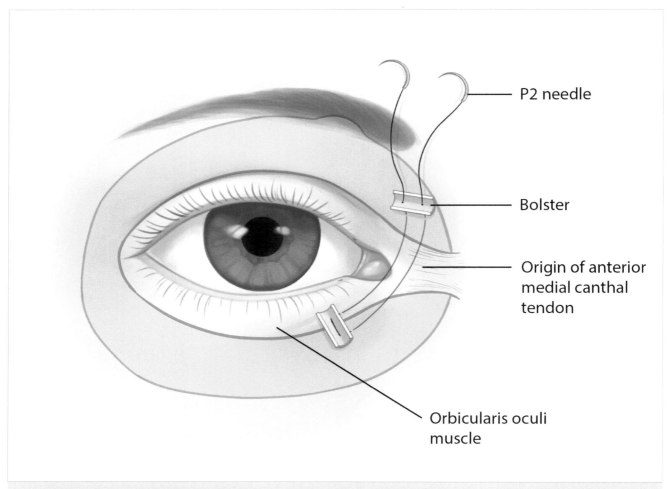

Fig. 5.6 A temporary bolster suture placed through the lower eyelid to provide support and a superior and posterior vector to the lower eyelid during the initial phase of healing. A 4–0 double armed silk suture is passed through a bolster in a horizontal mattress fashion through the lower eyelid skin and orbicularis muscle proximally, down to the periosteum of the nasal bone, then up through the skin over the origin of the anterior medial canthal tendon.

a 240 scleral buckle band cut into 1 cm segments (▶ Fig. 5.6). This temporary suture can be removed in 1 week, but helps support the lower eyelid and medial canthal complex and provides additional posterior and superior vector during the initial phase of healing.

- To further prevent medial ectropion, a supporting 4–0 polyglactin suture can be passed through the medial canthal tendon to reinforce this complex prior to performing pericanalicular repair.
- In situations where the surgeon is unable to locate both ends of the lacerated canaliculus, there are several techniques that can help:
  ○ In a monocanalicular laceration, viscoelastic or fluorescein dye can be injected slowly through the opposite, intact canaliculus while watching carefully for reflux through the proximal or medial lacerated end.
  ○ Methylene blue can also be used in a similar fashion, but carries the risk of staining surrounding tissues and making identification of the lacerated canaliculus more difficult.

  ○ 2.5% phenylephrine can also be applied to the lacerated tissue to cause local vasoconstriction. With the associated blanching of the pericanalicular tissues, it may become easier to identify the proximal cut end.
- If the stent cannot be located easily in the nose with the Crawford hook, several options exist:
  ○ Care should be taken not to search extensively with the Crawford hook as it can lead to trauma and bleeding from the highly vascularized nasal mucosa.
  ○ Awareness of the direction of the hook should be maintained, and initial efforts to make contact with the stent should be performed with the backside of the hook to minimize trauma. If difficulty is encountered, a blunt tipped instrument can be introduced beneath the inferior turbinate to search more gently and make contact with the stent. Once it is located, the surgeon can switch to the Crawford hook to gently retrieve it.
  ○ Placing oxymetazoline or epinephrine-soaked pledgets under the inferior turbinate can help reduce edema of the nasal mucosa, making the stent easier to locate.

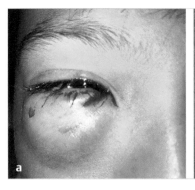
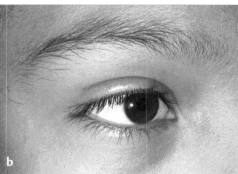

Fig. 5.7 **(a)** Preoperative photograph of a right lower eyelid canalicular laceration in a child. **(b)** Postoperative month 3 following repair. The footplate of the right lower eyelid monocanalicular stent is visible at the eyelid margin.

○ Sometimes, temporarily suspending nasal trauma, replacing the nasal packing, and briefly waiting for hemostasis and the reduction of edema, can help make anatomical landmarks more recognizable and stent retrieval more facile.

○ If contact with the stent cannot still be made, an endoscope can be used to directly visualize and retrieve the stent.

5.10 Complications

- Medial ectropion.
- Canalicular stenosis.
- Epiphora.
- Iatrogenic trauma to undamaged canaliculus.

5.10.1 Postoperative Care

Following repair of a canalicular laceration, the stent should be left in place a minimum of 6 weeks, although it is our practice to leave the stents for 4 to 6 months, provided they are well positioned and not causing ocular surface or nasal irritation to the patient. The stent may be removed from the nose, with the assistance of an endoscope when necessary. If the stent cannot be located in the nose, or was only placed in the upper nasolacrimal system, it can be removed by cutting the loop between the puncta and pulled through one of the puncta. Postoperatively, we prescribe patients topical steroid-antibiotic drops and oral antibiotics for 7 to 10 days. Antimicrobial therapy should be tailored to the circumstances and mechanism of injury for adequate coverage. Patients are typically seen at postoperative week 1, postoperative week 6, and then postoperative months 3 and 6. With observation of these principles, and anatomically successful primary repair, functional and aesthetic success of canalicular repair may approach 100% (▶ Fig. 5.7).

References

[1] Linberg JV, Moore CA. Symptoms of canalicular obstruction. Ophthalmology. 1988; 95(8):1077–1079

[2] Murgatroyd H, Craig JP, Sloan B. Determination of relative contribution of the superior and inferior canaliculi to the lacrimal drainage system in health using the drop test. Clin Exp Ophthalmol. 2004; 32(4):404–410

[3] Reed S, Lissner G. Clinical study on the effectiveness of tear drainage with a single canalicular system under environmental stress. Ophthal Plast Reconstr Surg. 1993; 9(1):27–31

[4] von Denffer H, Dressler J, Pabst HW. Lacrimal dacryoscintigraphy. Semin Nucl Med. 1984; 14(1):8–15

[5] White WL, Glover AT, Buckner AB, Hartshorne MF. Relative canalicular tear flow as assessed by dacryoscintigraphy. Ophthalmology. 1989; 96(2):167–169

[6] Chowdhury HR, Rose GE, Ezra DG. Long-term outcomes of monocanalicular repair of canalicular lacerations. Ophthalmology. 2014; 121(8):1665–6.e1

[7] Rosser PM, Burt B, Osborne SF. Determination of the function of a repaired canaliculus after monocanalicular injury by placing a punctal plug in the non-involved punctum on the affected side. Clin Exp Ophthalmol. 2010; 38 (8):786–789

[8] Yazici B, Yazici Z. Frequency of the common canaliculus: a radiological study. Arch Ophthalmol. 2000; 118(10):1381–1385

[9] Zoumalan CI, Joseph JM, Lelli GJ, Jr, et al. Evaluation of the canalicular entrance into the lacrimal sac: an anatomical study. Ophthal Plast Reconstr Surg. 2011; 27(4):298–303

[10] Dortzbach RK, Angrist RA. Silicone intubation for lacerated lacrimal canaliculi. Ophthalmic Surg. 1985; 16(10):639–642

[11] Kennedy RH, May J, Dailey J, Flanagan JC. Canalicular laceration. An 11-year epidemiologic and clinical study. Ophthal Plast Reconstr Surg. 1990; 6(1):46–53

[12] Murchison AP, Bilyk JR. Canalicular laceration repair: an analysis of variables affecting success. Ophthal Plast Reconstr Surg. 2014; 30(5):410–414

[13] Reifler DM. Management of canalicular laceration. Surv Ophthalmol. 1991; 36(2):113–132

[14] Chu Y-C, Wu S-Y, Tsai Y-J, Liao YL, Chu HY. Early versus late canalicular laceration repair outcomes. Am J Ophthalmol. 2017; 182:155–159

[15] Singh S, Ganguly A, Hardas A, Tripathy D, Rath S. Canalicular lacerations: factors predicting outcome at a tertiary eye care centre. Orbit. 2017; 36(1): 13–18

[16] Tavakoli M, Karimi S, Behdad B, Dizani S, Salour H. Traumatic canalicular laceration repair with a new monocanalicular silicone tube. Ophthal Plast Reconstr Surg. 2017; 33(1):27–30

[17] Naik MN, Kelapure A, Rath S, Honavar SG. Management of canalicular lacerations: epidemiological aspects and experience with Mini-Monoka monocanalicular stent. Am J Ophthalmol. 2008; 145(2):375–380

[18] Mauriello JA, Jr, Abdelsalam A. Use of a modified monocanalicular silicone stent in 33 eyelids. Ophthalmic Surg Lasers. 1996; 27(11):929–934

[19] Kersten RC, Kulwin DR. "One-stitch" canalicular repair: a simplified approach for repair of canalicular laceration. Ophthalmology. 1996; 103(5):785–789

[20] Lindsey JT. Lacrimal duct injuries revisited: a retrospective review of six patients. Ann Plast Surg. 2000; 44(2):167–172

[21] Anastas CN, Potts MJ, Raiter J. Mini Monoka silicone monocanalicular lacrimal stents: subjective and objective outcomes. Orbit. 2001; 20(3):189–200

[22] Lee H, Chi M, Park M, Baek S. Effectiveness of canalicular laceration repair using monocanalicular intubation with Monoka tubes. Acta Ophthalmol. 2009; 87(7):793–796

[23] Eo S, Park J, Cho S, Azari KK. Microsurgical reconstruction for canalicular laceration using Monostent and Mini-Monoka. Ann Plast Surg. 2010; 64(4): 421–427

[24] Chiang E, Bee C, Harris GJ, Wells TS. Does delayed repair of eyelid lacerations compromise outcome? Am J Emerg Med. 2017; 35(11):1766–1767

[25] Gonnering RS. Ocular adnexal injury and complications in orbital dog bites. Ophthal Plast Reconstr Surg. 1987; 3(4):231–235

[26] Herman DC, Bartley GB, Walker RC. The treatment of animal bite injuries of the eye and ocular adnexa. Ophthal Plast Reconstr Surg. 1987; 3(4):237–241

[27] Leibovitch I, Kakizaki H, Prabhakaran V, Selva D. Canalicular lacerations: repair with the Mini-Monoka® monocanalicular intubation stent. Ophthalmic Surg Lasers Imaging. 2010; 41(4):472–477

Part III

Lower Eyelid

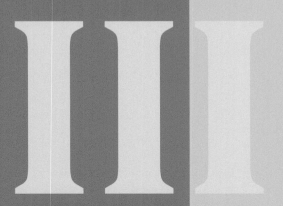

6 Entropion Repair

Brittany A. Simmons and Mithra O. Gonzalez

Summary

Entropion is an inverted malposition of the eyelid that, when left uncorrected by either surgical or nonsurgical means, can result in ocular surface irritation, infection, and even loss of vision. Entropion refers to the inward rolling of the eyelid margin. Its causes include involutional, spastic, cicatricial, and/or congenital factors. The etiology and severity of entropion determine the corrective approach. Correction of entropion ranges from eyelid taping or temporary sutures to incisional surgery. Adjunctive techniques include mitomycin C for advanced cicatricial disease and tarsal spacer grafts for markedly shortened posterior lamella. Beware of significant overcorrection that will induce ectropion.

Keywords: entropion, eyelid malposition, inverted eyelid, Quickert suture, lower lid retractor reinsertion, Weis procedure, tarsotomy, lateral tarsal strip

6.1 Goals

- To correctly understand the etiology and management of inwardly turned eyelids.

6.2 Advantages

Eyelid entropion can cause ocular surface irritation and predispose the eye to infections and corneal ulcers. If severe or longstanding, scarring of the cornea and loss of vision can occur. Return of the eyelid to its normal position, either by surgical or non-surgical means, resolves the ocular surface irritation that accompanies the malpositioned, inward-turned eyelid.

6.3 Expectations

- Durable restoration of normal eyelid anatomy and physiology.
- Determine the type of entropion to plan appropriate surgical correction.
- Involutional entropion requires lower lid retractor reinsertion with horizontal tightening with a lateral tarsal strip procedure to add stability, durability, and prevent overcorrection.[1]
- Spastic and cicatricial entropion necessitate increasing surgical intervention depending on severity.
- A small degree of intraoperative overcorrection results in an acceptable eyelid position.

6.4 Key Principles

Several types of entropion exist. The identification of its etiology and its corresponding anatomical defect determines the surgical correction of choice.

Involutional entropion occurs due to a combination of the weakening or dehiscence of the lower eyelid retractors, horizontal eyelid laxity, and orbicularis override.[1,2] Surgical lower eyelid retractor reinsertion coupled with a lateral tarsal strip operation address both retractor weakness and horizontal lid laxity. An initial subciliary skin incision may be used to induce scar formation that prevents overriding preseptal orbicularis oculi, while a transconjunctival dissection anterior to tarsus may be used to ablate or weaken the offending preseptal orbicularis oculi. Spastic entropion results from a sustained or recurrent spasm of the muscle of Riolan after a precipitating event such as recent eye surgery or eyelid inflammation,[2,3] and it likely shares the same mechanical factors as involutional entropion.[1] Eliminating the cause of the spasm often resolves the entropion. If this is not possible, Quickert sutures can be used to tighten the lower lid retractors and create scarring, which changes the eyelid vector and deters entropion. Cicatricial contraction of the posterior lamella—as seen with chemical or thermal injuries, autoimmune mucous membrane disorders like Stevens–Johnson Syndrome, ocular cicatricial pemphigoid, and trachoma—can also lead to entropion. Treatment may require lengthening the posterior lamella with or without a tarsotomy (or tarsal fracture) in mild cases, or lysis of any cicatrix with a posterior spacer graft in severe cases.

Congenital entropion arises from disinsertion of the lower lid retractor aponeurosis[4] and/or defects in the tarsal plate.[3] Repair is dependent on the anatomical defect, and is typically done by lower lid retractor reinsertion with or without horizontal tightening and/or posterior lamella grafting.

Prevailing surgical repairs are combination procedures that address the multiple anatomic abnormalities that produce entropion. Non-incisional repair includes the use of eyelid taping or a temporary suture. Common incisional options include reinsertion of the lower lid retractors with horizontal tightening of the lid and transverse tarsotomy (e.g., Weis procedure).

6.5 Indications

- Symptomatic ocular surface irritation.
- Keratopathy.
- Corneal ulceration.
- Corneal scarring.
- Persistent infectious keratitis.

6.6 Contraindications

- Acute flare of autoimmune or cicatricial lid disease.

6.7 Preoperative Preparation

Successful surgical repair of entropion requires appropriate identification of entropic vectors and their associated anatomic defects. Congenital entropion should be distinguished from epiblepharon and congenital distichiasis. Lower lid laxity should be quantified using snapback and distraction tests. Correction of involutional entropion is most successful when surgical repair includes horizontal eyelid tightening.[2,3,5,6] Autoimmune or inflammatory disease should be controlled, ideally with the help of the patient's primary care physician or rheumatologist, with immunosuppressant medications prior to surgical repair.

6.8 Operative Technique

6.8.1 Transverse Everting Sutures (Quickert Suture, Three-Suture Technique)

This is classically used for lower lid entropion. Three, double-armed, dissolvable sutures are passed full-thickness from the conjunctival cul-de-sac in the center, lateral, and medial aspects of the lower lid (avoiding the medial punctum and nasolacrimal duct system) and externalized 1 to 2 mm below the lower lashes, and tied to create eversion of the eyelid margin (Fig. 6.1).

6.8.2 Lower Lid Retractor Reinsertion

External Approach

A traction suture is placed through the gray line of the lower lid. A subciliary skin incision is made through the skin from the lateral canthus to the medial punctum along the inferior border of tarsus, after which a skin muscle flap is created and dissected

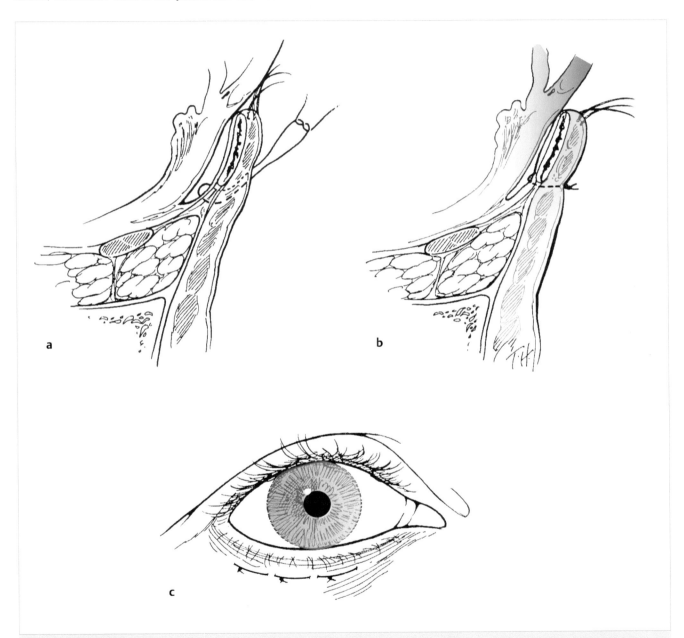

Fig. 6.1 Quickert sutures. **(a)** Double-armed sutures are placed starting in the inferior fornix, passing beneath the tarsus, and continuing in an upward vector exiting the skin about 3 mm below the cilia. **(b)** When tied, these sutures evert the lid margin and prevent the override of the preseptal orbicularis oculi muscle over the pretarsal portion. **(c)** Several sets of these sutures are placed along the width of the lower eyelid.

inferiorly toward the inferior orbital rim to expose the inferior orbital septum. The septum is entered and the underlying orbital fat is retracted to reveal the white fibrous band of the lower eyelid retractors. A combination of blunt and sharp dissection will free the retractors anteriorly from the orbital fat and posteriorly from the conjunctiva. The superior edge of the lower lid retractor is reattached to the anterior, inferior tarsal border using several interrupted buried sutures. The eyelid should be mildly overcorrected at this point. If horizontal lid tightening is required, attention should now be turned to completion of a horizontal tightening procedure, such as a lateral tarsal strip. (See below for details.) Skin incision(s) are closed with continuous running, dissolvable suture.

Internal Approach

The lower lid is everted and an incision is made through the palpebral conjunctiva inferior to the tarsus and extended to just lateral of the lower lid punctum. Dissection is carried down toward the inferior orbital rim to expose the lower lid retractors. The superior edge of the lower lid retractor is reattached to the anterior face of tarsus using several interrupted buried sutures. Attention is turned to horizontal tightening with completion of a lateral tarsal strip operation as discussed below.

6.8.3 Horizontal Tightening (e.g., Lateral Tarsal Strip Procedures)

- The patient is prepped and draped in the usual sterile manner for oculoplastic surgery. Local anesthetic such as 1% lidocaine with epinephrine is injected into the lateral canthal area and through the lateral commissure down to the lateral orbital rim periosteum. A scleral protecting shield is placed.
- Lateral canthotomy is performed with curved Stevens tenotomy scissors or alternatively Wescott scissors (Fig. 6.2a). The curve of the scissors is aimed inferiorly to parallel the lateral canthal rhytids and relaxed skin tension lines to minimize scarring. Some surgeons will make an initial skin incision with a #15 blade and then perform the canthotomy with scissors.
- Inferior cantholysis is performed to release the lid from the lateral orbital rim (Fig. 6.2b) by directing the scissors parallel to the plane of the patient's face and pointing the tips towards the patient's feet. It is common to inadvertently direct the scissors towards the globe and into the orbit, but this should be avoided to minimize risk of globe or orbital injury. The inferior crus of the lateral canthal tendon can be "strummed" and this firm tissue is sharply cut to free the lower lid from its attachment to the lateral orbital rim. If additional mobility of the lower lid is required, further release of connective tissue (lateral retinaculum and orbital

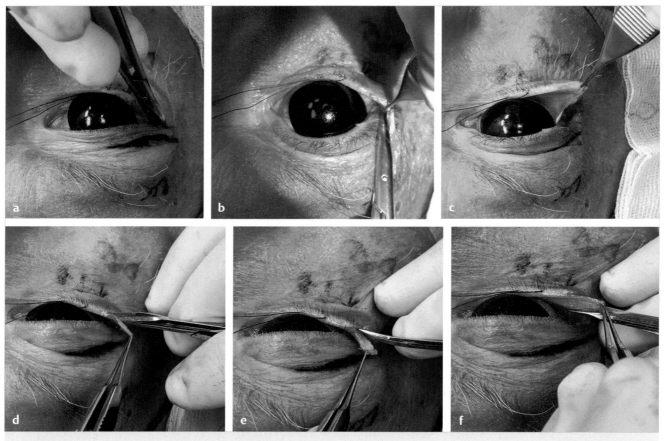

Fig. 6.2 (a) Lateral canthotomy is performed with curved Stevens tenotomy scissors. [Note: In this case silk traction suture is present in the lower lid to aid with subsequent posterior spacer graft placement a traction suture is otherwise not needed in a typical lateral tarsal strip procedure]. (b) Inferior cantholysis. (c) An Adson toothed forceps demonstrates a fully laterally released lower eyelid. (d) Wescott scissors excise the marginal epithelium above the tarsus. (e) The anterior lamella is separated from the tarsus (posterior lamella) using the Wescott scissors. (f) Wescott scissors make a small conjunctival cut at the inferior border of the tarsus to create a true strip. *(continued)*

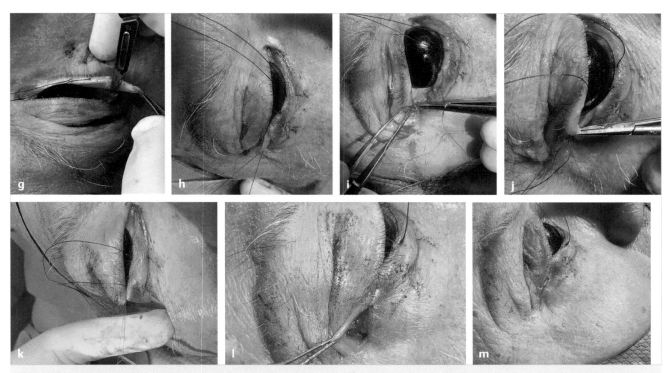

Fig. 6.2 (*continued*) **(g)** Palpebral conjunctiva of the tarsal strip is scraped away with a #15 blade. **(h)** Double-armed permanent suture is placed as horizontal mattress. **(i)** Tarsal strip suture is passed to the inner surface periosteum of the lateral orbital rim in an internal superior vector to complete the horizontal mattress, but not yet tied. **(j)** Lateral canthal angle cerclage is placed as a grey-line to grey-line suture with the knot buried in the lateral canthal wound. **(k)** Note sharp lateral canthal angle after tying of lateral canthal angle cerclage suture. **(l)** 4-0 lateral tarsal strip suture is tied within a submuscular pocket to prevent suture knot exposure. **(m)** Skin is closed with simple interrupted sutures placed to include skin and muscle. This canthal incision is much longer than usual as this patient simultaneously underwent lower lid posterior spacer graft surgery and upper lid retraction repair surgery.

septum) can be performed, and the lid can be freely moved from the lateral orbital rim (Fig. 6.2c).

- The margin of the lower lid is marked by scoring with a scissors the intersection point with the terminus of the lateral margin of the upper eyelid when the lower lid is distracted laterally under moderate tension. Wescott scissors are then used to remove the marginal epithelium above the tarsus up to this point (Fig. 6.2d).
- The anterior lamella (skin (including lashes) and orbicularis muscle) are separated from the tarsus (posterior lamella) using the Wescott scissors (Fig. 6.2e). It is helpful to press the curve of the scissors into the tarsus to aid with dissection.
- Wescott scissors are used to make a small cut at the inferior border of the tarsus to release conjunctiva, thus creating a true strip (Fig. 6.2f).
- A #15 blade is used to gently scrape the palpebral conjunctival epithelium away from the internal surface of the tarsal strip (Fig. 6.2g) with the goals of: a) creating a rough surface to aid with strip healing / adherence to the orbital rim and b) minimizing the risk of latent conjunctival inclusion cyst development postoperatively.
- Double-armed permanent suture, in this case 4-0 PTFE-coated braided polyester (silky PolyDek, Teleflex Medical OEM, Gurnee, Illinois, USA), is passed from posterior to anterior at the distal aspect of the tarsal strip in a horizontal mattress technique (Fig. 6.2h). The tarsal strip suture is then passed into the periosteum of the lateral orbital rim to

complete the horizontal mattress configuration (Fig. 6.2i). The superior arm of the suture is passed first, with the lateral orbital rim insertion point of the superior crus of the lateral canthal tendon used as a landmark for which to place the suture. The suture is placed such that it engages the periosteum from the inner / intra-orbital surface deep to the leading edge of the orbital rim itself; the needle then proceeds anteriorly along its natural curvature. Care is taken to avoid injury to the globe and to avoid incorporating the lacrimal gland (especially if the gland is prolapsed). The second arm of the suture is then passed just below the first. Once the sutures are placed they can be hand-tensioned to confirm appropriate positioning of the lateral canthal angle (generally approximately 2 mm superior to the medial commissure) and to confirm that the lower lid follows the curvature of the globe intimately and courses inwards towards the rim - if the lid is noted to pull away from the globe laterally the suture has been placed too anteriorly on the rim and the suture should be redone, this time being sure to engage the initial pass into the periosteum more deeply to ensure the lid maintains an inwardly directed tension vector. Once the positioning of the suture is confirmed to be satisfactory it is left untied to enable easier placement of the lateral canthal angle cerclage suture.

- A lateral canthal angle cerclage is performed (Fig. 6.2j) to promote a sharp lateral canthal angle and to maintain anterior-posterior alignment of the eyelid margin, i.e. to avoid override of one lid over the other, etc. To augment this effect, a small (1 mm or less) area of eyelid margin epithelium may be removed from the lateral upper eyelid with Wescott scissors. A fine suture such as 6-0 polyglactin or 6-0 chromic gut is then passed from the wound to the lid as a grey-line to grey-line simple interrupted suture with the knot buried within the lateral canthal wound. It is easiest to backhand the first pass of this suture. The lateral canthal cerclage suture is tied and the lateral commissure is noted to be sharp and properly aligned (Fig. 6.2k).

- The 4-0 tarsal strip suture can now be tied permanently. It is important to allow a submuscular pocket for the suture knot to sit in to avoid suture exposure subsequently (Fig. 6.2l). Additionally, the suture knot should be cut such that there is adequate tail to avoid loosening and to avoid a "stubble" effect from too short of a tail on a monofilament suture such as nylon or polypropylene that could become uncomfortable or poke through skin.
- Skin is closed with suture of the surgeon's preference to include skin and muscle with the aim of preventing tarsal strip suture knot exposure (Fig. 6.2m). The patient is then undraped, skin cleansed, the scleral shield is removed, and ophthalmic ointment is applied to the surgical site.

Pre- and post-operative photos are shown in Fig. 6.3.

6.8.4 Transverse Tarsotomy (Weis Procedure, Two-Snip Procedure)

Most commonly used for lower lid entropion, a transverse tarsotomy can also be employed for mild upper lid entropion. A full-thickness lid stab incision is created through the inferior edge of the tarsus (approximately 3 mm from the lid margin). The incision is extended medially and laterally. Horizontal mattress sutures are placed to approximate the conjunctiva and lid retractors to the infraciliary orbicularis and skin. Surgical results are more durable when this procedure is performed in conjunction with a lateral tarsal strip (Fig. 6.4).

6.8.5 Tarsal Spacer (Mucous Membrane) Grafts

The scarred conjunctiva is lysed along the horizontal length of the posterior lamella. A mucous membrane graft (commonly from buccal mucosa or labial mucosa of the lower lip) of a size similar to or just slightly larger than the newly created posterior lamellar defect is harvested and sewn into the posterior lamellar defect.

6.9 Tips and Pearls

- Consider the vectors that allow for the entropic lid.
- Quickert sutures do not address horizontal eyelid laxity, and recurrence of entropion is more likely when the sutures dissolve; thus, these are usually used as temporizing measures until either resolution of the spastic entropion or more definitive operative repair occurs.
- Quickert sutures should be considered for those patients who are poor surgical candidates.

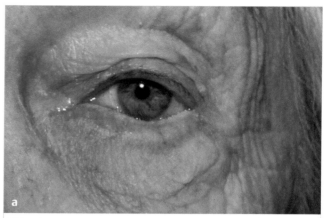

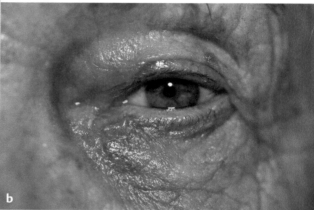

Fig. 6.3 (a) Pre-operative photograph demonstrating involutional entropion left lower eyelid in an elderly patient with significant horizontal eyelid laxity. (b) After undergoing lateral tarsal strip procedure, the lower eyelid is in normal position.

- During reinsertion of the lower lid retractors, advance the retractors as a whole; it is not necessary to separate the lower lid retractors into their voluntary and involuntary portions.
- During dissection before reinsertion of the lower lid retractors, the preseptal orbicularis oculi may be treated with gentle cautery or excised to attenuate overriding orbicularis.
- Mitomycin C can be used adjunctively in advanced cicatricial disease such as ocular cicatricial pemphigoid.
- Severe posterior lamellar contraction may require a spacer graft within the tarsus to lengthen the posterior lamella.
- Upper lid tarsotomy may benefit from a bandage contact lens in the postoperative period to prevent any sutures from irritating the ocular surface.
- Eye protection while sleeping may prevent wound dehiscence, particularly in patients with floppy eyelid syndrome or obstructive sleep apnea.

6.10 What to Avoid

Do not over-advance the lid retractor onto the tarsus, as this may cause lid retraction or ectropion. Avoid excising too much skin and orbicularis, as this can also lead to ectropion. If sutures are placed, ensure suture and knots are external to the conjunctival plane and do not come into contact with the ocular surface.

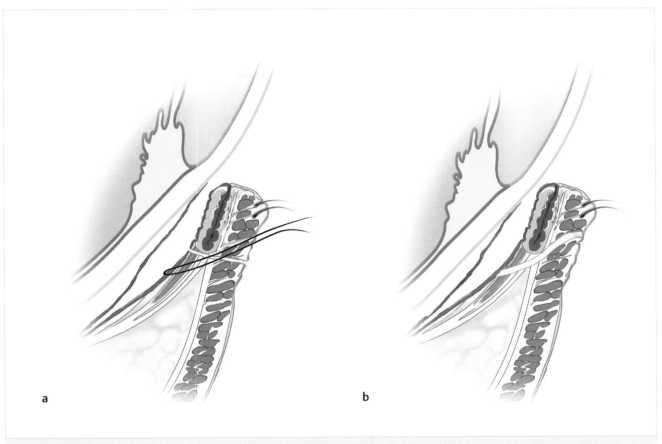

Fig. 6.4 **(a)** The Wies procedure: transverse tarsotomy and marginal rotation. **(b)** The resulting scar line after eyelid stabilization. From Codner M, McCord C. Eyelid & Periorbital Surgery. 2nd Edition. New York, NY: Thieme, 2016.

6.11 Complications/Bailout/Salvage

- Intraoperative hemorrhage, surgical site infection, wound dehiscence, scarring, corneal injury, and eyelid margin necrosis.
- Aggressive overcorrection (ectropion).
- Undercorrection (persistent entropion).
- Recurrence of entropion.
- Eyelid retraction.
- Eyelid asymmetry.
- Poor cosmesis including milphosis.
- Intraoperative hemorrhage is rare, and can often be controlled with local cautery. There are case reports of orbital hemorrhage after canthal surgery; thus, always employ meticulous hemostasis.
- Infection may be managed with topical antibiotics, systemic antibiotics, or, rarely, surgical washout and drainage.
- Advanced eyelid margin necrosis requires debridement of necrotic tissue, repair of any resultant defect, systemic antibiotics, and close monitoring.
- Superficial wound dehiscence may be observed and allowed to heal by secondary intention, depending on the size of the dehiscence. Internal wound dehiscence will likely require reoperation.
- Most overcorrection issues can be resolved by release of a suture in the office. If persistent overcorrection, undercorrection, or eyelid retraction is present, additional surgery may be required.

6.12 Postoperative Care

Antibiotic ointment is applied immediately postoperatively, as are chilled eye pads and protective eye shields. Chilled eye pads can be applied to the eyelid for 20 minutes of every hour while awake for the first 72 hours to decrease swelling and discomfort. Antibiotic ointment is applied several times per day, and an eye shield should be used while sleeping for the first 2 weeks after the procedure.

References

[1] Nerad JA. Techniques in Ophthalmic Plastic Surgery. Philadelphia, PA: Saunders Elsevier; 2010:99–112
[2] Cahill KV, Doxanas MT. Chapter 73: Eyelid abnormalities. In: Tasman W and Jaeger EA, eds. Duane's Clinical Ophthalmology Volume 5. Philadelphia, PA: Lippincott Williams & Wilkins; 2004:1–26
[3] Blaydon SM, Neuhaus RW. Entropion repair: anatomical approach. In: Fry CL and Faulkner AR, eds. Current Concepts in Aesthetic and Reconstructive Oculoplastic Surgery. The Hague/Netherlands: Kugler Publications; 2000:181–192
[4] Tse DT, Anderson RL, Fratkin JD. Aponeurosis disinsertion in congenital entropion. Arch Ophthalmol. 1983; 101(3):436–440
[5] Lance SE, Wilkins RB. Involutional entropion: a retrospective analysis of the Wies procedure alone or combined with a horizontal shortening procedure. Ophthal Plast Reconstr Surg. 1991; 7(4):273–277
[6] Scheepers MA, Singh R, Ng J, et al. A randomized controlled trial comparing everting sutures with everting sutures and a lateral tarsal strip for involutional entropion. Ophthalmology. 2010; 117(2):352–355

7 Ectropion Repair

Christina H. Choe

Summary

Lateral tarsal strip surgery has become the gold standard to treat eyelid ectropion. The reasons to perform lateral tarsal strip surgery are varied and it is useful as a primary or adjunctive surgery for many eyelid abnormalities. This chapter details the steps needed to successfully execute the surgery and other considerations to determine the best approach for ectropion repair.

Keywords: lateral tarsal strip, ectropion, lacrimal pump function, floppy eyelid syndrome, medial spindle

7.1 Goals

- To correct the outward turning of the eyelid.
- To tighten and stabilize the eyelid.
- To shorten the eyelid, which may become lengthened and lax with age.
- To help correct mild lid retraction and tearing due to poor lacrimal pump function.[1]

7.2 Advantages

The lateral tarsal strip procedure that was originally described by Anderson and Gordy has become the accepted gold standard for ectropion repair.[2] The lateral tarsal strip has the advantage of directly addressing the ectropion at the root cause: a lax lateral canthal tendon. Unlike approaches addressing ectropion via the central eyelid such as a tarsal wedge excision, it causes less rounding and medial displacement of the lateral canthal angle. It also has less risk of causing abnormal contour of the lid margin.[2]

7.3 Expectations

- Tightens and repositions a lax lower eyelid.
- Corrects ectropion, mild lid retraction, and decreased lacrimal pump function.
- With the improvement in eyelid position, it is common to note improved eyelid margin redness, irritation, and tearing.

7.4 Key Principles

Re-creating the appropriate curvature of the lower eyelid is required for successful ectropion repair. The normal lower eyelid wraps around the globe, and the lateral canthal tendon attaches to the periosteum on the inside of the lateral orbital rim at Whitnall's tubercle (▶ Fig. 7.1). Improper reattachment of the lower lid during ectropion repair may cause loss of lid/globe apposition, an abnormally rotated tarsal plate, or lateral canthal dystopia.

Reinsertion of the lower lid retractors is sometimes performed concurrently with the lateral tarsal strip if there is evidence of lower lid retractor disinsertion. Signs of lower lid retractor disinsertion include deepening of the inferior fornix, a higher lower eyelid resting position, reduced excursion in down gaze, and loss of the lower eyelid skin crease. Sometimes a white line may be visible on the conjunctival aspect of the eyelid representing the edge of the disinserted retractors.[3,4] Reinsertion of the lower lid retractors further stabilizes the eyelid by restoring the vector pull of the eyelid retractors.

Punctal ectropion may occur concurrently with general ectropion. Mild punctal ectropion will often be corrected by simple ectropion repair, but more severe punctal ectropion may require a medial spindle procedure to specifically address this issue.[5] This can be evaluated pre-operatively by applying lateral traction to the lower eyelid and evaluating how much correction of the punctal position is achieved.

Medial canthal laxity may be concomitantly found with lateral canthal laxity and it is important to evaluate for and address this if present. Medial canthal laxity can be diagnosed by applying lateral traction to the lower eyelid. If this results in displacement of the punctum past the medial limbus with the eye in primary gaze, significant medial canthal laxity is present and care must be taken to avoid excessively tightening the lower eyelid as this may displace the punctum into an abnormal position. Medial canthal plication to secure the medial canthal tendon can be performed concurrently when laxity is noted.

Any cicatricial or gravitational forces pulling the eyelid downward and contributing to the ectropion should be identified and addressed. Failure to do so will result in unsatisfactory results and risks early failure of the ectropion surgery. Be aware of any prior lid or facial surgeries (lower blepharoplasty, skin cancer resection and reconstruction, etc.) and note skin conditions like rosacea or actinic keratosis, which cause chronic inflammation and contraction of the anterior lamella. Evaluate the patient for involutional mid-face descent, which gravitationally pulls down the lower lid and contributes weight that the lateral canthal tendon must support. If present, it is recommended to address them concurrent to ectropion repair as well.

7.5 Indications

- Ectropion due to involutional changes, facial nerve paralysis, congenital abnormalities, and cicatricial changes.
- Excessive tearing that is felt to be due to loss of eyelid pump function.
- Chronic irritation from floppy eyelids. In severe cases of floppy eyelids, the lateral tarsal strip procedure may also be performed on the upper eyelids and is not limited to the lower eyelids.

7.6 Contraindications

- Cases with no or minimal lid laxity. In these cases, shortening the eyelid may result in excessive lid tightness, and lateral canthoplasty may be better able to address the displaced lateral canthal tendon without shortening the eyelid.

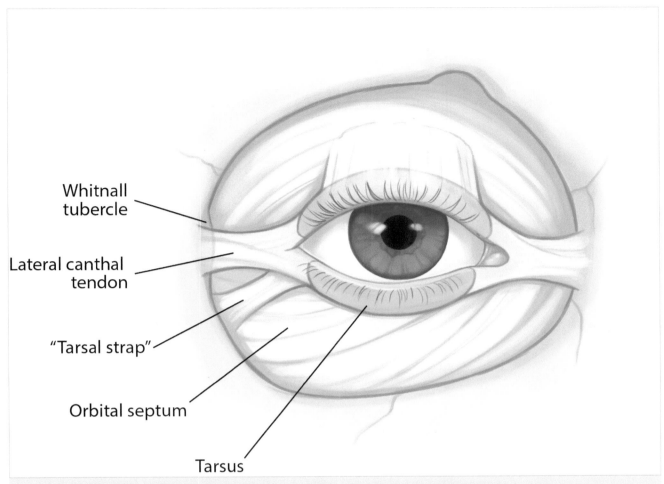

Whitnall tubercle

Lateral canthal tendon

"Tarsal strap"

Orbital septum

Tarsus

Fig. 7.1 The lateral canthal tendon attaches to the periorbita on the inside of the lateral orbital rim at Whitnall tubercle.

- Cases of ectropion with associated pathology in the central eyelid (lid mass, trichiasis, etc.). This is a relative contraindication. In these cases, doing a tarsal wedge excision would address both issues through one surgery and may be the preferred approach.

7.7 Preoperative Preparation

This surgery can be performed with sedation but may also be comfortably tolerated with local anesthetic. Local anesthetic is carefully infiltrated into surgical site taking care to inject around the lateral canthus, onto the lateral upper and lower eyelid, and down to the periosteum of the lateral orbital rim. Make sure to inject enough into the lower eyelid to cover the anticipated area of resection. Inject local anesthetic along the entire length of the lower eyelid if lower lid retractor reinsertion is needed and medially if medial spindle procedure for punctal ectropion is anticipated. Following the instillation of local anesthesia, a full-face surgical prep is done with dilute betadine, and sterile drapes are used to square off the face and allow visualization of both eyes for comparison of symmetry.

7.8 Operative Technique

First, a lateral canthotomy and inferior cantholysis is performed with Westcott scissors. The scissors are used to strum the canthal tendon until complete release of the lower eyelid is noted. If a medial spindle is required, this is best performed now as the medial conjunctiva may be difficult to access once the lid is tightened.

First a diamond of conjunctiva is excised with Westcott scissors just inferior to the punctum. This exposes the lower lid retractors, which are then imbricated with a double-armed 5–0 chromic gut suture. Both arms of the suture are then sequentially passed in a loop fashion through the inferior border of the tarsal plate before being externalized onto the skin in an inferior vector aiming toward the inferior orbit. The suture is tied. This full-thickness suture effectively reattaches the lower lid retractors while also providing an inverting vector (▶ Fig. 7.2).

If lower lid retractor reinsertion is required, this is also better addressed prior to completing the lateral tarsal strip procedure, as it is approached transconjunctivally. Cutting cautery is used to excise an ellipse of conjunctiva inferior to the tarsal plate along the horizontal length of the eyelid. The lower lid retractors are identified as a white band of tissue just deep to the

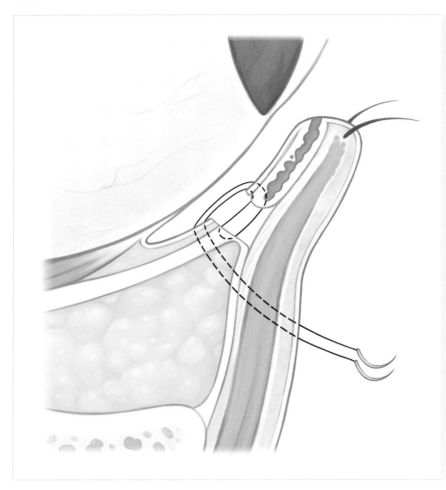

Fig. 7.2 The medial spindle procedure involves a full-thickness suture that provides an inverting vector for cases of punctal ectropion.

conjunctival layer. This can be differentiated from the septum by applying traction to the tissue and verifying that it is not attached to the orbital rim. In addition, the patient can be asked to look up and down and subtle pull on the tissue will be noted when the patient attempts to look in down gaze. 6–0 fast gut suture is used to attach the lower lid retractors to the inferior border of the tarsal plate.

Once the other elements of the surgery are addressed and stabilized, attention can then be turned to completing the lateral tarsal strip procedure. The lower eyelid is then placed on lateral traction to the desired tightness, and the point of overlap with the upper eyelid is noted. This point determines the length of the tarsal strip to be fashioned. The tarsal plate is then denuded of epithelium superiorly and anteriorly with scissors. The posterior epithelium is then denuded by scraping the conjunctiva off the tarsal tongue using either the flat part of a #15 blade or with diffuse gentle cautery. Once the tarsal strip is fashioned, the excess lateral tarsal plate and canthal tendon may be trimmed to avoid excessive bulkiness. A 5–0 polyglactin suture on a half-circle needle is passed through the tarsal strip and sutured to the periosteum on the inner aspect of the lateral orbital rim aiming slightly superiorly in order to approximate the position of Whitnall tubercle (▶ Fig. 7.3).

The 5–0 polyglactin suture is then used to re-create the lateral canthal angle by passing it through the gray line of the lateral upper and lower eyelid in a cerclage fashion with the knot buried in the incision. The canthotomy incision is then closed in layers. The orbicularis layer is closed using a buried interrupted 5–0 polyglactin suture. The skin is then closed with a 6–0 fast-absorbing gut suture or other dermal suture of your choice.

7.9 Tips and Pearls

- Attaching the tarsal strip to the periosteum can be a technically difficult maneuver. This is facilitated by holding the needle securely at the junction of posterior third and anterior two-thirds with the tip of a curved Castroviejo needle driver. It is also helpful to thin out the pre-periosteal tissue with cotton tip applicator in order to facilitate visualization of the needle as it exits the periosteum. In cases with a relatively posterior lateral orbital wall, it may be necessary to dissect the soft tissue away from the periosteum to allow more direct visualization of the needle tip as it exits the periosteum. Gently push the orbital tissue away from the orbital wall with the needle driver to expose the periosteum. The periosteum is engaged and a rotating motion of the wrist is used to gently nudge the needle forward until the tip can be retrieved.
- Tarsal ectropion is a particularly severe variant of eyelid ectropion to be aware of where the entire tarsus is everted

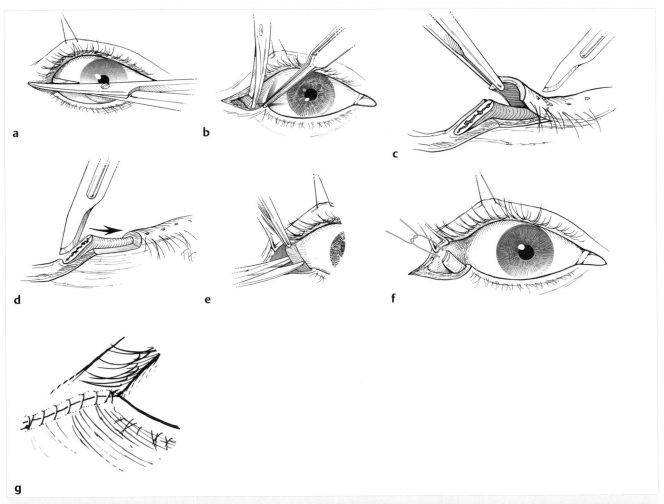

Fig. 7.3 (a–g) The lateral tarsal strip is fashioned by denuding the lateral tarsal plate superior, anteriorly and posteriorly before reattaching it to the periosteum on the inner aspect of the lateral orbital rim. From Cheney M, Hadlock T. Facial Surgery: Plastic and Reconstructive. 1st Edition. New York, NY: Thieme, 2014.

outward. This is typically associated with redness and follicular reaction of the exposed conjunctiva. In these cases, it is vital to perform both horizontal and vertical lid tightening. This is usually performed by reattaching the lower lid retractors to the inferior border of the tarsal plate in order to stabilize the eyelid along the vertical axis and performing the lateral tarsal strip to stabilize the eyelid along the horizontal axis.

- Chronic inflammation of exposed conjunctiva can result in cicatricial changes that may cause paradoxical marginal entropion and eyelash inversion after successful ectropion repair. Fortunately, this commonly self corrects once the lid is in proper position. However, additional surgical maneuvers including tarsal outfracture and anterior lamellar repositioning may be considered if it fails to resolve.[6]
- Avoid excessive shortening of the lower eyelid. This is especially important to consider in patients with a negative vector, where the globe protrudes more prominently than the malar eminence as it carries the risk of causing lower lid retraction if the lid slings under the globe. In addition, too much tension on the lid from aggressive lid shortening may

cause canthal dehiscence, resulting in an unattractive rounding of the lateral canthal angle. Finally, mismatch in the length of the upper lid compared to an excessively tightened lower eyelid can result in improper eyelid closure and lagophthalmos.

- Avoid lateralization of the punctum, which may occur when patients have significant medial canthal laxity. This may have negative consequences on tear drainage.
- When fashioning the tarsal strip, avoid excess dissection, which may devitalize the tissue, lead to necrosis, and increase the risk of wound dehiscence.

7.10 Complications/Bailout/Salvage

- Overcorrection. Secondary entropion may occur if excessive vertical tightening is performed. This is ideally appreciated intraoperatively and can be corrected by loosening the attachment of the retractors to the inferior tarsal plate.

- Undercorrection. Ectropion may persist after surgery. This may be temporary due to postoperative edema and weakness of the orbicularis muscle as it heals from the surgery. If this fails to self-correct after a few weeks, then identifying the cause of the failure and revision surgery is recommended. Potential causes of undercorrection include insufficient tightening of the lower eyelid, concomitant cicatricial or gravitational forces that were not addressed, failure to address the lower lid retractors, and improper attachment of the tarsal strip.
- Postoperative pain. Mild tenderness around the lateral canthal angle may occur and be normal in patients. This pain typically resolves after a few months when the suture dissolves.
- Wound dehiscence. It may be asymptomatic or cause pain, swelling, and sudden postoperative bleeding. Evaluation demonstrates loss of the lateral tarsal strip attachment to the orbital bone, and it must be surgically corrected.
- Pyogenic granulomas. These may also be asymptomatic or cause pain and bleeding. Evaluation demonstrates a red, pedunculated tumor. This most commonly occurs over the lateral canthal angle and can be easily removed surgically.
- Suture abscess. You may notice frank redness and purulent discharge or just mild fluctuance of the tissues overlying the lateral canthus. However, early infection should also be considered in cases of sudden worsening of pain after surgery. Antibiotics can be attempted to resolve infection but surgical removal of the suture may be required if it fails to respond or if the infection is advanced.

7.11 Postoperative Care

Postoperatively we request patients apply ice periodically for the first 2 days and attempt to sleep with the head elevated above the level of the heart for the first two nights. We also request that patients apply antibiotic ointment to the incision four times daily for 2 weeks and minimize their exertion for 2 weeks to help minimize bruising and swelling. We have a postoperative follow-up visit about a week after surgery to monitor for the development of complications, which is fortunately rare.

References

[1] Vick VL, Holds JB, Hartstein ME, Massry GG. Tarsal strip procedure for the correction of tearing. Ophthal Plast Reconstr Surg. 2004; 20(1):37–39
[2] Anderson RL, Gordy DD. The tarsal strip procedure. Arch Ophthalmol. 1979; 97(11):2192–2196
[3] Tse DT, Kronish JW, Buus D. Surgical correction of lower-eyelid tarsal ectropion by reinsertion of the retractors. Arch Ophthalmol. 1991; 109(3):427–431
[4] Shah-Desai S, Collin R. Role of the lower lid retractors in involutional ectropion repair. Orbit. 2001; 20(2):81–86
[5] Kam KY, Cole CJ, Bunce C, Watson MP, Kamal D, Olver JM. The lateral tarsal strip in ectropion surgery: is it effective when performed in isolation? Eye (Lond). 2012; 26(6):827–832
[6] Hatt M. Treatment of the paradoxic inversion of the lashes in ectropion. Ophthal Plast Reconstr Surg. 1992; 8(3):178–181, discussion 182

8 Epiblepharon Repair

Livia Teo

Summary

Lower eyelid epiblepharon is a common condition that can affect up to 46% of Asian children. It is believed to be a result of a horizontal fold of redundant skin and orbicularis oculi muscle that pushes and tilts the eyelashes toward the globe, resulting in cilia-ocular surface contact. This can result in ocular surface irritation and compromise.

Keywords: lower lid epiblepharon, epicanthoplasty, epicanthal fold

8.1 Goals

- Epiblepharon is when a horizontal fold of redundant skin and the orbicularis oculi muscle push against the eyelashes and tilt them toward the globe (▶ Fig. 8.1a).[1]
- Other possible contributing factors include a failure of the lower eyelid retractors to make contact with the skin, or a failure of interdigitation of septae in the subcutaneous plane.[2,3]
- A weak attachment of the pretarsal orbicularis muscle and skin to the tarsal plate can also lead to a redundant skin muscle fold that pushes the eyelashes against the cornea.
- Hypertrophy of the orbicularis oculi muscle is also thought to be a possible etiologic factor.[4]
- These contributing factors should be addressed in order to correct lower lid epiblepharon.[5]
- In the presence of epiblepharon, the cilia ocular surface contact can lead to corneal and conjunctival complications (e.g., punctate epitheliopathy and abrasions on the cornea and conjunctiva) and in severe cases it may even lead to scar and pannus formation on the cornea.
- The aim of epiblepharon repair is to externally rotate the row of lashes to prevent cilia-ocular surface touch and the complications that arise from it.

8.2 Advantages

Epiblepharon repair will correct or minimize cilia-ocular surface contact, ocular surface irritation, and erosions.

8.3 Expectations

- The surgery should provide eversion of the lashes to prevent cilia-ocular surface contact.

8.4 Key Principles

The key principles in epiblepharon correction are to correct the vertical misdirection of the lashes by debulking the pretarsal orbicularis oculi muscle, removing the redundant skin, and providing tarsal fixation of the lash bearing pretarsal skin and orbicularis oculi flap.

8.5 Indications

- In a study conducted in Japan, the incidence of epiblepharon in newborns was 46% and this decreased to 2% by 12 years of age.[6] It has been well described that most children will outgrow this condition and hence the decision to proceed with surgery should depend on the patient's age and the severity of symptoms and clinical signs of ocular surface complications.
- These should be weighed against the risks of surgery.
- The symptoms that are frequently encountered include eye redness, epiphora, irritation, photophobia, and discharge.
- On clinical examination, the presence of cilia-ocular surface touch should be assessed in both primary gaze and downgaze (▶ Fig. 8.1b).
- The horizontal extent of the lower eyelid where the lashes are in contact with the ocular surface should be noted as this would guide the surgeon on where to focus the surgical correction (medial, central, or lateral).
- The presence of a prominent medial epicanthal fold and its relation to the lashes in the medial aspect of the eyelid should also be recorded (▶ Fig. 8.2).
- The ocular surface must be assessed for cornea and conjunctival punctate epithelial erosions, abrasions, infectious keratitis, scars or Salzmann nodules, and pannus formation. This can be further documented with the help of fluorescein staining of the ocular surface.

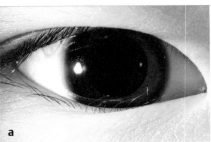 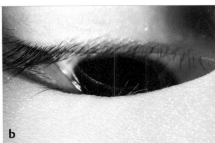

Fig. 8.1 (a) Clinical photograph of lower eyelid epiblepharon with overriding of the redundant skin and orbicularis oculi muscle with resultant vertical misdirection of the lashes. **(b)** Demonstration of cilia-ocular surface contact in downgaze during clinical examination.

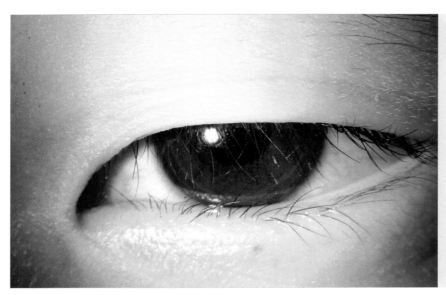

Fig. 8.2 A prominent medial epicanthic fold involving the lower lid, contributing to medial lower lid epiblepharon.

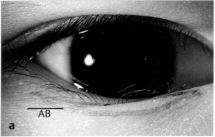
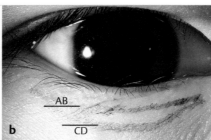

Fig. 8.3 **(a)** An intraoperative photograph of how much skin and orbicularis to excise. The upper edge of the ellipse is formed by a line drawn 2 mm below the lash line (AB). **(b)** The projection of this line onto the overriding redundant skin will form the lower edge of the ellipse (CD). The ellipse as seen when the lower lid is retracted downwards to expose it. The upper and lower edges of the ellipse are joined at the medial and lateral ends to complete the ellipse.

- If the patient is symptomatic and/or clinical signs of ocular surface compromise are documented, they can be offered the option of surgical correction of the epiblepharon.

8.6 Contraindications

- The relative contraindications for epiblepharon repair include patients who have eyelid eczema or allergic eye disease. These patients tend to be chronic eye rubbers and it is thought that eye rubbing might contribute to the development or recurrence of epiblepharon.[7]
- Patients with eyelid eczema have a poor skin texture that might result in poor wound healing. This can result in a cosmetically unacceptable scar.
- Surgery should be avoided in patients who have a strong keloidal tendency as the surgery might lead to an unacceptable scar.

8.7 Preoperative Preparation

The age of the patient will determine the type of anesthesia selected. In young children or uncooperative adult patients, general anesthesia is preferred. Surgeons should be aware that the severity of epiblepharon is significantly reduced by the induction of general anesthesia and when patients are in the supine position.[8]

In older children or cooperative adults, regional anesthesia can be used. For the skin marking, an ellipse is drawn as shown in the diagram. The upper edge of the ellipse is a horizontal line 2 mm below the lower eyelid lash line or following the natural lower lid crease (Line AB). The length of the ellipse can extend from the inferior lacrimal punctum till the lateral end of the lower eyelid. A shorter ellipse can be drawn if the epiblepharon is limited to the medial end of the lower eyelid. The lower edge of the ellipse is drawn on the fold of skin that lies on top of the upper edge that was previously drawn. This line (Line CD) is a projection of the previous line (AB) drawn. The skin is then pulled down and the medial and lateral ends of the ellipse are joined together (▶ Fig. 8.3).

8.8 Operative Technique

Currently described methods include the lid crease and capsulopalpebral fascia repair, modified Hotz procedure, everting suture technique, and cilia rotational suture with minimal skin excision.[9,10]

A local anesthetic that can be used is Marcaine with 1:100,000 dilution epinephrine. Two milliliters of this can be injected into each lower eyelid after the skin marking, prior to performing the skin incision. A 4–0 traction suture is placed in the lower lid margin and held down with an artery clamp. Incision of the upper edge and lower edge of the ellipse is performed with a number 15 blade. The ellipse of skin and pretarsal orbicularis is excised with Westcott scissors. The tarsal

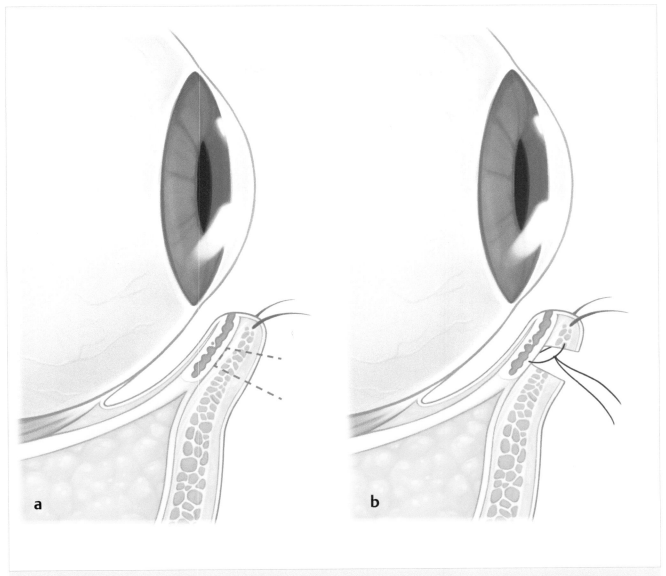

Fig. 8.4 **(a)** A wedge of tissue as delineated by the red lines will be excised. **(b)** A suture is placed for external rotation and tarsal fixation of the cilia bearing anterior lamellar.

plate is exposed and a wedge of pretarsal orbicularis is excised (▶ Fig. 8.4 x2 cross-section). For tarsal fixation and external rotation of the anterior lamella, a 6–0 nylon suture is used to attach the upper edge of the ellipse (remaining pretarsal orbicularis) to the tarsal plate. The lower edge of the ellipse is draped over the upper edge to assess if there is any redundant skin and orbicularis. Any additional skin and orbicularis is debulked if there is significant overriding of the lower edge of the skin-orbicularis fold. Skin closure is performed with an absorbable suture like 7–0 Vicryl in children or non-absorbable suture like 7–0 nylon in adults.

8.9 Tips and Pearls

- Removing an adequate amount of skin and orbicularis muscle without causing lid retraction and ectropion is crucial for the success of this surgery.

- Intraoperatively, if the patient is able to cooperate, he is first asked to look straight ahead and downward to assess for cilia-ocular surface touch. If redundant skin and orbicularis still push the lashes against the ocular surface, further debulking of the skin and orbicularis muscle is performed.
- To avoid excessive skin removal, the patient is asked to look up while opening the mouth. The upper and lower edges of the skin should maintain apposition in this instance. It is better to be conservative in skin removal.
- The correction of epiblepharon without addressing the prominent medial epicanthal fold may result in persistent cilia-ocular surface contact in the medial half of the lower eyelid.[11] Many methods address this medial epiblepharon by performing medial epicanthoplasty[12] and the skin redraping technique.[11]
- The skin incision should not be more than 2 mm below the lid margin as it might leave a cosmetically unacceptable scar. If

the patient has a natural lower lid skin crease, it should be incorporated into the upper edge of the ellipse to minimize skin tension and scarring.

- In addressing the medial lower lid epiblepharon, care should be taken to avoid the inferior canalicular system. The surgeon should always remain lateral to the lacrimal punctum during the dissection. A bowman probe can also be inserted into the lower canalicular system to serve as a guide during the surgery.
- Excessive skin and orbicularis removal should be avoided as this might lead to lower lid retraction or ectropion.

8.10 Complications/Bailout/Salvage

- If the inferior canaliculus is transected intraoperatively, repair of the canaliculus should be performed. This can be done with a monocanalicular stent like the Mini monoka stent (see Chapter 5, Canalicular Laceration Repair and Medial Canthal Tendon Avulsion Repair, for details).
- During the dissection down to the tarsus, a buttonhole through the tarsus can occur, especially if dissection is performed with a Colorado needle. The damaged tarsus can be apposed using 6–0 or 7–0 Vicryl suture. If a buttonhole through the conjunctiva or lower lid retractors occurs, and if the defect is small, it can be left alone. However, if large, it should be repaired using 7–0 Vicryl suture.

8.11 Postoperative Care

During the postoperative period, wound care is important to prevent unsightly scar formation. A topical steroid-antibiotic ointment can be applied for at least 2 weeks. An anti-scarring cream may also be prescribed if the individual is prone to keloid formation or might be expected to have poor wound healing.

The use of topical lubricants can minimize any ocular surface irritation. If the patient has allergic eye disease, the use of anti-allergy eyedrops will help to minimize any eye itching and an eye shield can help to prevent eye rubbing. The patient should be advised not to engage in any exercise or vigorous activity for at least 1 week postoperatively. A cold compress can be applied to help with resolution of the postoperative edema.

References

[1] Johnson CC. Epiblepharon. Trans Am Ophthalmol Soc. 1968; 66:74–81

[2] Jordan R. The lower-lid retractors in congenital entropion and epiblepharon. Ophthalmic Surg. 1993; 24(7):494–496

[3] Millman AL, Mannor GE, Putterman AM. Lid crease and capsulopalpebral fascia repair in congenital entropion and epiblepharon. Ophthalmic Surg. 1994; 25(3):162–165

[4] Choo C. Correction of oriental epiblepharon by anterior lamellar reposition. Eye (Lond). 1996; 10(Pt 5):545–547

[5] Kakizaki H, Leibovitch I, Takahashi Y, Selva D. Eyelash inversion in epiblepharon: is it caused by redundant skin? Clin Ophthalmol. 2009; 3:247–250

[6] Noda S, Hayasaka S, Setogawa T. Epiblepharon with inverted eyelashes in Japanese children. I. Incidence and symptoms. Br J Ophthalmol. 1989; 73(2):126–127

[7] Simon JW, Williams KH, Zobal-Ratner JL, Barry GP. Conservative management of lower eyelid epiblepharon in children. J Pediatr Ophthalmol Strabismus. 2017; 54(1):15–16

[8] Rhiu S, Yoon JS, Zhao SY, Lee SY. Variations in the degree of epiblepharon with changes in position and induction of general anesthesia: Graefe's archive for clinical and experimental ophthalmology. Albrecht Von Graefes Arch Klin Exp Ophthalmol. 2013; 251(3):929–933

[9] Woo KI, Yi K, Kim YD. Surgical correction for lower lid epiblepharon in Asians. Br J Ophthalmol. 2000; 84(12):1407–1410

[10] Woo KI, Kim YD. Management of epiblepharon: state of the art. Curr Opin Ophthalmol. 2016; 27(5):433–438

[11] Jung JH, Kim HK, Choi HY. Epiblepharon correction combined with skin redraping epicanthoplasty in children. J Craniofac Surg. 2011; 22(3):1024–1026

[12] Ni J, Shao C, Wang K, Chen X, Zhou S, Lin H. Modified Hotz procedure combined with modified Z-epicanthoplasty versus modified Hotz procedure alone for epiblepharon repair. Ophthal Plast Reconstr Surg. 2017; 33(2):120–123

9 Repair of Lower Eyelid Retraction

Nora K. Siegal and Christopher B. Chambers

Summary

Lower eyelid retraction can result in exposure keratopathy and significant morbidity. The expectations of eyelid retraction repair include restoring normal function and cosmesis to the eyelids. Repair of lower eyelid retraction involves evaluation of the scarring, and specifically, identifying the cause(s) of eyelid shortening. This chapter will review the preoperative assessment and surgical tools required for retraction repair.

Keywords: eyelid retraction, retraction repair, lower eyelid scarring

9.1 Goals

- This chapter will review eyelid anatomy and the myriad causes of lower lid retraction.
- Understanding eyelid anatomy and the relationship between its structure and function is requisite both for determination of the *cause* of cicatrix and for *repair* of retraction.
- This chapter will outline the operational techniques used in retraction repair.

9.2 Advantages

Periorbital scarring with eyelid retraction can have serious implications on morbidity and contribute to vision loss. Eyelid scarring can result in tissue contracture, ectropion, and entropion, all of which alter normal anatomic eyelid position and prevent protection of the cornea.[1] Retraction repair can restore both function and cosmesis of the eyelids.

9.3 Expectations

- The expectations of eyelid retraction repair include restoring normal function and cosmesis to the eyelids. Often, due to preoperative limitations of the existing eyelid structure, excellent cosmesis may not be possible. This should be discussed in detail with the patient in order to avoid postoperative dissatisfaction.
- Eyelid retraction repair may require a multistaged series of surgeries, and the patient should be counseled regarding expectations of each intervention.

9.4 Key Principles

The eyelids function to protect the anterior globe and to provide lubrication for the cornea and conjunctiva. The upper eyelid should sit 1 to 2 mm below the superior limbus and the lower eyelid should sit at the inferior limbus. Positioning above (or below, in the case of the lower lid) those landmarks is considered eyelid retraction. Malposition of the eyelids can induce exposure keratopathy due to improper maintenance of the tear film.

The eyelid is typically delineated into two layers, the *anterior* and *posterior lamellae*, but some refer to it as trilaminar. The *anterior lamella* is composed of skin (which does not contain subcutaneous fat) and orbicularis oculi muscle. The orbicularis is innervated by CN7 and functions to close the eyelids; the pretarsal and preseptal portions are responsible for involuntary closure and the orbital portion is responsible for purposeful, forced closure. Scarring of the anterior lamella leads to eyelid retraction and/or eyelid ectropion. The *posterior lamella* includes the tarsus and conjunctiva. The tarsus is made up of dense connective tissue, measuring between 8 to 12 mm in the upper eyelid and 3.5 to 5 mm in the lower eyelid.[2] These connective tissue plates are continuous with the medial and lateral canthal tendons, providing structure and support for the eyelids. The conjunctiva lines in the inner surface of the eyelid and the globe; it is composed of a non-keratinized mucous membrane that contains both goblet cells and accessory tear glands that secrete the mucin and aqueous components of tears, respectively. Scarring of the posterior lamella can lead to symblepharon, entropion, or eyelid retraction. The *middle lamella* of the lower lid refers to the tissue in between the two aforementioned layers below the inferior border of the tarsus. This layer includes the orbital septum, preaponeurotic fat pad, and lower eyelid retractors. Scarring of this layer, usually in the setting of previous surgery or trauma, can cause eyelid retraction, entropion, or ectropion.

The eyelids are suspended and supported by the medial and lateral canthal tendons that attach to periosteum of the orbital rim. The medial canthal tendon separates into *anterior* and *posterior* portions that surround the lacrimal sac within the lacrimal fossa. The anterior portion attaches to the anterior lacrimal crest of the frontal bone and the posterior portion attaches to the posterior lacrimal crest. While the anterior portion functions to support the medial canthal angle, the posterior portion remains firmly apposed to the globe.[3] The lateral canthal tendon attaches to Whitnall tubercle on the lateral orbital rim approximately 10 mm inferior to the frontozygomatic suture. The insertion of the tendon is approximately 4 mm posterior to the lateral palpebral raphae. The position of the lateral canthal angle is typically 2 mm superior to the medial canthal angle. This anatomic relationship should attempt to be restored in repair after trauma or scarring.

9.5 Indications

- The goals of eyelid retraction repair are to restore function and cosmesis.
- The first step in retraction repair involves evaluation of the scarring, and specifically, identifying the cause(s) of eyelid shortening.
- Scarring may result from anterior, middle, or posterior lamellar shortening, and ectropion/entropion may be the result of canthal tendon laxity. Often, eyelid retraction is a result of an amalgamation of the above anatomic changes.

9.6 Contraindications

- Eyelid retraction repair should not be performed in patients who have active eyelid/palpebral conjunctival inflammation, if possible (ocular cicatricial pemphigoid, Graves disease, or Stevens–Johnson syndrome).
- It is also suggested that in cases of retraction caused by burns, retraction repair be postponed until at least 12 months after the initial traumatic insult.

9.7 Preoperative Preparation

A few easy tests can be performed in order to garner information about the cause of eyelid retraction. The *lower lid distraction test* involves grasping the lower eyelid and pulling it anteriorly away from the globe. Distraction of more than 6 mm is considered abnormal and represents lid laxity and often canthal tendon weakness. The snapback test, which also involves pulling the lid off the globe, assesses the speed with which the lid returns to its normal anatomic position. If the patient needs to blink in order to bring the eyelid back into apposition with the globe, the test is abnormal.

The *2-finger test* can also be used to determine the cause of eyelid retraction. In this test, two fingers are placed below the eyelid margin and moved superiorly. If retraction is resolved with this movement, the anterior lamella has likely shortened. If the retraction is unchanged, the scarring is likely in the middle or posterior lamellae (▶ Fig. 9.1, ▶ Fig. 9.2, ▶ Fig. 9.3, ▶ Fig. 9.4).[1]

Using two fingers to put lateral traction on the eyelid can be a useful tool to determine the cause of entropion or ectropion. r/f results when the lid margin rolls posteriorly, usually secondary to involutional changes but also as a result of orbicularis spasm or scarring. The inward turning of the lid can result in trauma to the cornea. If the entropion is unchanged after the 2-finger test, the cause is likely middle or posterior lamellar scarring and will require repair with lysis of scar tissue and with use of a lamellar graft. If the entropion is improved with the 2-finger test plus lateral tension on the eyelid, it can often be corrected with a procedure that achieves lid tightening (▶ Fig. 9.5).[1]

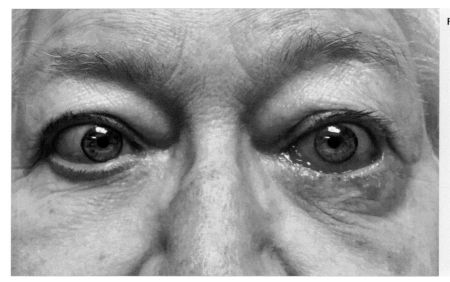

Fig. 9.1 Left lower eyelid retraction.

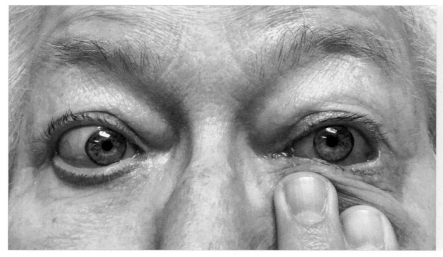

Fig. 9.2 Two-finger test with no eyelid elevation suggesting posterior lamellar shortening.

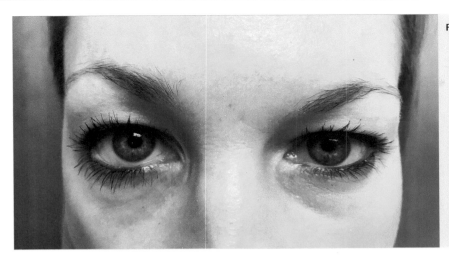

Fig. 9.3 Right lower eyelid retraction.

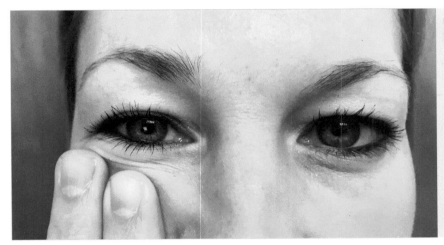

Fig. 9.4 Two-finger test with elevation of eyelid suggesting anterior lamellar shortening.

Cicatricial ectropion is common in the setting of eyelid retraction due to scarring and involves eversion of the margin away from the globe. This results in evaporation of tears, exposure of the palpebral conjunctiva, and epiphora. If the ectropion is unchanged by the 2-finger test, the cause is likely middle or posterior lamellar shortening and, as aforementioned, requires augmentation of the lamella and scar lysis. If the retraction can be improved with the 2-finger test but not with lateral tension on the lid, ectropion is usually the result of anterior lamellar shortening and requires full-thickness skin grafting. If the eyelid margin can be elevated with the two-finger test and the ectropion resolves with lateral traction, the retraction can be repaired with a tendon tightening procedure (▶ Fig. 9.1).[1]

9.8 Operative Technique

Retraction repair requires separate reconstruction of the anterior and posterior lamella. Anterior lamellar repair often requires full-thickness skin grafting, which is best achieved when the skin of the donor site matches the color and texture of the recipient site. The contralateral eyelid skin is typically the best option, as posterior auricular and supraclavicular skin grafts are often more thick and less well-matched. The graft should be hairless and *full* thickness, as partial-thickness grafts are more prone to contraction. Care should be made to avoid removing orbicularis tissue in the setting of scarring and retraction in order to preserve muscular (i.e., closure) function. Posterior lamellar reconstruction involves augmentation of the structural and lubricating functions of the eyelid; a buccal mucosal graft or a synthetic graft (such as Acellular dermis matrix allografts [AlloDerm; LifeCell Corporation, Branchburg, NJ] or Xenografts [EnduraGen; Stryker Corporation, Newnan, GA EnduraGen]) can be used. See section 9.8.1, #7.

9.8.1 Cicatricial Retraction with Ectropion

Anterior lamellar skin grafting is the procedure of choice. Below is a stepwise procedure for retraction repair.
1. After identifying the scar tissue to be lysed, mark a subciliary incision, taking care to extend the lysis beyond the cicatrix.
2. Inject local anesthetic with epinephrine into the eyelid using a 30-gauge needle.

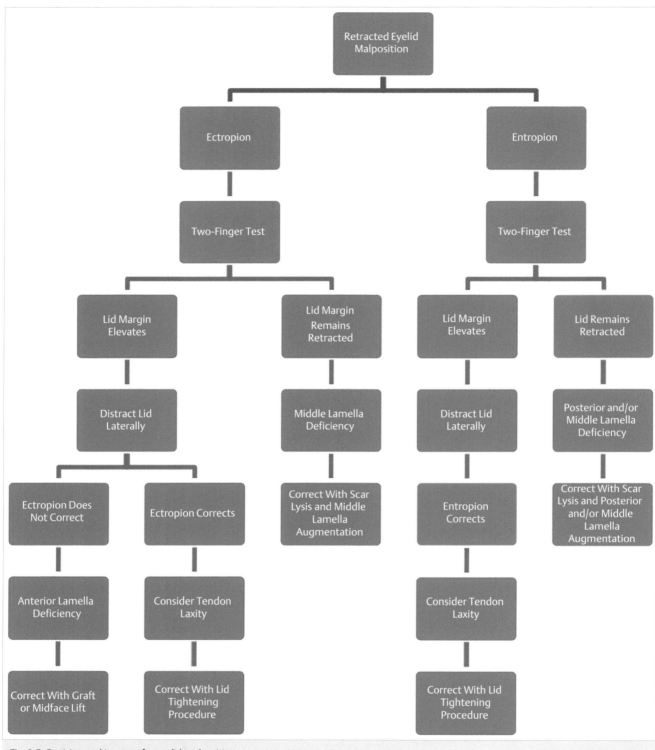

Fig. 9.5 Decision-making tree for eyelid malposition.

3. Place two 4.0 silk sutures in the lid margin to provide traction.
4. Using a number 15 Bard-Parker blade, create a subciliary incision.
5. Lyse all scar tissue using Westcott scissors.
6. Using the silk sutures to pull the eyelid on traction, mark a template for the full-thickness skin graft.
7. Harvest a full-thickness skin graft from the contralateral upper eyelid, supraclavicular skin, or posterior auricular skin.
8. Thin the graft, removing any subcutaneous fat with scissors.
9. Suture the graft in place using 5.0 fast gut suture or 6.0 nylon suture and cover the graft with ophthalmic antibiotic ointment.
10. Tape the 4.0 traction silk sutures to the forehead to provide traction.
11. Tie a bolster over the graft with 4.0 silk sutures.
12. If there is any eyelid laxity, a lid-tightening procedure such as a lateral tarsal strip should be performed (see section 9.8.5). This procedure also provides tension during the healing process to decrease further cicatrix. A similar procedure could be performed with a pedicle flap from the ipsilateral upper eyelid.

Adapted from Chambers CB, More KS. Periorbital scar correction. Facial Plast Surg Clin North Am. 2017; 25(1):25–36.

9.8.2 Cicatricial Retraction with Entropion

Posterior lamellar shortening with entropion can be the result of trauma/previous surgery, chemical injury, ocular cicatricial pemphigoid, trachoma, Stevens–Johnson syndrome, and chronic inflammation. Posterior lamellar augmentation is best achieved with a free tarsal graft from the contralateral eyelid. In this setting, the tarsal graft is lined with conjunctiva and is symmetric in its size and thickness. Hard palate is another option that provides both structural rigidity and mucosal lining. The mucosal lining of hard palate is keratinized, however, and this can irritate the cornea. In a patient who cannot provide adequate donor tissue, a Xenograft (EnduraGen; Stryker Corporation, Newnan, GA) or Acellular dermis matrix allograft (Allo-Derm; LifeCell Corporation, Branchburg, NJ) can be used. These grafts are associated with higher rates of contraction. Below is a stepwise procedure for graft harvesting and retraction repair with lamellar augmentation.

9.8.3 Free Tarsal Graft Harvesting

1. Inject local anesthetic with epinephrine into the pretarsal orbicularis of the donor eyelid. Evert the eyelid and inject local anesthetic into the conjunctiva and Müller muscle.
2. Place a 4.0 silk suture through the eyelid margin to provide traction and evert the eyelid using a Desmarres retractor.
3. Using Calipers mark 4 mm above the eyelid margin and draw a line at this level parallel with the margin. This line is marked because 4 mm of tarsus should be left in the donor eyelid.
4. Using a number 15 Bard-Parker blade incise the conjunctiva and tarsus along the line previously marked 4 mm above the

eyelid margin. Take care not to go full thickness with this incision and preserve the overlying orbicularis muscle. Make vertical incisions superiorly along the conjunctiva and tarsus medially and laterally.
5. Free the tarsal graft from the overlying levator aponeurosis and orbicularis muscle using a combination of sharp and blunt dissection with Westcott scissors.
6. Use Westcott scissors to cut the conjunctiva and Muller muscle on the superior boarder of tarsus and remove the tarsal graft from the eyelid.
7. Place the tarsal graft on the Mayo stand in a damp sponge until the recipient site is prepared.
8. Remove the traction sutures and place the eyelid to its natural position. The graft donor site will re-epithelialize and does not need to be closed.

Retraction repair and lamellar augmentation:
1. Inject local anesthetic with epinephrine into the conjunctival side of the eyelid.
2. Place two 4.0 silk sutures into the lid margin to provide traction.
3. Incise the conjunctiva below the tarsal plate with a number 15 Bard-Parker blade, lysing the cicatricial bands with Westcott scissors. If there is also scarring of the middle lamella, lyse it using sharp dissection. Avoid cautery to decrease the chance of recurrent cicatrix.
4. Put tension on the silk traction sutures and use palpation to feel for any remaining cicatrix. Once the scar bands have been lysed and the lid can protract freely, suture the free tarsal graft into place with the conjunctival side facing the fornix. Running 6.0 gut sutures can be used to secure the graft to the wound edges.
5. Tape the 4.0 traction silk sutures to the forehead in order to keep the lid on stretch. These traction sutures should be removed at the post-op week 1 visit.
6. If there is any eyelid laxity, a lid-tightening procedure, such as a lateral tarsal strip, should be performed.

Apply ophthalmic antibiotic ointment to the wound three times per day for 10 days.
Adapted from Chambers CB, More KS. Periorbital scar correction. Facial Plast Surg Clin North Am 2017; 25(1):25–36.

9.8.4 Horizontal Lid Tightening

If at the end of either ectropion or entropion repair it is apparent that lid laxity is contributing to poor eyelid positioning, a lateral tarsal strip should be performed. In this procedure, the lower lid is shortened and then reattached to the lateral orbital rim.

9.8.5 Lateral Tarsal Strip

1. Inject local anesthetic with epinephrine into the lateral canthal area, infiltrating the lateral third of the lower lid and down to the orbital rim at the lateral canthus.
2. Incise the skin at the lateral canthus using a number 15 Bard-Parker blade, starting at the lateral canthal angle and continuing laterally for 0.5 to 1 cm.
3. Perform a canthotomy/cantholysis using Westcott scissors; place one blade into the fornix at the lateral canthal angle and one blade through the skin incision created. Pull the

lower lid anteriorly using Adson forceps and then strum the inferior crus of the lateral canthal tendon. Cut the tendon to release the lid of the lateral orbital rim (▶ Fig. 9.6).

4. Hemostasis with cautery should be performed in order to decrease the chance of intraorbital hematoma formation.

5. Pull the freed eyelid laterally and estimate the amount of redundant tissue. Using Westcott scissors, excise the eyelid margin mucocutaneous junction, leaving the superior border of tarsus (▶ Fig. 9.7). Then separate the anterior and posterior lamella between the tarsus and orbicularis muscle. At this point you can cut along the inferior border of the tarsus laterally to remove the lower eyelid retractors.

6. Reflect the strip anteriorly and denude the conjunctival epithelium from the posterior border of the tarsus using a number 15 Bard-Parker blade (▶ Fig. 9.8).

7. Pull the tarsal strip laterally and evaluate lid position and tension. The strip can be shortened if necessary.

8. Pass a 4.0 double-armed Mersilene suture on a P-2 needle in a mattress fashion from posterior to anterior through the tarsal strip (▶ Fig. 9.9). The two ends of the suture can then be passed through the periosteum at the level of the superior crus of the lateral canthal tendon and approximately 4 mm posterior to the lateral orbital tubercle of Whitnall tubercle from posterior to anterior. A robust periosteal bite is made with both passes. The position of the eyelid on the globe is then evaluated using the *distraction test* (▶ Fig. 9.10). The sutures can be loosened or tightened prior to being tied down. The lid should not be distracted more than 3 mm.

9. Trim the excess anterior lamella (including eyelashes, skin, and orbicularis).

10. Use a 6.0 Vicryl suture to re-create the canthal angle: pass the suture through the cut edge of the upper lid through the gray line of the eyelid margin. Then pass the suture through the gray line of the lower lid and out of the wound edge (▶ Fig. 9.11). The skin overlying the incision can then be closed using interrupted 6.0 gut sutures.

Apply ophthalmic antibiotic ointment to the wound three times per day for 10 days.

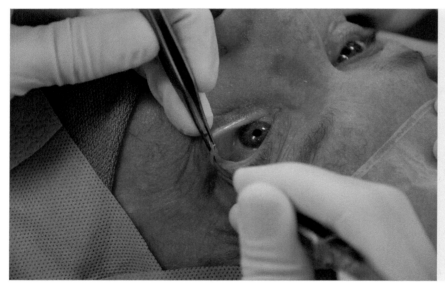

Fig. 9.6 Canthotomy/Cantholysis.

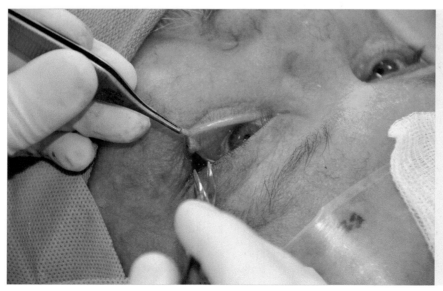

Fig. 9.7 Excision of the eyelid margin mucocutaneous junction.

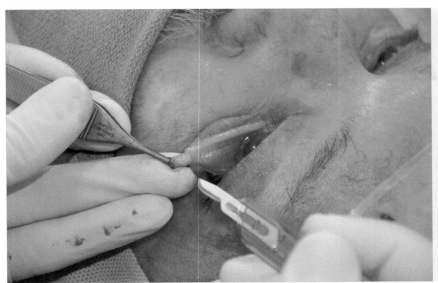

Fig. 9.8 Denuding of conjunctival epithelium from posterior border of tarsus with #15 blade.

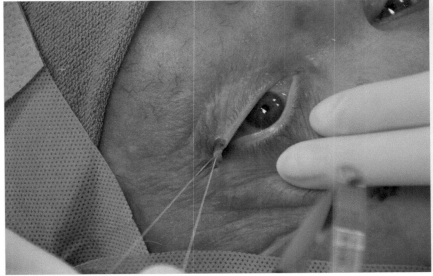

Fig. 9.9 Passing of a 4.0 double armed nonabsorbable suture through tarsal strip.

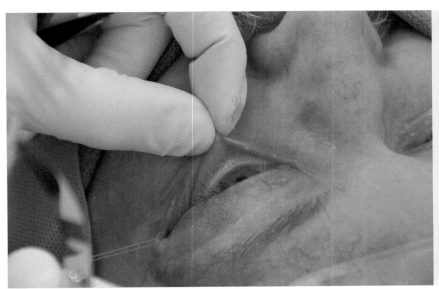

Fig. 9.10 Distraction test.

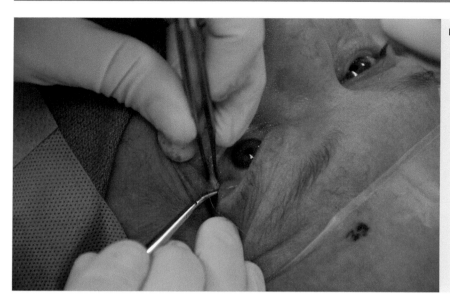

Fig. 9.11 Reconstruction of lateral canthal angle.

Adapted from Chambers CB, More KS. Periorbital scar correction. Facial Plast Surg Clin North Am 2017; 25(1):25–36.

9.9 Tips and Pearls

- In some cases, retraction repair may need augmentation with medical treatments. Classically, steroids have been the treatment of choice for modulation of scarring. Intralesional Kenalog inhibits the expression of genes involved in collagen synthesis, which reduces the production of collagen and increases its degradation.[4] Steroids may induce depigmentation and skin atrophy, so the patient should be counseled on these risks.[4]
- Injection of 5-fluorouracil (5-FU), a pyrimidine analogue with antimetabolite activity, has become a popular means of modulating scarring. 5-FU inhibits fibroblast proliferation and collagen synthesis.[5] As long as 5-FU is not injected intravenously (and the upper limit of dosing is not reached), the adverse hematologic effects including leukopenia, anemia, and thrombocytopenia can be avoided.[5] Intralesional side effects are rare but include erythema and ulceration/scar dehiscence.[6]
- For periorbital scarring, Massry has reported excellent results using a 1:3 mixture of Kenalog (5 mg/mL) with 5-FU (50 mg/mL) injected every 3 weeks for a total of three injections.[6] He also suggested that the combination may prevent tissue atrophy (seen with steroid injections) and inflammation (seen with 5-FU injections).
- Medical treatment of scarring/retraction is often combined with surgical reparation, but the most important intervention is proper reconstruction during the initial repair.

9.10 Complications/Bailout/Salvage

- Complications of retraction repair are usually the result of improper preoperative assessment. If both anterior and posterior lamellar shortening are present but only one is addressed, the surgery will not be successful.
- It is also advisable to over-correct lower eyelid retraction as both autogenous and synthetic grafts contract during the postoperative period.
- If in the weeks following repair that scarring appears to be antagonistic, authors would recommend prompt treatment with intralesional steroids.

9.11 Postoperative Care

Eyelid retraction repair should be performed unilaterally if possible. At the end of the retraction repair, it is recommended to place the lower eyelid on stretch for up to 1 week. This can be achieved with the use of the Frost suture, which provides upward tension on the lower lid through its connection to the brow. A bandage contact lens can be placed for patient comfort. The eyelids should be lubricated with antibiotic ointment and patched at the end of the repair. Patients are counseled to leave the patch in place until the first postoperative appointment. At that time, the Frost suture can be removed and the patient can begin application of antibiotic ointment three to four times daily. Close follow-up is required to monitor for the development of antagonistic scarring.

References

[1] Chambers CB, Moe KS. Periorbital scar correction. Facial Plast Surg Clin North Am. 2017; 25(1):25–36
[2] Goold LA, Casson RJ, Selva D, Kakizaki H. Tarsal height. Ophthalmology. 2009; 116(9):1831–1831.e2
[3] Anderson RL. Medial canthal tendon branches out. Arch Ophthalmol. 1977; 95(11):2051–2052
[4] Son D, Harijan A. Overview of surgical scar prevention and management. J Korean Med Sci. 2014; 29(6):751–757
[5] Khan MA, Bashir MM, Khan FA. Intralesional triamcinolone alone and in combination with 5-fluorouracil for the treatment of keloid and hypertrophic scars. J Pak Med Assoc. 2014; 64(9):1003–1007
[6] Massry GG. Cicatricial canthal webs. Ophthal Plast Reconstr Surg. 2011; 27 (6):426–430

10 Transconjunctival Lower Eyelid Blepharoplasty

Mica Y. Bergman and Sandy Zhang-Nunes

Summary

Lower eyelid transconjunctival blepharoplasty is a commonly performed aesthetic procedure with numerous technique nuances and adjuncts which when properly performed results in high patient satisfaction. This chapter will discuss the various surgical options along with an explanation of their goals, including fat repositioning and adjunctive skin pinch. There are many possible pitfalls and complications that can occur if the surgeon is not well versed in the regional anatomy, makes unwise decisions regarding the approach or fails to address all of the related anatomic factors. Special attention is also directed to management of complications including retrobulbar hemorrhage, diplopia and eyelid retraction.

Keywords: lower eyelid blepharoplasty, cosmetic surgery, aesthetic surgery, aging face, facial rejuvenation, oculoplastic surgery, oculofacial plastic surgery

10.1 Goals

- Goals of lower eyelid blepharoplasty:
  - Rejuvenate the lower eyelids and mid-face.
  - Improve the appearance of the lower eyelids and mid-face.
  - Restore a more youthful appearance by addressing signs of aging.
- Signs of aging in the lower eyelid:
  - Herniation of orbital fat ("under eye bags").
  - Accumulation of excess skin.

10.2 Advantages

Aging changes of the lower eyelid and mid-face may be approached surgically, as will be elucidated in this chapter, or by nonsurgical mechanisms including botulinum toxin, filler, chemical peeling, or laser treatments. There are two primary advantages of a surgical approach. First, it directly addresses the underlying etiology, by removing or repositioning herniated orbital fat, or by excising excess skin. The nonsurgical alternatives can enhance the appearance of the aberrant tissue, but do not correct the inciting issue. Second, surgical approaches tend to confer longer lasting results of 10 to 15 years or more in comparison to filler injections (9–18 months). Botulinum toxin injections, laser resurfacing, or chemical peels all are adjuncts to surgery, not alternatives.

10.3 Expectations

- Safe and effective operation.
- Long-term cosmetic enhancement of the lower eyelid.
- Bias toward undercorrection:
  - Generally may be successfully addressed with in-office enhancement.
- Avoidance of overcorrection:
  - Complications can be devastating:
    - Lower eyelid retraction and ectropion (▶ Fig. 10.1).
    - Double vision.
    - Blindness.
    - Severe dry eye.
    - Periorbital hollowing.

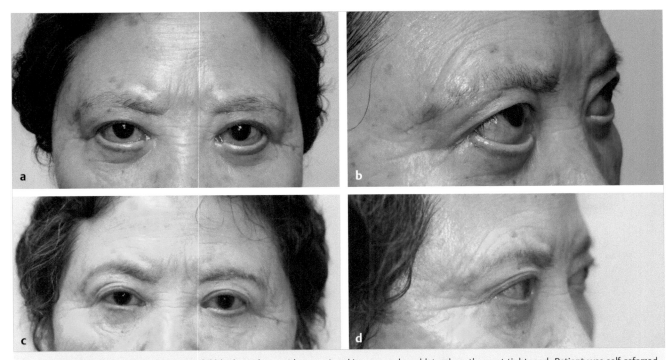

Fig. 10.1 (a,b) One month after lower eyelid blepharoplasty with excessive skin removed, and lateral canthus not tightened. Patient was self-referred in for excessive dryness of the eyes, lagophthalmos and a new angry appearance to her face. **(c,d)** She was treated with 5-fluorouracil to the dermal ciatrix, hyaluronic acid filler to stent up the eyelid, and may need further therapy.

10.4 Key Principles

10.4.1 Relevant Anatomy

The lower eyelid consists of seven layers (▶ Fig. 10.2), the composition of which depends on the level within the eyelid. From anterior to posterior, these are skin, orbicularis oculi muscle, orbital septum, orbital fat, lower eyelid retractors, tarsus, and conjunctiva. Near the orbital rim, all layers are present except for tarsus. More superiorly, the septum and retractors condense and insert into the tarsus. There is no orbital fat present above this condensation. Moving more superiorly, near the eyelid margin, only skin, orbicularis, tarsus, and conjunctiva are present.

The lower eyelid skin, like the upper eyelid skin, is the thinnest skin of the body. With age, it loses elasticity. The orbicularis oculi is the primary eyelid protractor. It is a circumferentially oriented muscle that is responsible for voluntary and involuntary eyelid closure. The orbital septum is a thin, but firm, connective tissue, which originates from the arcus marginalis at the inferior orbital rim and combines with the capsulopalpebral fascia just inferior to the tarsus such that they insert together onto the inferior tarsal border. It is an important landmark, in that it separates the anterior eyelid structures from the posterior orbital structures. Orbital fat lies just posterior to the septum, and is divided into three distinct fat pads (▶ Fig. 10.3, ▶ Fig. 10.4). The medial and central pads are divided by the inferior oblique muscle, whereas the central and lateral pads are divided by the same muscle's arcuate expansion. Posterior to the orbital fat are the eyelid retractors: the capsulopalpebral fascia, which is analogous to the levator palpebrae superioris in the upper eyelid, and the sympathetically innervated inferior tarsal muscle, which is analogous to Müller muscle in the upper eyelid. The tarsus is a dense connective tissue that confers structural support to the eyelid, and the most posterior layer is the conjunctiva, which is contiguous with the conjunctiva of the globe itself.

Fat Repositioning

Oftentimes with aging, herniation of orbital fat arises in concert with infraorbital hollowing, which occurs when the sub-orbicularis oculi fat (SOOF) descends below its native position at the inferior orbital rim. When this occurs, the surgeon may consider using the fat that would otherwise be removed to add volume to the nearby atrophic area.

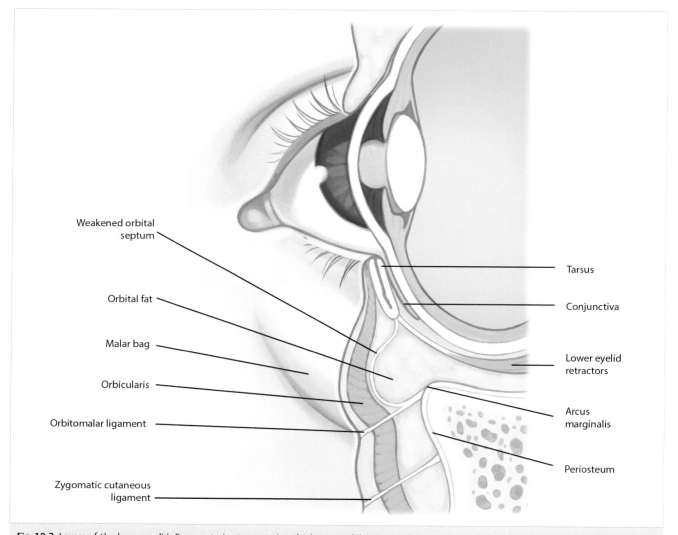

Fig. 10.2 Layers of the lower eyelid. From anterior to posterior, the lower eyelid consists of skin, orbicularis oculi muscle, orbital septum, orbital fat, lower eyelid retractors, tarsus, and conjunctiva. Depending on the level relative to the margin, some layers are not present. In this diagram, note the features of the aging face: the weakened orbital septum, allowing the orbital fat to herniate forward, resulting in the presence of a malar bag.

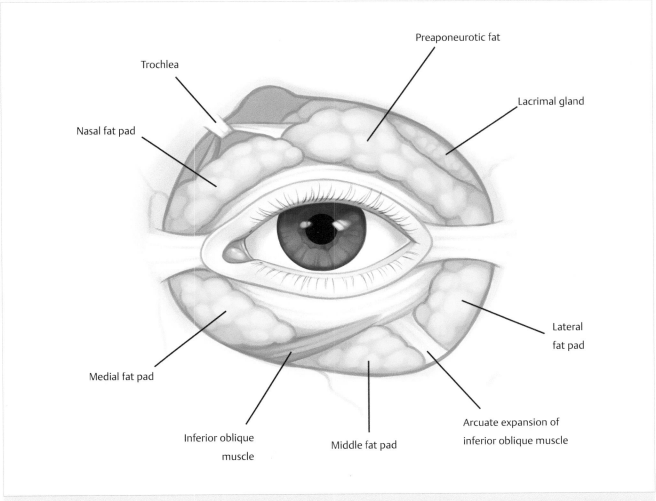

Fig. 10.3 Fat pads of the upper and lower eyelid. Lower eyelid orbital fat is divided into three distinct fat pads. The medial and central pads are divided by the inferior oblique muscle, whereas the central and lateral pads are divided by the same muscle's arcuate expansion. Blood vessels tend to be more prominent in the medial fat pad.

10.4.2 Indications

- Specific indications:
  - Herniation of orbital fat ("bags" under the eyes).
  - Excess or sagging lower eyelid skin.
  - Descent of the mid-face tissues (► Fig. 10.5).
- Overarching considerations:
  - Patient should desire aesthetic enhancement or rejuvenation of the lower eyelids.
  - Patient and surgeon should agree on intended aesthetic outcome.
  - Surgeon must reasonably believe that the intended outcome may be achieved surgically.

10.4.3 Contraindications

- Absolute contraindications:
  - Patients with unrealistic expectations:
    - The only true measure of success in a cosmetic procedure is the patient's satisfaction.
    - Failure to align patient and surgeon views of an optimal result preoperatively virtually guarantees an unhappy postoperative patient.
- Relative contraindications:
  - Overly picky, demanding, critical, or particular patient:
    - Extreme care should be taken preoperatively to review goals, risks, and plan for addressing postoperative dissatisfaction.
  - High bleeding risk (intrinsic coagulopathy, patient in whom it is unsafe to discontinue anticoagulation):
    - Given the potentially devastating consequences of intra-orbital hemorrhage, caution should be exercised in these patients.

10.5 Preoperative Preparation

Preoperative preparation for lower eyelid blepharoplasty is similar to that for any oculoplastic procedure.

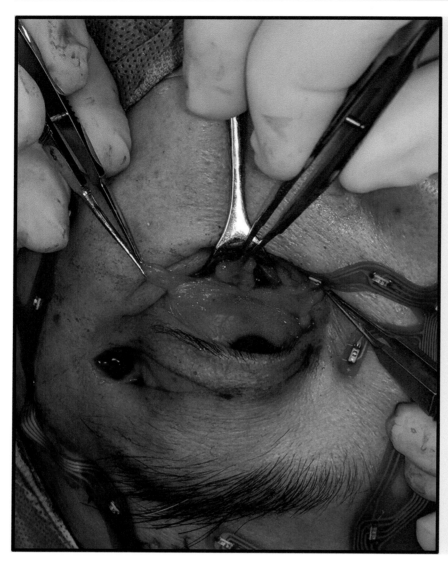

Fig. 10.4 Fat pads of the lower eyelid. Intraoperative photograph demonstrating the three lower eyelid fat pads of the left eye. The inferior oblique can be seen dividing the medial and the central fat pads, and the arcuate expansion dividing the central and lateral fat pads.

10.5.1 Operative Setting

The procedure may be performed in an ambulatory surgery center or in the office setting. It is important to note, however, that manipulation of fat is painful, and as such, discretion in patient selection is advised if choosing the office setting, with careful attention to both the personality of the patient and the intended surgical plan. If fat repositioning is to be employed, an ambulatory surgery center is recommended. If the office setting is chosen, the surgeon should consider preoperative treatment with oral pain medication and anti-anxiolytic agents.

10.5.2 Preoperative Marking

It is useful to mark the location of the orbital fat pockets with the patient sitting upright, as the fat tends to retract posteriorly when the patient is supine.

10.5.3 Local Anesthesia

The choice of local anesthesia is according to surgeon preference. These authors recommend a 50/50 mixture of a short-acting anesthetic (e.g., xylocaine 1–2%) and a long-acting anesthetic (e.g., bupivacaine 0.25–0.5%) with total 1:100,000–1:200,000 epinephrine, mixed with hyaluronidase (2–3 USP units/cc) for improved tissue spread. Local anesthesia should be injected subcutaneously in the skin and the inferior conjunctival fornix, being careful to avoid any orbital structures such as extraocular muscles and, the globe. An infraorbital block may also be performed particularly if fat transposition is to be performed, although injury to the infraorbital nerve should be avoided.

10.5.4 Facial Preparation

The eyelids and face should be prepared with 5% betadine. Careful attention should be paid to preparation of the eyelid margins and the eyelashes, where meibum and debris can accumulate, and the ocular surface itself should be irrigated with the solution. Saline should then be used to irrigate the eyes to avoid betadine toxicity to the ocular surface. It is important that higher concentrations are not used, as these may be toxic to the cornea. In iodine-allergic patients, low-dose hypochlorous acid solution 0.01 to 0.02% may be used to clean the eyes and lashes.

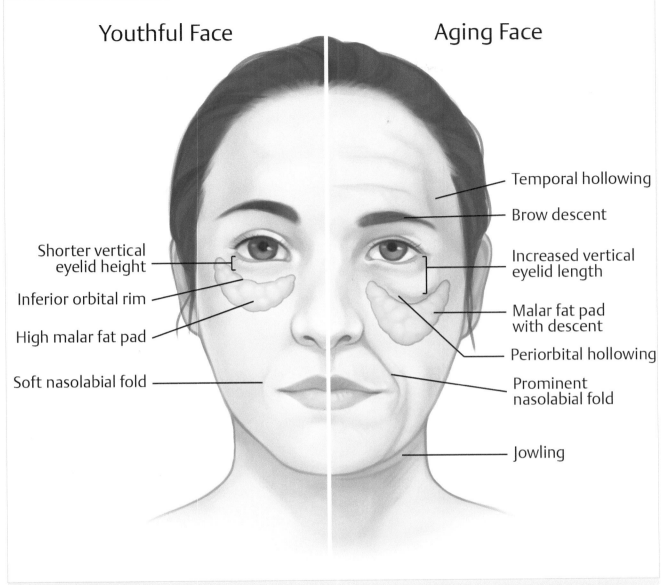

Youthful Face

Aging Face

Shorter vertical eyelid height

Inferior orbital rim

High malar fat pad

Soft nasolabial fold

Temporal hollowing

Brow descent

Increased vertical eyelid length

Malar fat pad with descent

Periorbital hollowing

Prominent nasolabial fold

Jowling

Fig. 10.5 Aging changes of the lower eyelid and mid-face. Diagram illustrates facial changes associated with aging (right side) compared to the youthful face (left side). Particularly relevant to lower eyelid blepharoplasty are the descent of the malar fat pad and the periorbital hollowing.

If this is unavailable, one may have to consider using chlorhexidine on the face, being careful to not let it enter the eye, and the eyes should be irrigated copiously with saline. In such a scenario, the patient needs to understand the theoretically higher risk of infection.

10.6 Operative Technique

10.6.1 Transconjunctival Subtractive Blepharoplasty

1. A traction suture (4–0 silk) is placed in the lower eyelid tarsus near the lash line, and the eyelid is everted over a Desmarres retractor or cotton tip applicator.

2. An incision is made through the conjunctiva and lower eyelid retractors using monopolar cautery or Westcott scissors. This incision is made approximately 2 mm inferior to the inferior tarsal border (▶ Fig. 10.6). If Westcott scissors are used, it is often helpful to cauterize any visualized conjunctival vessels prior to proceeding.

3. A second traction suture (4–0 silk or 6–0 Vicryl) is placed through the proximal cut edge of conjunctiva and lower eyelid retractors and clamped superiorly to the drape. To aid in exposure, it can be helpful to weave this suture in and out such that it encompasses the medial-lateral extent of the eyelid, or to place one suture medially and one suture laterally.

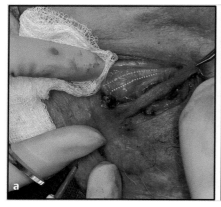 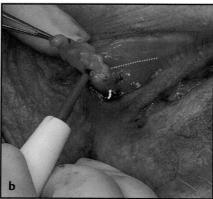

Fig. 10.6 Lower eyelid transconjunctival incision. The lower eyelid tarsus extends 4 mm from the eyelid margin and is usually appreciated intraoperatively as a function of its more yellow color and firm appearance. For a preseptal approach, an incision is made transconjunctivally approximately 2 mm inferior to the inferior tarsal border (blue line). For a postseptal approach, the incision is made further inferiorly, approximately 3 to 5 mm inferior to the inferior tarsal border (yellow line).

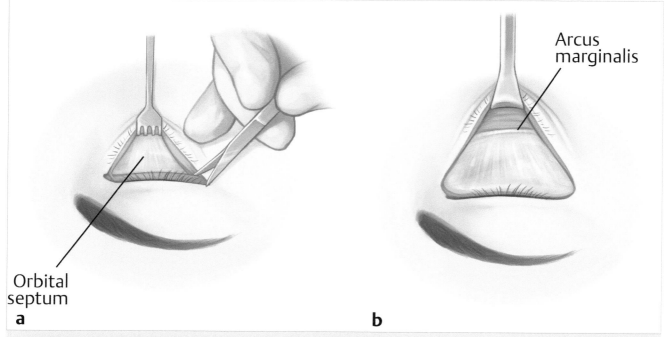

Fig. 10.7 Preseptal approach to lower eyelid fat. **(a)** The preseptal (postorbicularis) plane is developed using Westcott scissors or monopolar cautery. To aid in establishing this plane, the assistant retracts the lower eyelid using a lacrimal rake then a Desmarres retractor, pulls the cheek inferiorly using a finger, and pulls the tarsal edge of the conjunctiva anteriorly using a forcep. **(b)** After expanding the incision medially and laterally, dissection is carried inferiorly to the arcus marginalis and inferior orbital rim.

4. Careful dissection is carried out in the preseptal (postorbicularis) plane using cotton tips, Westcott scissors, and monopolar cautery. To assist in this dissection, the assistant holds a blunt, four-prong rake first, then a Desmarres retractor in the lower eyelid, a finger to pull the cheek down, and q-tip dissection to open up the preseptal plane. The dissection is carried out to the inferior orbital rim. (▶ Fig. 10.7).

5. The septum is opened anterior to each of the fat pads using monopolar cautery or Westcott scissors. Orbital fat is prolapsed through these buttonhole(s), aided by gentle massage with cotton tip applicators and gentle digital palpation of the globe. If the patient is awake, additional local anesthesia should be injected into the fat pads prior to manipulation.

6. The desired amount of fat is removed from each pocket using monopolar cautery, or bipolar cautery, then cutting with scissors. It is often effective to cauterize circumferentially around the base of the fat to be removed prior to amputating it. Meticulous hemostasis is critical at this point to avoid postoperative hemorrhage. Furthermore, care should be taken to avoid injury to the inferior oblique muscle.

7. Additional fat that will not be removed is returned to its original position with gentle cautery.

8. Conjunctiva may be left to close by secondary intention, but if desired, it may be closed with buried, interrupted sutures (6–0 plain gut or 8–0 Vicryl) medially and laterally to realign the conjunctiva.

[A step-by-step photo series is available in a chapter written by one of these authors.[1]]

10.6.2 Transconjunctival Blepharoplasty with Fat Repositioning

1. Steps 1 to 5 above are performed.
2. Fat pedicles are mobilized in a manner similar to that for fat removal.
3. The arcus marginalis and orbitomalar ligament are released from the inferior orbital rim using a Freer elevator. The same instrument is then used to create a subperiosteal plane, which will receive the mobilized fat.
4. Often, a combination of fat removal and fat repositioning will be employed.
5. Typical areas of hollowing are the medial and central infraorbital areas (tear trough), and sometimes more laterally (orbitomalar groove). The fat pedicles are imbricated with double-armed suture (4–0 polypropylene), and suture ends externalized through the overlying cheek tissue to fill in the areas of hollowing. A large Desmarres retractor is used to aid in this. A polypropylene suture on a free needle can be used for this step as well if a double-armed version with a large enough needle is not available.

The sutures arms are then tied over a bolster (silicone or foam) (▶ Fig. 10.8).

10.6.3 Pinch Blepharoplasty

1. After completing the transconjunctival portion of the blepharoplasty, preparation for skin excision may be undertaken. The superior portion of the excision is made 2 to 3 mm below the lash line. The inferior extent of the excision is determined by using forceps to pinch excess skin (▶ Fig. 10.9). To guard against excessive skin removal, the pinch is often undertaken with the patient opening his or her mouth and looking upward to ascertain maximum tension on the lower eyelid. The medial extent of the excision is approximately 2 mm lateral to the punctum, and the lateral extent is at the lateral canthus.
2. Skin is excised with Westcott scissors, with or without scoring first with a number 15 blade.
3. Skin closure is with a running suture such as 6–0 plain gut, again using care to minimize vertical tension on the wound.

10.6.4 Modifications

1. The transconjunctival approach above describes a preseptal approach to the fat pockets. The fat pockets may, alternatively, be approached transconjunctivally in the postseptal plane. The advantage of this approach is that it is more direct and does not compromise the integrity of the septum. The disadvantage may be that it can be cumbersome in patients with large amounts of fat because access is immediate rather than graded. As a result, this approach

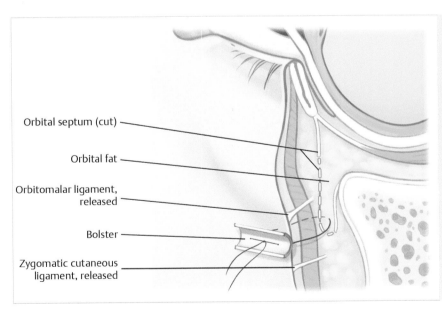

Orbital septum (cut)

Orbital fat

Orbitomalar ligament, released

Bolster

Zygomatic cutaneous ligament, released

Fig. 10.8 Lower eyelid fat repositioning. After mobilizing the fat pedicles, the arcus marginalis and orbitomalar ligament are released from the inferior orbital rim, and a subperiosteal plane is established. The fat pedicles are imbricated with double-armed suture and transposed into this subperiosteal plane. The sutures are then externalized through the overlying cheek tissue and tied over a bolster.

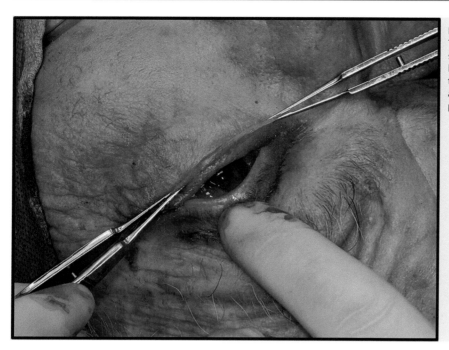

Fig. 10.9 Lower eyelid skin pinch blepharoplasty. Two pairs of forceps are used to pinch up excess skin only. If the patient is awake, he or she should be asked to open the mouth in order to ensure no tension is placed on the lower eyelid. This helps to assure a safe amount of skin is excised, preventing postoperative lower eyelid retraction.

tends to be employed in younger patients with less fat herniation.

2. Fat repositioning may be in the pre-periosteal plane rather than the subperiosteal plane. In this case, the fat is reposited between the SOOF and the orbicularis. Suturing of the fat may be as described for subperiosteal repositioning, or it may be sutured directly to the orbicularis muscle anteriorly or SOOF or periosteum posteriorly.

3. The entire lower eyelid blepharoplasty may be performed anteriorly via a subciliary incision. This technique is described in detail in the next chapter.

10.7 Tips and Pearls

10.7.1 Older patient with lower eyelid laxity:

- Lid tightening procedure should be performed during the same operation to avoid postoperative lower eyelid retraction:
  - ○ Typically achieved with canthotomy, inferior cantholysis, and lateral tarsal strip.
    - – This procedure will also allow more ready access to the fat pads.
  - ○ May be achieved with closed canthoplasty or canthopexy through an upper blepharoplasty incision (if being simultaneously performed) in patients with mild lower eyelid laxity.
    - – Beyond the scope of this chapter, but described in detail in reference [1]

10.7.2 Patient with globe prominence or mid-face retrusion (▶ Fig. 10.10):

- Complexity of anatomy should be explained to the patient.
- This anatomic profile results in inadequate support of the eyelids.
- Patient's complaints will be inadequately addressed if mid-face is not simultaneously addressed.
- Anatomy may be addressed with a cheek implant or complementation of the surgery with pre- or postoperative cheek fillers.
- In severe cases, orbital decompression may need to be considered (beyond the scope of this chapter).

10.7.3 Patient selection is a critical component determining success of lower eyelid blepharoplasty:

- If questions exist as to whether the patient's expectations will be met, surgery should not be offered.

10.8 What to Avoid

Measures should be taken during the pre-, intra-, and postoperative periods to avoid untoward results. Preoperatively, care should be taken to ensure that the patient's expectations are consistent with the surgeon's expectations and the limits of surgery. Surgery should not be undertaken until these goals are aligned. Intraoperatively, it is critical for the surgeon to strike

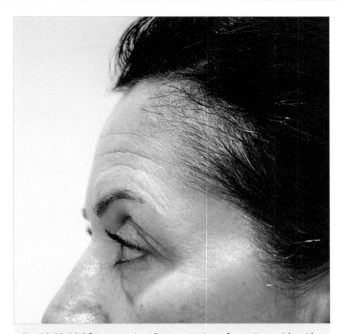

Fig. 10.10 Mid-face retrusion. Demonstration of a patient with mid-face retrusion. Note the inferoposterior slope of the patient's mid-face, which makes her lower eyelid fat appear more prominent than it would appear in a patient with a less acute angle. This is a patient where cheek filler or implant would help support the lower eyelid. A traditional subtractive lower eyelid blepharoplasty may not achieve the desired outcome in this patient. Furthermore, over-tightening of the lower lid under a prominent globe can also lead to sliding of the lower eyelid beneath the globe.

an appropriate balance between removing sufficient fat and/or skin and removing excessive tissue. Of the three lower eyelid fat pads, the lateral one is most commonly neglected during blepharoplasty, resulting in an incomplete and heterogeneous improvement. On the opposite end of the spectrum, overly aggressive fat removal can result in a "hollowed" appearance, and overly aggressive skin removal can result in eyelid retraction. Meticulous hemostasis throughout, and particularly at the conclusion of surgery is imperative to avoid postoperative hemorrhage. Postoperatively, the surgeon must be attentive to patient concerns such that any complications can be managed appropriately and expeditiously.

10.9 Complications/Bailout/Salvage

10.9.1 Orbital hemorrhage:

- Ocular emergency that, if untreated, can quickly lead to orbital compartment syndrome and permanent blindness.
- Signs/symptoms:
  - Severely edematous and ecchymotic eyelids (▶ Fig. 10.11).
  - Pain.
  - Decreased vision.
  - Motility disturbances.
  - Pupillary disturbances.
  - Increased intraocular pressure.
- Treatment:
  - Must be treated immediately on recognition.
  - Release of incisions.

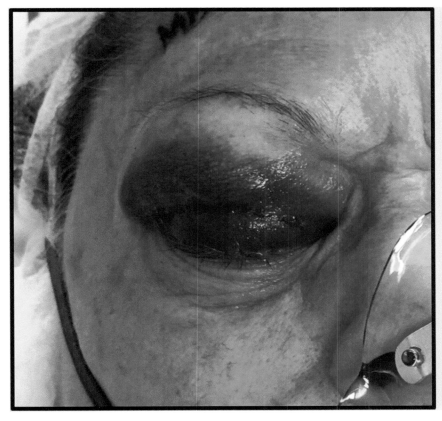

Fig. 10.11 Orbital hemorrhage. Clinical photograph of a patient with an (upper eyelid) orbital hemorrhage. Note the profound edema and ecchymoses and tense appearance to the eyelid, which is better appreciated clinically.

- If release of incisions is insufficient, immediate lateral canthotomy and inferior cantholysis.
  - Local anesthesia is injected into lateral canthus and lower eyelid.
  - Using Stevens tenotomy scissors, lateral canthus is cut down to the lateral orbital rim.
  - With one hand tenting up the lower eyelid, Stevens tenotomy scissors in the other hand are used to cut the inferior crus of the lateral canthal tendon.
  - Multiple cuts may be necessary to completely release the lower eyelid.
  - The eyelid is completely released when it can be lifted off the globe and the eyelid completely everted.
  - If the bleeding vessel can be identified, it should be cauterized.
  - Repair is not typically undertaken in this setting, and the eyelid usually heals nicely. If revision surgery is necessary, it may be performed in the future.
  - Ensure the intraocular pressure has normalized and the vision has returned by the end of the release. Using a formal tonometer is recommended.

10.9.2 Injury to the inferior oblique muscle:

- To avoid injury, this muscle should be identified intraoperatively prior to removing or repositioning the neighboring fat pads.
  - Inferior oblique travels between the medial and central fat pads as it courses from its origin on the maxillary bone to its insertion on the posterior globe.
- If injury is noted intraoperatively, a surgeon familiar with eye muscle surgery can attempt reapproximation of the inferior oblique muscle with 6-0 or 5-0 vicryl suture. Prompt referral should be arranged.
- Patients with injury to the inferior oblique will present with binocular vertical or oblique diplopia.
  - Should be referred to a strabismus surgeon for further management.

10.9.3 Lower eyelid retraction (▶ Fig. 10.1):

- Can occur when too much skin is removed during lower eyelid blepharoplasty.
- Cosmetically unacceptable.
- Puts cornea at risk of exposure and keratopathy.
- Can lead to lagophthalmos and severe recalcitrant dry eye long term.
- Treatment depends on the degree of retraction.
  - In the early post-op period, 5-fluorouracil may be injected to reduce the cicatrization.
    - We recommend approximately 0.2 to 0.6 mL of a 50 mg/mL preparation every 2 weeks.
  - In mild cases, or in patients reluctant to undergo further surgical procedures, hyaluronic acid filler may be injected to provide appropriate lift.[2]

- Safe and effective remedy.
- May need to be repeated as the filler resorbs.
  - In patients with more severe retraction, lower eyelid tightening, often with a posterior lamella graft (e.g., hard palate, post-auricular cartilage), and mid-face lifting should be employed.[3,4]
    - When anterior lamellar shortening is severe, a skin graft may even be required.

10.9.4 Over-hollowing:

- May result if fat removal is performed overzealously.
- Volume can be replaced by injection with either hyaluronic acid filler or autologous fat.

10.9.5 Undercorrection:

- Insufficient fat removal.
  - Reoperation may be pursued.
    - Typically at least 3 months after the initial operation to ensure tissues have assumed their postoperative position and edema has resolved.
- Insufficient skin removal.
  - Reoperation may be pursued.
    - Risk of eyelid retraction (see above) increases with successive operations, and thus should be undertaken judiciously.
  - In cases where excess skin is mild, skin resurfacing with laser or chemical peeling may be effective and obviate the need for further operative intervention.

10.10 Postoperative Care

Postoperatively, patients should be treated with combination steroid-antibiotic treatment. Drops are preferable to ointment to reduce blurring of the vision during the day. Ointment should be used externally if a skin incision is made, as well as in the eye at night during early recovery. Patients who underwent extensive dissection intraoperatively may be treated with a short course of oral steroid taper, if desired. Frequent application of ice and mild compression for the first 48 hours postoperatively is recommended to minimize edema, though patients should be informed that swelling is expected, and may worsen prior to improving.

References

[1] Zhang-Nunes S, Foster J, Czyz CN, Nabavi C, Massry GG. Lower eyelid blepharoplasty and lateral canthoplasty. Chapter 15 In: Sataloff RT, Facial Plastic and Reconstructive Surgery (Sataloff's Comprehensive Textbook of Otolaryngology: Head and Neck Surgery), 1st Edition

[2] Goldberg RA, Lee S, Jayasundera T, Tsirbas A, Douglas RS, McCann JD. Treatment of lower eyelid retraction by expansion of the lower eyelid with hyaluronic Acid gel. Ophthal Plast Reconstr Surg. 2007; 23(5):343–348

[3] Ben Simon GJ, Lee S, Schwarcz RM, McCann JD, Goldberg RA. Subperiosteal midface lift with or without a hard palate mucosal graft for correction of lower eyelid retraction. Ophthalmology. 2006; 113(10):1869–1873

[4] Pak J, Putterman AM. Revisional eyelid surgery: treatment of severe postblepharoplasty lower eyelid retraction. Facial Plast Surg Clin North Am. 2005; 13 (4):561–569, vi–vii

11 Transcutaneous Lower Blepharoplasty

Bradford W. Lee

Summary

Transcutaneous lower lid blepharoplasty is a surgical approach to lower lid rejuvenation that utilizes a subciliary incision to remove lower lid dermatochalasis and manage orbital fat prolapse and/or infraorbital hollowing. This chapter details which patients are appropriate candidates and how to optimize outcomes and minimize the risk of complications with this procedure.

Keywords: lower blepharoplasty, transcutaneous, subciliary incision, dermatochalasis, orbital fat prolapse, infraorbital hollowing

11.1 Goals

- Transcutaneous lower blepharoplasty facilitates surgical removal of excess skin on the lower lids through a subciliary incision.
- When necessary, orbital fat prolapse can be addressed via the subciliary surgical approach. This may include fat excision and/or fat repositioning below the inferior orbital rim to address infraorbital hollowing and to create a smooth transition at the lid-cheek junction.

11.2 Advantages

The primary advantage of the transcutaneous approach is the ability to excise excess skin on the lower eyelids, which is not feasible from a purely transconjunctival approach. When performed correctly, the incision is hidden just beneath the lash line on the lower lid and blended into a crow's feet line at the lateral canthus.[1,2]

11.3 Expectations

- Patient expectations are aesthetic rejuvenation of the lower eyelids while maintaining an anatomically correct position and function of the lower eyelids.
- Every patient's lower eyelids age differently, but common goals are to address excess skin and wrinkles on the lower lid, address any orbital fat prolapse, and to create a vertically short lower lid that transitions gracefully into the cheek.
- If there are any pre-existing lid malpositions such as ectropion, entropion, or eyelid retraction, these should be discussed and addressed simultaneously.

11.4 Key Principles

A customized lower blepharoplasty evaluation should provide an individualized assessment of the patient's lower lid anatomy and a surgical plan that addresses specific issues. There are various approaches to lower blepharoplasty (transconjunctival, transconjunctival with skin pinch excision, and transcutaneous), and

various adjuncts such as fat repositioning, mid-face lifting, autologous fat grafting, and laser resurfacing. Every patient deserves consideration as to which technique would be most appropriate.

Transcutaneous lower blepharoplasty involves a subciliary incision for surgical access as well as for removing excess skin. When performing subcutaneous dissection, preservation of the pretarsal orbicularis neuromuscular anatomy by incising the orbicularis and septum more inferiorly down the lid helps to minimize weakening the orbicularis oculi muscle, which can lead to ectropion, lagophthalmos, and exposure keratopathy.

Management of fat should include reducing any prolapsed orbital fat but should not be overaggressive such that the patient looks hollowed or "skeletonized." Fat repositioning can be performed to address infraorbital hollowing along the orbital rim and to smooth the transition zone of the lid-cheek junction.

11.5 Indications

- Dermatochalasis of the lower eyelids.
- Desire for aesthetic rejuvenation of the lower lids and lid-cheek junction.
- Orbital fat herniation on the lower eyelids.
- Periorbital hollowing along the lower lids.

11.6 Contraindications

- Paralytic lagophthalmos due to facial nerve palsy or multiple prior surgeries.
- Pre-existing cicatricial ectropion or eyelid retraction.
- Unrealistic patient expectations.
- Inability to stop blood thinners.

11.7 Preoperative Preparation

To minimize intraoperative bleeding and reduce the risk of postoperative bruising and bleeding complications, the surgeon should discuss stopping anticoagulants, vitamins, and supplements with patients, pending approval by the patient's cardiologist or primary physician. Ideally, blood thinners such as aspirin, ibuprofen, and other vitamins and supplements can be stopped 7 to 14 days prior to surgery, although certain anticoagulants can be stopped safely within 2 to 5 days prior to surgery. Before surgery, patients should receive a thorough history and physical and medical clearance from their primary care physicians.

In the preoperative area, with the patient sitting in an upright position, the periorbital grooves can be marked along the inferior orbital rim, above which the orbital fat prolapse can be visualized (▶ Fig. 11.1a). Having patients supraduct their eyes helps to accentuate orbital fat prolapse. The surgeon can annotate on the eyelids which fat pads are most herniated to help guide an individualized approach to fat reduction and redraping (▶ Fig. 11.1b).

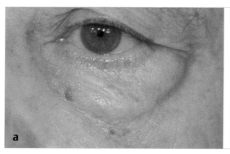
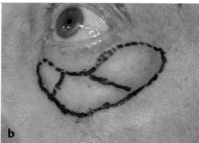

Fig. 11.1 (a) Preoperative photo demonstrating lower lid dermatochalasis, lower lid fat prolapse, and a periorbital groove along the orbital rim. (b) With the patient looking upward, the lower lid is marked, demarcating the prolapsed fat pads and the groove along the orbital rim.

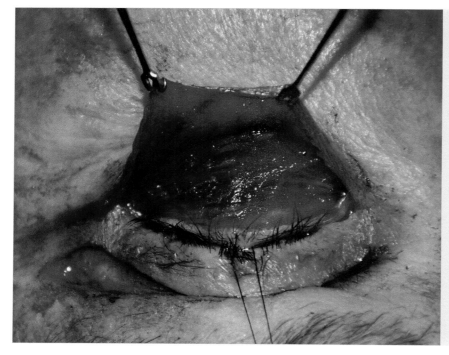

Fig. 11.2 After placing a 6–0 silk traction suture, a subciliary incision is created and a skin-flap is raised.

A subciliary incision can be marked, if desired, prior to injection of local anesthetic. Some surgeons prefer to mark the amount of skin to be excised preoperatively, whereas others prefer to determine the amount of skin to be excised after undermining, managing the orbital fat, and redraping the skin. Local anesthetic containing epinephrine is infiltrated into the lower lids and lateral canthal regions with sufficient time given for hemostasis.

11.8 Operative Technique

Prior to making the subciliary incision, it can be helpful to place a 6–0 silk traction suture through the lower lid margin for superior lid traction. A subciliary incision is performed with Westcott scissors 1 mm below the lashes. Subcutaneous dissection is performed over the pretarsal orbicularis (▶ Fig. 11.2). Below the pretarsal orbicularis, the orbicularis is incised and dissection is continued inferiorly in a preseptal plane down to the orbital rim (▶ Fig. 11.3).

At this point, the orbital septum is opened across the eyelid, and the medial, central, and lateral fat pads are pedicalized and prolapsed outward. Care is taken to avoid injury to the inferior oblique muscle located between the medial and central fat pads (▶ Fig. 11.4). The fat pads are conservatively debulked as needed. To determine the amount to be excised, the eye can be manually retropulsed and the fat pedicles trimmed flush with the surface of the lower lid. To treat infraorbital hollowing, the fat pads can be redraped after creating a preperiosteal dissection plane below the orbital rim (▶ Fig. 11.5). The fat pedicle is redraped below the orbital rim using a 5–0 monocryl suture that is passed in a horizontal mattress fashion through the fat pedicle, through a slip of periosteum below the infraorbital rim, and back up through the fat pedicle (▶ Fig. 11.6). The suture is tied off, and this *preperiosteal* fat redraping results in correction of infraorbital hollowing and blending of the lid-cheek junction (▶ Fig. 11.7). Alternatively, the fat can be redraped in a *subperiosteal* plane. In this technique, a subperiosteal dissection plane is created below the orbital rim. A double-armed 5–0 prolene or gut suture can be passed through the fat pedicle, and the needles are externalized through the skin below the orbital rim and tied off on the skin or over a bolster.[3] Finally, the orbital septum is evaluated and any necessary further septal release is performed to ensure the septum and lower lid retractors are not being tethered downwards by the redraped fat pads.

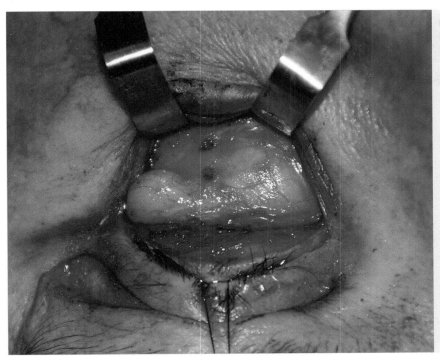

Fig. 11.3 The orbicularis is incised below the pretarsal orbicularis and a preseptal dissection plane is carried down below the orbital rim.

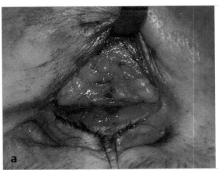
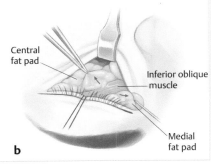

Central fat pad

Inferior oblique muscle

Medial fat pad

a

b

Fig. 11.4 (a,b) After opening the orbital septum across the lower lid, the three fat pads are now visible with the inferior oblique muscle separating the medial and central fat pads.

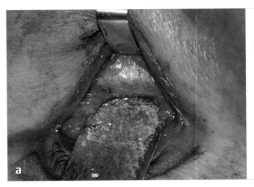
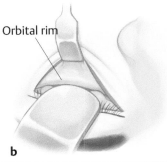

Orbital rim

a

b

Fig. 11.5 (a,b) With a malleable retractor holding back the orbital fat, a pre-periosteal dissection plane is used to expose the area below the orbital rim in preparation for fat redraping.

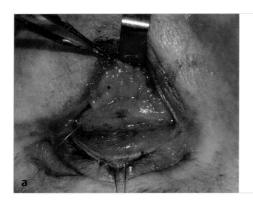

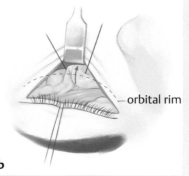

Fig. 11.6 (a,b) The fat pad to be redraped is mobilized in horizontal mattress fashion below the infraorbital rim.

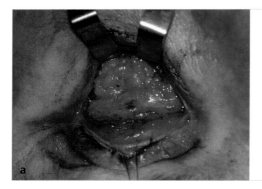

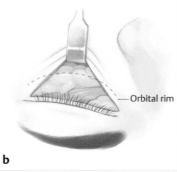

Fig. 11.7 (a,b) Once the fat has been repositioned, there should be a smooth contour on the lower lid created by the fat pedicle bridging the orbital rim.

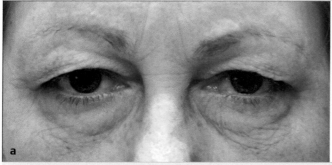

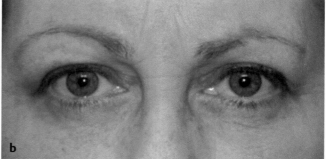

Fig. 11.8 (a) Before and **(b)** after photos of a 57-year-old female who underwent an upper blepharoplasty and lower blepharoplasty with fat repositioning and subciliary skin excision.

After addressing the fat, any further lid tightening or supportive procedures can be performed as needed or desired. Options include a simple canthoplasty for horizontal lid tightening, or additional adjunctive measures that can provide more robust support, such as orbitomalar ligament release with orbicularis-pexy or a sub-orbicularis oculi fat (SOOF) lift. The orbicularis-pexy and SOOF lift are helpful in preventing post-blepharoplasty eyelid retraction in patients with significant mid-face descent or who are at high risk of eyelid retraction due to a negative vector.[4]

Finally, the skin is redraped, and a conservative amount of skin is excised. Typically, more skin is excised laterally than medially along the subciliary incision. After ensuring hemostasis, the subciliary incision is closed in running fashion using 6–0 fast-absorbing gut suture from lateral to medial. This concludes the transcutaneous lower lid blepharoplasty procedure (► Fig. 11.8, ► Fig. 11.9).

11.9 Tips and Pearls

- Identify patients who are at high risk for post-blepharoplasty lid malpositions, such as those with significant lid laxity, heavy mid-faces, or negative vectors. In these patients, consider a transconjunctival blepharoplasty approach or robust SOOF lift with canthoplasty to help support the lower lid and avoid postoperative lid malpositions.[5] A facelift or mid-face lift can be another powerful means to use the mid-face to support the lower lid, thereby mitigating the risk of post-blepharoplasty eyelid retraction.

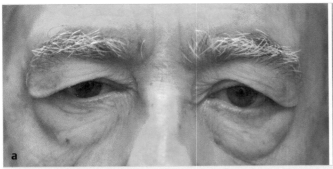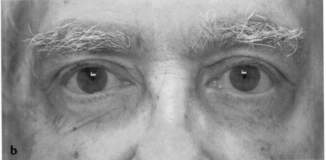

Fig. 11.9 (a) Before and (b) after photos of a 76-year-old male who underwent an upper blepharoplasty, lateral direct brow lift, and lower blepharoplasty with subciliary skin excision.

- For patients with mild-to-moderate skin laxity, consider performing transconjunctival blepharoplasty with a skin pinch excision and/or ablative laser resurfacing. The skin pinch excision results in less trauma and denervation to the orbicularis oculi muscle than performing the entire surgery transcutaneously, which requires skin undermining and incising through the orbicularis oculi muscle.[6]
- In patients with concomitant festoons or malar mounds, ablative laser resurfacing can be a helpful adjunct for tightening the skin and preventing fluid reaccumulation.
- In patients who have significant hollowing with minimal orbital fat prolapse, inform them preoperatively that to efface the periorbital hollows, they may need further volume augmentation that can be achieved surgically via autologous fat transfer or nonsurgically via injection of dermal fillers. In fact, some of these may not need any surgical blepharoplasty and may be candidates for volume augmentation only.
- In younger patients in their 30 s to 50 s, there is often minimal fat prolapse but significant periorbital hollowing, resulting in "dark circles" and shadowing along the lower eyelids. In these patients, it is important to efface the periorbital hollowing via fat repositioning and/or volume augmentation.
- In older patients in their 60 s to 80 s, there is a greater tolerance for mild concavity of the lower lids, and these patients are typically pleased as long as the orbital fat prolapse is reduced. If they desire comprehensive smoothing of the lid-cheek junction, periorbital volume augmentation is oftentimes necessary with or without a mid-face lift.
- In patients who are younger and have tighter lids, subperiosteal fat redraping with externalization of sutures through the skin can result in easier fat redraping and fat can be redraped further down below the orbital rim. In more senior patients with greater lid laxity, pre-periosteal fat redraping is easier and does not require externalized sutures.
- The subciliary incision should be gently tapered inferiorly at its most lateral extent beyond the lateral canthus. This follows the expression lines of the lateral canthal region (i.e., crow's feet) and helps conceal the incision.
- Take care to preserve the pretarsal orbicularis muscle, which has an important role in eyelid closure. Excessive trauma to the orbicularis muscle can result in lagophthalmos,

denervation, and weakening of the muscle, and resultant dry eyes.
- Lower lid tightening or suspension is often indicated to help support the lower lid and prevent post-blepharoplasty ectropion and eyelid retraction.

11.10 What to Avoid

- Avoid making the subciliary incision too far from the lashes, since this results in a visible scar and is a stigma of poor incision planning.
- Avoid overaggressive fat debulking to prevent an excessively hollowed appearance. If planning to redrape the fat pedicles, one can excise less fat so that there is sufficient fat to reposition below the orbital rim.
- Avoid inadequate debulking of the lateral fat pad. This fat pad is commonly undercorrected. If the orbital septum is not fully opened laterally, the lateral fat pad will not prolapse forward in its entirety and the resulting undercorrection of lateral fat prolapse may necessitate revisional surgery. Releasing the arcuate expansion of Lockwood ligament helps to facilitate complete prolapse of the lateral fat pad while communicating it with the central fat pad.
- Avoid excessive skin resection, especially over the central and medial lower eyelid, which can lead to cicatricial ectropion.
- Close the subciliary incision laterally to medially with the needle passes directed superiorly. This helps to conceal any "dog ears" in the concavity of the nasojugal groove and prevents incarcerating lashes within the suture line.

11.11 Complications/Bailout/ Salvage

- Retrobulbar hemorrhage is a vision-threatening complication that can be minimized by properly reviewing and stopping anticoagulants perioperatively and by ensuring careful hemostasis intraoperatively. If it occurs, the incision should be immediately opened, the clot evacuated, and cautery applied for hemostasis.
- Injury to the inferior oblique muscle can occur either during dissection and fat excision or by incarcerating the muscle during fat repositioning.

- Chemosis is not uncommon and typically resolves over the first couple weeks. However, in certain cases, chemosis can be exuberant or prolonged. In these cases, topical steroid drops, a short course of oral steroids, lubrication of prolapsed conjunctiva, and a pressure patch can be helpful.
- Infections such as orbital cellulitis or suture granulomas can occur postoperatively and should be addressed using systemic antibiotics, drainage of any pustules or abscesses, and removal of foreign body/suture material.
- Lower lid retraction typically occurs from excessive cauterization of the orbital septum and lower lid retractors, or from tethering the orbital septum and lower lid retractors inferiorly in the process of redraping the fat pads.
- Lower lid ectropion can occur from overaggressive skin excision or from unaddressed or undercorrected horizontal lid laxity. Typically, it is advisable to wait at least 6 to 12 weeks postoperatively and instruct the patient to perform eyelid massage, since ectropion can sometimes spontaneously improve as eyelid edema regresses. However, revisional surgery may be necessary in the form of mid-face lifting, horizontal lid tightening, or even full-thickness skin grafting.
- Lateral canthal dystopia can occur due to suboptimal technique in lid tightening, canthal angle reformation, and/or reinsertion of the canthal complex on the lateral orbital rim.
- Inadequate or excessive fat excision can result in residual fat prolapse or hollowed appearing lids, respectively. The former can be addressed by revisional surgery to excise additional fat, whereas the latter can be addressed via injection of dermal fillers or autologous fat grafts.

11.12 Postoperative Care

Patients are instructed to apply ice packs intermittently for the first 48 to 72 hours, keep the head elevated while sleeping, and avoid strenuous activity, bending, and Valsalva maneuver. Ophthalmic antibiotic or steroid-antibiotic ointment is applied twice daily to the incisions for 1 to 2 weeks. In cases of significant chemosis or eyelid edema, a short course of oral steroids can be prescribed.

References

[1] Kikkawa DO. Lower eyelid blepharoplasty. Oculofacial Plastic Surgery Education Center. https://www.aao.org/oculoplastics-center/lower-eyelid-blepharoplasty. Accessed November 17, 2017

[2] Marrone AC. Lower eyelid blepharoplasty. In: Tse DT, ed. Color Atlas of Oculoplastic Surgery. Philadelphia: Lippincott Williams & Wilkins; 2011: 111–119

[3] Goldberg RA. Transconjunctival orbital fat repositioning: transposition of orbital fat pedicles into a subperiosteal pocket. Plast Reconstr Surg. 2000; 105 (2):743–748, discussion 749–751

[4] Korn BS, Kikkawa DO, Cohen SR. Transcutaneous lower eyelid blepharoplasty with orbitomalar suspension: retrospective review of 212 consecutive cases. Plast Reconstr Surg. 2010; 125(1):315–323

[5] Griffin G, Azizzadeh B, Massry GG. New insights into physical findings associated with postblepharoplasty lower eyelid retraction. Aesthet Surg J. 2014; 34(7):995–1004

[6] Kim EM, Bucky LP. Power of the pinch: pinch lower lid blepharoplasty. Ann Plast Surg. 2008; 60(5):532–537

Part IV

Upper Eyelid

IV

12 External Ptosis Repair

Omar Dajani and Alison Callahan

Abstract

External ptosis repair is a crucial tool in any ophthalmic plastic surgeon's practice. It is used when a patient requires elevation of a ptotic eyelid to improve superior visual field defects or even cosmesis of a droopy lid. As with any surgery, there are primary indications and advantages to this approach, but one must also be aware of the contraindications and disadvantages. Preoperatively, a surgeon must analyze the lid height, etiology of the ptosis, and also the patient's preferences for the end result. This chapter will highlight all of the above, as well as the operative technique, what to avoid, and other tips for successfully utilizing external ptosis repair surgery.

Keywords: blepharoplasty, ptosis, levator dehiscence

12.1 Goals

- To discuss external ptosis repair as a cornerstone of the ophthalmic plastic surgeon's repertoire for elevating a ptotic eyelid to improve superior visual field defects as well as cosmesis of a droopy upper eyelid.
- Using an external skin incision placed within the upper eyelid crease to access the underlying levator superioris tarsi muscle.
- Enhance eyelid elevation by reanchoring a plicated or resected levator muscle to the tarsal plate, thereby strengthening its effect.

12.2 Advantages

External ptosis repair is a powerful approach to elevating the eyelid in patients with a healthy levator having normal or near-normal function. The approach involves direct visualization of the levator muscle, allowing for visual confirmation of levator dehiscence when this etiology is suspected or for biopsy if clinically indicated. External ptosis repair can be considered even in cases of an abnormal muscle, if sufficient levator function is measured preoperatively. The procedure can often be performed with only local anesthesia and proper monitoring of the patient. If local anesthesia is used, adjustments can even be made intraoperatively as the patient is awake and can help in the assessment of proper lid height and contour. In addition, an upper eyelid blepharoplasty of variable size may easily be performed in conjunction as it does not require a separate incision. Finally, a major benefit is that recovery is quick, with patients often seeing improvements just days after surgery once most swelling has resolved.

12.3 Expectations

- Patients should be aware that the anticipated improvement in vision is related to an improved superior visual field; other underlying visual issues will not be improved with this surgery.

- While the aim is for both lids to appear symmetric, there is some degree of inherent surgical and healing variability that can lead to asymmetry; the surgeon needs to discuss this with the patient preoperatively.
- In cases of reduced levator function or histologically abnormal levator muscle, the degree and predictability of elevation are reduced.
- Patients should be counseled to be patient as the eyelids heal and in the postoperative use of ice, and elevation and activity limitation to minimize edema and ecchymosis.

12.4 Key Principles

External ptosis repair allows for direct visualization and anatomic correction of the most common cause of ptosis, namely dehiscence of the levator aponeurosis. It offers a powerful elevation of the upper eyelid in an otherwise normal functioning levator muscle. The external upper eyelid crease incision is the same as that of an upper blepharoplasty and therefore these procedures can easily be coupled without additional surgical time. Patient cooperation during surgery will help achieve both appropriate lid height and contour.

12.5 Indications

- External ptosis repair is intended to correct blepharoptosis due to defects of the levator palpebrae superioris.
- The most common indication is a dehiscence of the levator aponeurosis from its normal position. This is often seen due to involutional changes over time, but can occur in patients with a history of trauma or repetitive traction on the eyelid, due to either rubbing or long-term use of rigid contact lenses.[1,2]
- Other indications:
  ○ Superior visual field impairment (functional).[1]
  ○ Poorly fitting prosthesis in setting of anophthalmic socket (functional).[1]
  ○ Asymmetry of eyelid contour and height (cosmetic).[1]

12.6 Contraindications

- External ptosis repair requires some degree of levator excursion/function and therefore is relatively contraindicated in cases of severely reduced levator function.[1,3]
- Less than 5 mm of function should prompt consideration of other surgical approaches.
- Relative contraindications include the following:
  ○ Severe congenital ptosis.[2]
  ○ Ptosis due to third nerve palsies in which the levator muscle lacks innervation.[1,4]
  ○ Myopathies such as central progressive external ophthalmoplegia and oculopharyngeal dystrophy.[4]
  ○ Neuromuscular disease such as myasthenia gravis.[4]
  ○ Severe dry eyes and corneal disease.

- Variability of measurements during an examination or across separate examinations should raise suspicion and prompt further investigation before contemplation of surgical repair.
- Consideration should be given to whether patients will be able to cooperate during surgery if local anesthesia is being utilized, as they will need to open their eyes to help the surgeon assess for proper lid height and contour.
  - While external levator resections are performed under general anesthesia in cases of congenital ptosis, the external approach is best suited to local anesthesia in which patients are able to participate in opening and closing their eyes throughout the surgery.

12.7 Preoperative Preparation

Prior to proceeding with external ptosis repair, a thorough preoperative evaluation is crucial. History should seek to elucidate the underlying etiology (and rule out relatively contraindicated diagnoses mentioned above) as well as any history of dry eye disease. A slit lamp exam should be performed to further assess corneal health. Eyelid measurements that should be performed include the margin reflex distance–1 (MRD1) and levator function/excursion. Other helpful measurements include palpebral fissure height and the location of the upper eyelid crease relative to eyelid margin.

The **MRD1** is the distance between the upper lid margin and the corneal light reflex of a pen light when the patient is fixating. A normal MRD is approximately 4 to 4.5 mm.[1,4] **Levator function** is the total excursion of the eyelid, assessed by measuring the excursion of the upper lid margin from downgaze to upgaze.[4] It is absolutely critical that when measuring levator function, the frontalis muscle is immobilized by firmly pressing down on the brow. Normal levator function is approximately 15 mm.[4] Reduced levator function introduces further variability in elevation and surgical predictability that should be discussed with the patient preoperatively. Consensus regarding the minimum levator function required for successful repair via external approach is somewhat contentious, but certainly any excursion less than 5 mm should cause strong consideration of alternate approaches (e.g., frontalis fixation).

Palpebral fissure height measures the distance between the upper and lower lid margins, and the distance is measured in the pupillary plane. The height is approximately 8 to 10 mm in men and 8 to 12 mm in women.[4] **Upper lid crease** is the distance from the upper lid margin to the lid crease in downgaze.[4] A high crease suggests a possible aponeurotic dehiscence as described previously. In an occidental population, a normal crease is 8 to 10 mm in men and slightly higher in women, approximately 10 to 12 mm.[4] In an Asian eyelid, specific notation of the eyelid crease presence or absence as well as its height should be made. Patient should be informed about incision placement and its implications for eyelid crease placement.

Preoperative photographs in primary and oblique positions should be taken both for intraoperative reference and postoperative comparison. It is not uncommon for patients to quickly forget their old appearance or have overlooked small skin imperfections that become more salient in the postoperative period. Old photographs are also often helpful in determining what the patient looked like prior to the development of ptosis

as there is a range of natural eyelid position. Examining old photographs with the patient can be a useful tool in preoperative planning, counseling and expectation setting.

If assessing for a functional deficit in visual field, a visual field test can be performed with the upper eyelid at rest and taped. This will not only verify the potential visual improvement, but also allow the patient to see what they can expect postoperatively.

12.8 Operative Technique

1. Prior to surgery, the surgeon should discuss with the anesthesiologist about the need for an alert patient who can participate and follow commands throughout the surgery.
2. An ellipse is marked using the intended upper eyelid crease as the inferior marking. The upper marking of the ellipse is drawn at the discretion of the surgeon depending on the amount of preferred skin resection.
3. Local anesthetic is injected into the upper lid just under the skin, being careful not to penetrate posterior to the septum, as the epinephrine in anesthetics can potentially blunt the levator muscle function by acting upon sympathetic receptors in Müller muscle.
4. Corneal shields may be inserted.
5. A skin incision is made with a #15 blade along the previously made markings on the eyelid.
6. Westcott scissors or a form of cautery and toothed forceps are used to excise the skin +/− orbicularis muscle (surgeon preference).
7. Sharp, Westcott scissor dissection inferiorly and posteriorly exposes the superior border of the tarsal plate and continued dissection of the tarsal plate also disinserts the attachments of the levator aponeurosis.
8. A suborbicularis dissection is carried out superiorly and posteriorly to expose the orbital septum, often demarcated by the visualization of underlying preaponeurotic fat.
9. Orbital septum is opened with Westcott scissors and preaponeurotic fat is carefully dissected away from the underlying levator aponeurosis. A Desmarres retractor may be inserted under preaponeurotic fat to facilitate its separation from the underlying levator aponeurosis.
10. Attention should be paid at this point to the contour of the tarsus. It is often possible to find a natural peak in the tarsus that alludes to the natural peak of the lid from the patient's original contour and thus where the suture should be placed. A double-armed suture is then placed partial thickness through the anterior surface of the tarsus. This should be placed about 2 to 3 mm inferior to the superior border of the tarsus (▶ Fig. 12.1a). Prior to pulling the needle through, the lid is everted to verify that the pass was not full thickness (▶ Fig. 12.1b). Suture choice varies by surgeon, often either 6–0 Prolene or silk.
11. Each arm of the suture is then passed through the advanced levator (▶ Fig. 12.1c). For simple levator dehiscence, this is usually at the junction where aponeurosis becomes muscle, thereby restoring its anatomic attachment to tarsus. A temporary tie is then placed (▶ Fig. 12.1d).
12. While firmly disengaging the frontalis muscle by pressing down on the brow, the surgeon should ask the patient to

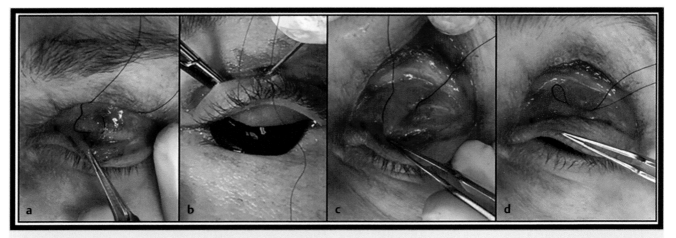

Fig. 12.1 Careful dissection as described exposes the tarsal plate inferiorly and the levator superiorly. **(a)** The natural peak of the tarsus is identified and a double-armed suture placed in a partial-thickness fashion through the anterior surface of tarsus. **(b)** With the needle still in its lamellar pass, the eyelid is everted to ensure the pass was not full thickness. Each arm of the suture is then placed through **(c)** advanced levator and a **(d)** temporary knot tied. Once contour and height are deemed correct, the suture is then permanently tied.

open their eyes. This can be done either sitting up or lying down as long as the frontalis is disengaged. The height of the upper lid as well as contour should be assessed and readjusted depending on the appearance. For alterations of elevation, the temporary tie is undone and each arm (one at a time so initial placement may be gauged by the remaining arm) is backed out of the levator and repassed through more or less of the muscle/aponeurosis. For alterations of contour, the placement of the suture on tarsus may be changed or additional double-armed sutures passed in a similar fashion to elevate more lateral or medial aspects of the eyelid.

13. Once the contour and height are deemed correct, the temporary tie should be converted to a permanent tie.
14. Excess advanced levator may be excised if pathology is desired.
15. Skin is then closed as one would close a blepharoplasty wound.

12.9 Tips and Pearls

- It is imperative that prior to surgery you discuss with the anesthesiologist the need for patient cooperation throughout surgery. Over-sedation can drastically alter the patient's ability to open their eyes and thus the perceived effect of the advanced levator. The authors' preference is to completely avoid the use of midazolam for this reason, despite its fast washout time.
- Make sure to discuss eyelid crease placement with patients preoperatively, especially when there is an anatomic question, for example, some Asian eyelids or eyelids with prior blepharoplasty incisions.
- Adequate manual blocking of the frontalis intraoperatively is crucial for a good outcome. The surgeon must be aware and prevent brow use so that when the patient opens their eyes, the lid height is in fact due to the levator without involvement of frontalis.

- Be consistent! Judging the appropriate intraoperative height at which to leave the upper eyelid takes practice and experience. Numerous steps of the surgery can slightly alter intraoperative eyelid height, including sedation, type of local injection (i.e., concentration of epinephrine), and amount of injection. You will not be able to make appropriate adjustments in your technique if you are not performing these steps in the exact same manner in each surgery.

12.10 What to Avoid

External ptosis repair is not recommended for patients with severely reduced levator function in whom this approach is ineffective. In those who do undergo surgery, one should be cautious of over-elevation in patients who cannot tolerate a fully open aperture due to dry eye, ocular surface disease, or low-lying blebs after glaucoma surgery.

When using local anesthesia, be careful not to use an excessive amount because this might block the levator function, making it harder to accurately assess the true height of the lid during surgery. At minimum, be consistent in the amount delivered and refine where *you* should leave the intraoperative height based on your compilation of postoperative results. The authors find that approximately 2 mL/side is more than sufficient.

In addition, after each lamellar pass, be sure to evert the eyelid to confirm a partial-thickness lamellar pass. An inadvertent full-thickness suture will likely abrade the cornea and potentially require later surgical revision and/or vision-threatening corneal damage. Prolonged surgical time and manipulation can potentially lead to undesirable results. The more adjustments the surgeon performs, the more swelling can be expected during and after surgery. This ultimately will make it harder to assess the actual height of the eyelid during surgery and will prolong recovery.

12.11 Complications/Bailout/Salvage

- Most severe, though exceedingly rare, complication is that of retrobulbar hemorrhage.
  - Always inquire about anticoagulants (by name) in the preoperative evaluation.
  - It is the authors' opinion that this type of elective surgery should not be performed on anticoagulated patients due to this remote risk; if unable to discontinue them, surgery should ideally be postponed.
- Most common complications after external ptosis repair are related to contour abnormalities and/or height asymmetries.
  - Minimized with intraoperative patient cooperation, careful use of local and intravenous anesthesia, and manual blocking of the frontalis.
- Dry eye is another common complication.
  - Be cautious in patients with known history of dryness.
- If, despite all these efforts, the upper eyelid height is incorrect or has an abnormal contour, one may adjust the height in the office with relative ease at approximately 2 weeks.
  - Additional double-armed sutures may be placed and/or old sutures removed.
    - Best to place new sutures first utilizing the old as landmarks in conjunction with the identified error (rather than removing the suture first and losing that reference point).
- If an in-office adjustment fails to elevate an eyelid, one should consider a different surgical approach.
  - Posterior approaches and frontalis fixations may both be performed after failed external ptosis repair.

12.12 Postoperative Care

After surgery, physical activity should be limited for the first week so as to avoid retrobulbar hemorrhage. Patients should be informed of the need to apply ice as much as possible to help reduce swelling during the first 2 to 3 days. If possible, they should also sleep at an angle to reduce edema around the eyes and make-up should be avoided around the eyes for 2 weeks. Antibiotic ointment can be applied 2 to 4 times per day to each area of suture for 7 to 10 days. Patients should be aware that while pain and swelling are to be expected, they should never experience severe swelling such that their eyelids are swollen shut after the first 48 hours. Follow-up is usually within 1 to 2 weeks depending on skin closure, with non-absorbable sutures removed at approximately 1 week.

References

[1] Bowling B. Kanski's Clinical Ophthalmology: A Systematic Approach. Elsevier; 2016: 38–45

[2] Baldwin HC, Manners RM. Congenital blepharoptosis: a literature review of the histology of levator palpebrae superioris muscle. Ophthal Plast Reconstr Surg. 2002; 18(4):301–307

[3] McDonald H. Minimally invasive levator advancement: a practical approach to eyelid ptosis repair. Semin Plast Surg. 2007; 21(1):41–46

[4] Nerad J. Techniques in Ophthalmic Plastic Surgery: A Personal Tutorial. Saunders Elsevier;2010: 149–55

13 Internal Ptosis Repair

Nora Siegal and Christopher B. Chambers

Summary

Conjunctival Müller muscle resection (CMMR) is a reliable and technically facile approach to ptosis repair. Based on results of the phenylephrine test during a preoperative evaluation, surgical outcome can be highly predictable. For patients who require eyelid elevation of up to 3 mm, CMMR (internal ptosis repair) is an excellent surgical option. The success of the CMMR is manifest in its wide adoption by oculoplastic surgeons who had previously favored an external approach to ptosis repair.

Keywords: ptosis, conjunctiva Müller muscle resection, internal ptosis repair

13.1 Goals

- To provide a step-by-step approach to preoperative evaluation of ptosis.
- To provide the surgical steps necessary to complete internal ptosis repair.
- To provide tips and pearls regarding surgical technique and postoperative management.

13.2 Advantages

Patients with small amounts (<3 mm) of involutional ptosis and good levator function (LF) who have a good response to phenylephrine may benefit from internal ptosis repair. The advantages of the conjunctival Müller muscle resection (CMMR) involve its predictability, ease of operation, and lack of an external incision. Results of external levator advancement vary considerably, and the need for reoperation may be as high as 8.7%.[1] Tarsal removal in the Fasanella–Servat procedure can lead to tenting, abnormal lid contour, and conceivably keratitis sicca via its removal of Meibomian glands.[2] The success of the CMMR is manifest in its wide adoption by oculoplastic surgeons who had previously favored an external approach to ptosis repair.[3]

13.3 Expectations

- To elevate the upper eyelid so that it may clear the visual axis.
- To determine the amount of ptosis, measured by the MRD1, in order to decide on an approach for treatment.
- Internal ptosis repair is typically chosen for cases in which the eyelid requires up to 3 mm of elevation.
- If the amount of required elevation significantly exceeds 3 mm, ptosis repair by external levator advancement is preferred.

13.4 Key Principles

The eyelids serve to protect and lubricate the globe. Normal positioning of the eyelids is important in maintaining these functions. The upper lid has a more arched contour than the lower lid, with the peak of the upper lid located just nasal to the pupil.[4] The palpebral fissure, the distance between the upper and lower eyelids, is approximately 9 to 10 mm. The position of the upper eyelid is measured using the MRD1 which represents the number of millimeters between the corneal light reflex and the upper lid margin, a measurement that is integral to the identification and management of ptosis. The average measurement is between 4 and 5 mm.

There are two muscles that elevate the upper eyelid: the levator muscle and the Müller muscle. The levator is a voluntary, skeletal muscle innervated by the oculomotor nerve and it is the main retractor of the upper eyelid. The levator courses anteriorly from the orbital apex to below the orbital roof where it subsequently becomes an aponeurosis that extends inferiorly into the eyelid, inserting onto the anterior aspect of the tarsus. Several extensions of the aponeurosis extend anteriorly through the orbicularis muscle to create the upper eyelid crease.

Müller muscle is a diaphanous structure that has an *involuntary* eyelid elevation function. The muscle is located under the levator aponeurosis and anterior to the conjunctiva, beginning at the superior border of the tarsal plate and extending to Whitnall ligament. The Müller muscle is not as powerful as the levator in terms of its elevating capacity; it is, however, innervated by sympathetics, and contributes to the eyelid changes associated with a 'fight or flight' response.[4] Loss of sympathetic tone, which is seen in Horner syndrome, results in a mild ptosis and would not cause a complete ptosis.

Ptosis refers to drooping of the upper eyelid. Although there are many different types of ptosis, most cases can be classified as *congenital*, *involutional*, or as a result of trauma/associated medical condition. The amount of ptosis, measured by the MRD1, helps to determine the approach for surgical treatment. The other important factor in determining the surgical plan is the amount of LF; this is defined as the amount of movement (measured in millimeters) of the eyelid from extreme downgaze to extreme upgaze and is normally 14 to 16 mm.[4] Congenital ptosis is associated with poor LF, and therefore usually requires treatment with a frontalis sling. Involutional ptosis, which is the cause of the majority of adult-onset ptosis, is typically associated with normal or near-normal LF. In the setting of good LF, surgical options include an external levator advancement (ELA) or internal ptosis repair known as a conjunctival Müller muscle resection (CMMR).

This chapter will help guide the identification of cases in which internal ptosis repair is appropriate and provide surgical pearls for excellent function and cosmesis.

13.5 Indications

- Internal ptosis repair is indicated for mild ptosis (<3 mm) in patients who show a positive response to the phenylephrine test which is discussed below.
- Internal ptosis repair does not require suturing of the skin, so for patients concerned about postoperative scarring and recovery, this may also be indicated.

13.6 Contraindications

- Internal ptosis repair is typically not performed on patients who do not show a positive response to the phenylephrine test.
- Other contraindications are patients who have evidence of posterior lamellar abnormalities such as those on the palpebral conjunctiva (e.g., scarring or persistent inflammation).
- Reserve caution in patients who have had glaucoma filtering surgery, especially in patients with a cystic bleb. Postoperatively, the posteriorly placed suture can rub on the filtering bleb.

13.7 Preoperative Preparation

As mentioned earlier, the LF and MRD1 are the most important measurements when evaluating a patient with ptosis. It is important to have the patient relax during these measurements, and it is often necessary to stabilize the patient's brow. Recruitment of the frontalis muscle is very common in patients with ptosis and it may cause eyelid measurements to be inaccurate.

Before proceeding with ptosis repair, it is important to determine whether elevation of the lid would result in improper lid closure and/or corneal exposure. The following quick tests will help in this assessment:

1. Check for lagophthalmos (ask patient to close their eyelids gently and lift their chin to examine if there is any scleral show). In the presence of preexisting lagophthalmos or orbicularis weakness in diseases like Myasthenia Gravis, consider conservative elevation of the eyelid.
2. Instill fluorescein to examine the cornea and do a Schirmer test: patients may experience dry eye after eyelid surgery, and this can be significant in the setting of preexisting tear film inadequacy.
3. Evaluate the *Bell phenomenon* (the palpebral oculogyric reflex): when closing one's eyes there is an upward and outward movement of the eyes. This phenomenon is likely a defense reflex that protects the cornea. It is important to make sure this is present as elevation of the eyelids will increase the palpebral fissure and may contribute to corneal exposure.

Success of the Müller muscle resection is suggested by a good response to the phenylephrine test. Preoperative evaluation includes measurement of MRD1. The number of millimeters (usually measured with a small ruler held next to the eye) from the corneal light reflex (from a muscle light held at the patient's eye level) to the upper eyelid margin is noted. One to two drops of 2.5% phenylephrine are then placed in conjunctival fornix of the ptotic eye. After approximately 5 to 10 minutes, the eyelid position using the same technique as above is measured. A response of lid elevation of greater than 1 mm is typically deemed a good response. The amount of lid elevation is used to determine the number of millimeters of conjunctival and Müller muscle resection; a relationship is based on the original description of the procedure (see below). According to Dresner, a 4 mm resection of conjunctiva and Müller muscle reliably elevates the eyelid 1 mm, and so a standard resection of 8 mm typically achieves a 2 mm lift.[5]

13.8 Operative Technique

The seminal paper by Putterman and Urist[2] describing a technique for internal ptosis repair was created after Fasanella and Servat developed a procedure in which both the conjunctiva–Müller muscle complex and part of the tarsus were removed. Putterman had suggested that the success of the Fasanella–Servat operation was a result of strengthening of the Müller muscle (through its shortening and advancement). In this manuscript, Putterman and Urist revealed successful lid elevation with cosmetically appealing lid contour in patients whose eyelids elevated in response to 10% phenylephrine. Authors showed that an 8 mm Müller muscle–conjunctival resection (MMCR) led to a predictable amount of lid elevation based on the response to phenylephrine during preoperative testing.

The following is a step-wise approach to internal ptosis repair that the authors feel is safe and effective. A small amount (approximately 0.5 mL of 1% lidocaine with epinephrine—1:100,000) is injected into the central portion of the upper lid just below the skin (▸ Fig. 13.1). A 4–0 silk suture is placed through the gray line of the upper lid, and with the help of a Desmarres retractor, the upper lid is everted (▸ Fig. 13.1). Another injection of local anesthetic (approximately 0.5–1 mL)

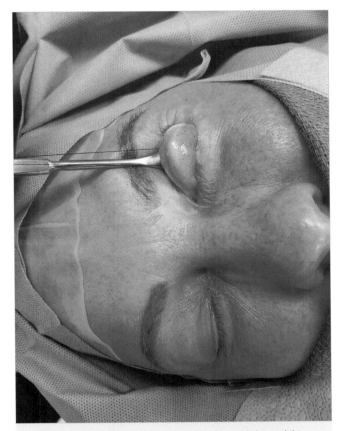

Fig. 13.1 Silk suture is passed through gray line and the eyelid is everted on a Desmarres retractor.

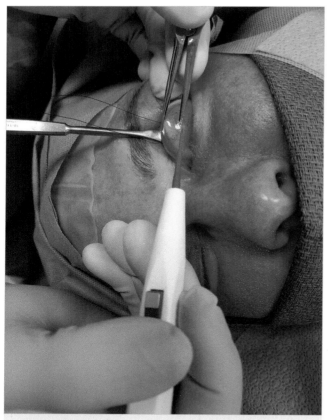

Fig. 13.2 Bovie cautery is used to mark points on the conjunctiva measured with calipers.

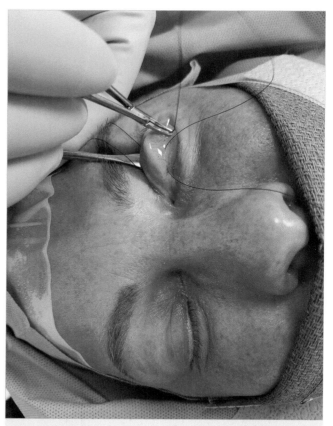

Fig. 13.3 A 4.0 silk suture is passed through conjunctiva and Müller muscle.

is injected transconjunctivally and then massaged into the lid with a cotton-tip applicator. A caliper is then set at half of the desired resection amount (a value which is determined in the preoperative evaluation). Using a sterile marking pen or cautery, the tips of the caliper are marked and then three points on the conjunctiva are made above the tarsus. These marks represent the medial, central, and lateral portions of the tissue to be excised (▶ Fig. 13.2). A study by Carruth and Dale revealed that using only two central markings in the vertical meridian superior to the tarsus could achieve excellent functional and cosmetic success.[6] Another 4–0 silk suture is then passed through conjunctiva and Müller muscle at these markings. The loops of suture are left long and grasped together once the last suture is passed. Using two hands, the silk loops are then elevated away from the patient and the Desmarres retractor is removed from the upper lid (▶ Fig. 13.3). Using counter traction, an assistant can hold down the eyelid margin superiorly as the silk sutures are pulled inferiorly elevating the conjunctiva and Müller muscle (▶ Fig. 13.4). The müllerectomy clamp is used to grasp the conjunctiva and underlying Müller muscle under the silk suture loops. Once the clamp is closed, the silk suture can be pulled laterally and removed (▶ Fig. 13.5).

While elevating the ptosis clamp away from the cornea, a double-armed 6–0 pain gut suture is passed in a running horizontal mattress fashion from lateral to medial and then back laterally, passing approximately 1 mm below the clamp. Each

stitch should be placed 2 to 3 mm from the next. Once the suturing is complete, the two ends of the double-armed suture are pulled laterally to create tension. The suture is then tied and cut. The suture can be externalized and tied down at the lid crease to decrease the chance of corneal irritation postoperatively. An assistant can stabilize the Putterman clamp. Using counter traction from the plain gut sutures, a 15 Bard Parker Blade is then used to excise the tissue within the clamp. Care is made to angle the blade towards the base of the clamp so as not to cut the suture (▶ Fig. 13.6). The clamp can then be removed. The two suture ends are then externalized through the skin laterally and tied down at the lid crease. Gentle pressure is held on the eyelid for 1 to 2 minutes. A small amount of antibiotic ointment is then placed under the eyelid.

13.9 Tips and Pearls

- Some surgeons may elect to provide anesthesia via a frontal nerve block. Another option is to instill local anesthetic in both the preseptal and post-tarsal planes.
- Once the suture has been passed under the Putterman clamp, the knot can be tied laterally (i.e., within the conjunctiva) or externalized to the skin. In the latter case, the knot can be buried in the lid crease for better cosmesis.

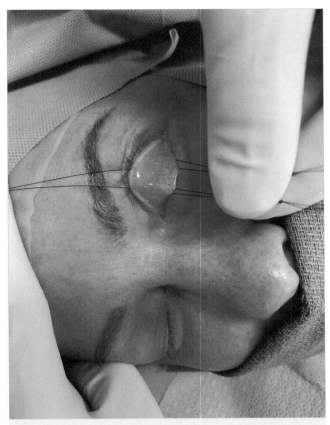

Fig. 13.4 Silk sutures are pulled inferiorly to elevate the conjunctiva and Müller muscle from the eyelid.

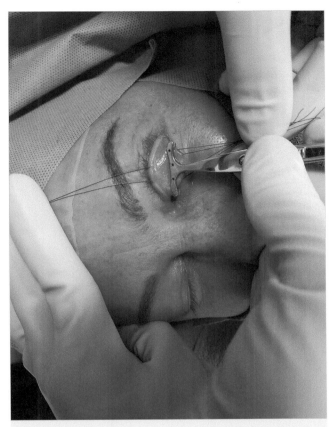

Fig. 13.5 Müllerectomy clamp is used to grasp the conjunctiva and Müller muscle.

13.10 Complications/Bailout/ Salvage

- Although abnormal contour is an infrequent occurrence in CMMR, if an uneven amount of tissue is excised medially or laterally, the contour may be altered. It is therefore important to pause after the müllerectomy clamp is closed and evaluate whether the tissue within the clamp is evenly distributed throughout the clamp.
- Each of the suture passes under the clamp should be equal in terms of its distance from the clamp. Care should be taken not to unintentionally capture tarsus in the suture pass. This will help prevent uneven elevation of the eyelid.
- Dry eye is a possible consequence of ptosis surgery, so it is important to treat symptoms both pre- and postoperatively and sometimes even to under-correct during ptosis repair.

- Surgeons should refrain from everting the eyelid for at least 2 to 3 weeks after surgery to avoid breaking the suture.
- Surgeons should also be aware of the possibility of a postoperative corneal abrasion from the suture. If this occurs, a bandage contact lens can provide symptomatic relief.

13.11 Postoperative Care

Antibiotic ophthalmic ointment should be used for at least 1 week three to four times daily after CMMR. Patients are instructed to instill a small amount (about the length of a grain or two of rice) into the inferior fornix. Ice packs should be used 20 minutes on and 20 minutes off for the first 48 hours to reduce pain and postoperative ecchymosis and edema. Warm compresses can be used starting on day 3. Patients should also be instructed not to rub the eye and to refrain from intense physical activity and swimming for at least 1 week.

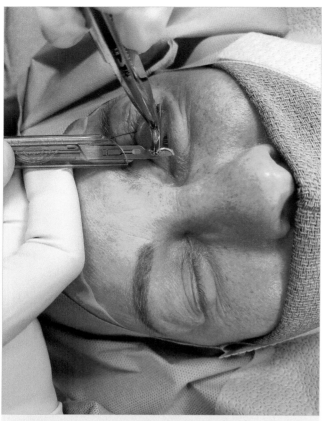

Fig. 13.6 A 15 Bard Parker blade is used to excise the tissue below the müllerectomy clamp.

References

[1] McCulley TJ, Kersten RC, Kulwin DR, Feuer WJ. Outcome and influencing factors of external levator palpebrae superioris aponeurosis advancement for blepharoptosis. Ophthal Plast Reconstr Surg. 2003; 19(5):388–393

[2] Putterman AM, Urist MJ. Müller muscle-conjunctiva resection: technique for treatment of blepharoptosis. Arch Ophthalmol. 1975; 93(8):619–623

[3] Allen RC, Saylor MA, Nerad JA. The current state of ptosis repair: a comparison of internal and external approaches. Curr Opin Ophthalmol. 2011; 22(5): 394–399

[4] Nerad JA. Techniques in Ophthalmic Plastic Surgery.1st ed. Saunders: Elsevier; 2009:205, 30, 41

[5] Dresner SC. Further modifications of the Müller's muscle-conjunctival resection procedure for blepharoptosis. Ophthal Plast Reconstr Surg. 1991; 7(2): 114–122

[6] Carruth BP, Meyer DR. Simplified Müller's muscle-conjunctival resection internal ptosis repair. Ophthal Plast Reconstr Surg. 2013; 29(1):11–14

14 Frontalis Suspension Ptosis Repair

Julius T. Oatts and Alexandra T. Elliott

Summary

Frontalis suspension ptosis repair is required in cases of complete or near complete absence of levator function. This occurs in congenital ptosis, congenital fibrosis of the extraocular muscles (CFEOM), blepharophimosis, chronic progressive external ophthalmoplegia (CPEO), third nerve palsy, oculopharyngeal dystrophy, and Marcus Gunn jaw winking syndrome. The incidence of childhood ptosis has been estimated at 7.9 per 100,000 children (< 19 years). When the levator palpebra is too weak to oppose gravity and orbicularis tone, severe ptosis is the result. In many cases in which levator function is < 5 mm, frontalis suspension is the only option to improve lid height. In this technique, implant material effectively suspends the upper eyelid margin from the brow to oppose the action of gravity and antagonistic orbicularis tone. Suspension materials can be autogenous, alloplastic, or synthetic. Silicone rods tend to last as long as if not longer than banked fascia lata; use of the latter actually results in more initial lag and a less stable long-term effect. Autogenous fascia lata can last a lifetime, but it places the patient at risk for exposure to keratopathy, particularly in environments known to cause tear breakdown (e.g., high altitudes, low humidity, or airplane travel). Also unknown is the long-term effect of childhood fascia lata harvest on the aging knee.

Keywords: frontalis suspension, congenital ptosis, blepharophimosis, congenital fibrosis of the extraocular muscles, chronic progressive external ophthalmoplegia, Marcus Gunn jaw wink, third nerve palsy, oculopharyngeal dystrophy, silicone rods, banked fascia

14.1 Goals

- Elevate the ptotic eyelid(s).
- Minimize amblyopia in infants and children.
- Improve peripheral visual fields in all patients.
- Provide reconstruction in those with facial deformity or asymmetry (▶ Fig. 14.1, ▶ Fig. 14.2).

14.2 Advantages

Frontalis suspension techniques offer a more certain postoperative elevation of the eyelid than maximal levator resections in those with very poor or absent levator function. Silicone, in particular, offers some elasticity,[1] lessening the degree of lagophthalmos. In addition, frontalis suspension does not disrupt the underlying levator anatomy and, with certain materials, can be reversible and/or adjustable.

14.3 Expectations

- Postoperative improvement in ptosis is immediate.
- The procedure induces some lagophthalmos with sleep and downgaze, the degree of which varies based on sling material, sling tension, and individual facial characteristics (such as brow prominence).
- Postoperative subjective and objective blink will be less robust, stiffer, or in some cases nearly absent.
- Lid height and symmetry in primary gaze will be improved.

14.4 Key Principles

All non-autogenous materials will likely need to be replaced during a patient's lifetime, especially in congenital ptosis or ptosis acquired in childhood. The material requiring fewest revisions is autogenous fascia lata,[2] but using this material requires longer surgical time and can lead to harvest site pain, infection, or scarring. Another theoretical risk that has yet to be explored in the orthopedic literature is the long-term sequelae of fascia lata harvesting on the aging knee or hip. The fascia lata and associated iliotibial (IT) band support the knee, extend from the iliac crest to the lateral condyle of the tibia, and function as a hip abductor (used in activities such as soccer and horseback riding). Unknown long-term effects of removal of the central strip of this band—especially for the youngest patients, in whom a more substantial section of fascia will be harvested—merit mention in preoperative discussions with patients and families (▶ Fig. 14.3). In practice, the advantages of silicone over fascia lata are reversibility, adjustability within the first year, and ability to stretch.

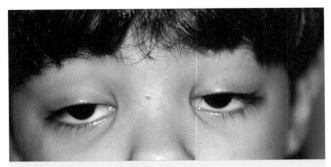

Fig. 14.1 Preoperative patient with congenital ptosis and no frontalis function.

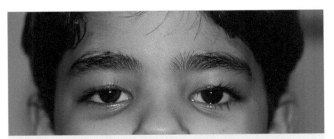

Fig. 14.2 Same patient after frontalis suspension with autogenous fascia.

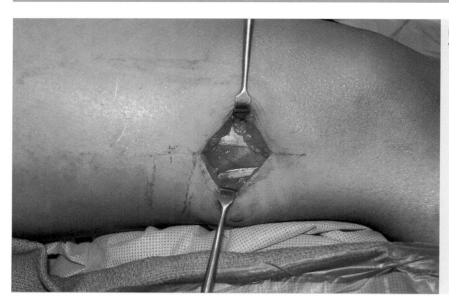

Fig. 14.3 Gap left in fascia after harvest of 6-mm-wide strip. Note fullness of underlying muscle.

For temporizing repair, such as in an infant with complete ptosis, silicone rods offer reversibility if the levator improves during the first year of life. Silicone rods come swedged onto straight needles that are smaller in caliber than Wright fascia needles, so these cause less trauma to the infant's pretarsal anatomy. Another advantage of silicone is that it can be adjusted with relative ease during the first 1 to 2 postoperative years. After that point, it becomes increasingly brittle and develops calcifications, which increase the likelihood of breakage during adjustment. The elasticity of silicone renders less postoperative lagophthalmos, which is helpful in those patients with poor tear film (e.g., mature adults with oculopharyngeal dystrophy and patients with poor Bell phenomenon due to third cranial nerve palsy, CFEOM, or CPEO). This elasticity also tends to slightly reduce the severity of the wink in patients with Marcus Gunn jaw winking. Finally, the decreased lagophthalmos with sleep and downgaze associated with the elasticity of silicone is far less troubling to parents than the stiff lid seen with fascia lata (although the initial lagophthalmos with fascia lata does typically improve after the first 6 months).

The importance of managing patient and parental expectations preoperatively cannot be overemphasized. It is helpful to frame this procedure as a structural bypass of a defective or functionally absent muscle rather than a physiologic repair of a stretched or weak muscle.

14.5 Indications

Frontalis suspension for ptosis repair is the procedure required in absent or near complete absence of levator function.
- Severe ptosis with < 5 mm of levator function.
- Acquired or congenital complete third nerve palsy.
- Oculopharyngeal dystrophy.
- CFEOM.
- Marcus Gunn jaw winking (both to improve baseline ptosis and decrease the severity of retraction wink). Patients with this condition have good levator function, but aberrant innervation between the levator and usually the lateral

pterygoid muscle renders anomalous and variable lid positioning dependent on jaw position. In cases with severe ptosis, a sling (with or without extirpation of the levator) is warranted.

14.6 Contraindications

- Patients with a poor Bell reflex, such as CFEOM or extraocular muscle limitation, should be approached with caution. In these patients, conservative and reversible sling tension should be employed so that exposure does not occur postoperatively.
- Patients with some levator function but ipsilateral amblyopia may benefit more from a maximal levator procedure or a Whitnall suspension, since they are less likely to have spontaneous brow elevation.[3]
- Patients with underlying poor or absent frontalis function should be counseled that they may be disappointed with frontalis suspension, and that Whitnall suspension may be a better choice.[4]

14.7 Preoperative Preparation

It is important to confirm the presence of Bell reflex, without which postoperative exposure keratopathy is more likely to occur. This can be well assessed in infants > 18 months. Another predictive assessment should include testing for amblyopia. Preoperative phenylephrine testing should be performed by placing 1 drop of 2.5% phenylephrine and assessing eyelid position 10 minutes later. This medication, a sympathetic agonist, stimulates Müller muscle and can provide an approximation or estimation of the results of a Müller muscle conjunctival resection.

Patients and their families tend to find the aftereffects of delayed blink and lagophthalmos while sleeping most troubling. It is important to discuss these and to explain that some degree of persistent ptosis when the brow is relaxed is likely and expected. Patients should also be made aware of variable lid crease appearance, as often a lid crease forms from the folds of skin after sling placement, but this is not an active fold and has a static appearance.

In addition, physiologic movements such as smooth blink response and symmetric downgaze relaxation will not be possible, and this must also be discussed. Disclosure of these limitations improves patient satisfaction. Ptosis with lack of frontalis function is a lifelong condition. Early in the patient's amblyogenic period, silicone or banked fascia can be implanted, with the expectation that a revision will be required in future. This contingency often happens a decade after initial procedure, at which time the child can be involved in discussions regarding autogenous harvest for a more permanent result versus replacing worn out or stretched silicone or other non-autogenous materials.

14.8 Operative Technique

14.8.1 Operative Technique: Ptosis Repair

If using banked fascia, confirm the correct length and appropriate expiration date prior to bringing patient into the OR. Soak the fascia in bacitracin irrigating solution early, as this can be the rate-limiting step of the procedure. The fascia should be pliable after 20 minutes of soaking. Mark for incisions. While making planned incisions, palpate the supratrochlear notch and note the location of the neurovascular bundle. In some cases, the bundle is displaced somewhat laterally, in which case the implant material will pass above it, and therefore the stab incision and sling pass should be more shallow than usual. Infuse bupivacaine with epinephrine subcutaneously into incision sites using a 30-gauge needle. Prep and drape the entire upper face and eyelashes in usual sterile fashion using betadine and ensure the drape aperture reveals 1 cm above the brows. Use a #15c blade to create five stab incisions—three on the brow and two at the lid margin. Lid margin incisions in the skin just superior to the lash line should correspond to the medial and lateral limbi. Brow incisions should correspond to the medial and lateral canthi, with the third incision centered above the pupil. The depth of these incisions should be to the tarsus in the eyelid

and the dermis in the brow. Hold pressure until bleeding stops. Thread sling material (either silicone or fascia) along the lid margin using the attached needle (in case of silicone rod) or the Wright fascia needle (in the case of fascia and other unswedged strips). Needle should be just anterior to the tarsus. In cases of prior lid crease incision, form a lid crease incision again and pass needle inferior to it along the margin, through undissected pretarsal orbicularis rather than through lid margin stab incisions.

Pass the Wright fascia needle perpendicular to the lateral brow incision and then inferiorly over the arcus marginalis. The needle will enter through the septum into the preaponeurotic fat. There are variable amounts of resistance in different individuals based on age and tissue composition, so it is critical to protect the underlying globe at all times with a Jaeger (lid plate) lid plate placed under the lid and held firmly against the superior orbital rim by your assist. During passage through the preaponeurotic fat pad, keep needle tip up and be aware of its depth. If the overlying skin begins to pull, reposition the needle tip slightly deeper. When passing the area where the lid crease should be, a band of resistance is often encountered, presumably due to the needle tip exiting the preaponeurotic fat pad and encountering the projections from levator aponeurosis to the skin. Since this is a thin part of the pass, take care to keep the preseptal skin taut so the needle does not perforate overlying skin. Direct the needle through pretarsal orbicularis and exit via the lateral lid margin incision. Thread the lateral end of the sling material into the eye of the fascial needle and withdraw the needle through tract. Confirm the Jaeger (lid plate) lid plate is in the correct position prior to withdrawal. See ▶ Fig. 14.4. Create a symmetric medial brow incision, as above, taking care to avoid disruption of the previously identified neurovascular bundle. Widen the central brow incision with blunt Westcott scissors deeply in superior and lateral directions. This creates a pocket for the knot or silicone sleeve.

Insert the fascial needle into the middle brow incision and direct it laterally through the lateral brow incision. Thread the sling material into the fascial needle and retrieve it through the central brow incision. Repeat this on the medial side. Close lid margin or crease incisions with 6–0 fast-absorbing gut suture

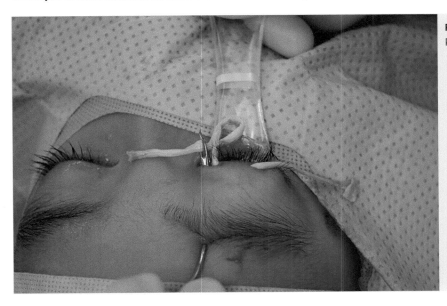

Fig. 14.4 Jaeger lid plate in position during passage of Wright fascial needle.

prior to tightening the sling, because access to them after tightening is limited. Connect the two ends of sling material in the central brow incision (with fascia, tie the two ends; with silicone, thread in opposing directions through the silicone sheath using a Watzke spreader).

In bilateral cases, lubricate the first eye, place a tegaderm or wet gauze over it with the lid closed, and repeat the procedure in second eye. Adjust eyelid height by altering the amount of tension on the sling material. Lid height should be as high as possible when there is an intact Bell reflex, ideally placing the lid margin at the superior limbus. In some patients, maximal lid height may result in 3 or more millimeters of scleral show. Adjusting to limbus height rather than maximal lift results in good cosmetic outcomes. The lid position is expected to drop a couple of millimeters once the orbicularis muscle is active. In some cases, no matter how tight sling material is pulled, the margin does not rise to the limbus. In these cases, relax the sling material, as over-tightening the sling will lead to earlier cheesewiring and excessive lagophthalmos. Always confirm that sling tension is not causing eyelid distraction from the globe. Reposit ends of the sling material into central brow incision and confirm lid height. In patients with thicker brow tissue, there may be a substantial drop on reposition that requires further tightening of the knot. In bilateral cases, do this simultaneously before finalizing knot to optimize likelihood of symmetry. Reinforce knots or sling with 6–0 vicryl suture. Close all wounds with buried 6–0 vicryl suture and superficial 6–0 fast-absorbing gut sutures. Cover with steristrips and antibiotic ointment.

14.8.2 Operative Technique: Fascia Lata Harvest

Mark and prep leg from knee to thigh with a slight bend to knee, supported by bolster, and toes pronated slightly inward to put stretch on fascia lata. Incise skin starting 4 cm superior to lateral condyle of the femur and extending 4 cm upward parallel to fibers of underlying fascia lata in the direction of the greater trochanter of the hip. Dissect bluntly down to fascia

and, using peanuts, clean fascia until it glistens. With a long Metzenbaum scissors, dissect 15-cm subcutaneous tissue from underlying fascia toward hip. Create a 6-mm-wide strip in the center of the fascia starting 4 cm above lateral condyle with two parallel incisions through fascia only. Take care not to incise underlying muscle. Incise parallel with muscle fibers freehand as far as possible under direct visualization.

Place tips of long Metz under fascia and dissect upward, releasing fascia from underlying muscle. Thread strip through stripper and grasp free end with clamp. Advance stripper up the length of fascia while holding tension on developing strip (▶ Fig. 14.5). Once stripper is advanced sufficiently (15 cm is ideal, but as little at 10 cm is acceptable), cut and harvest strip. Clean strip of attached fat and prepare strip for lid. If doing both eyes, strip can be divided in half to render two 3-mm lengths, one for each eyelid. Close leg in two layers.

If there is insufficient length of fascia for formation of a pentagon, a double triangle can be formed with shorter lengths. Otherwise, proceed with Fox pentagon technique (described in 14.8.1) using a square knot reinforced with vicryl suture to secure.[5] Place steristrip, antibiotic ointment, and a tegiderm over leg incision. Wrap leg from heel to thigh with ace bandage for 3 to 4 days.

14.9 Tips and Pearls

- Always get consent for silicone or banked fascia lata in an autogenous fascia lata case, in case you are unable to get a good strip.
- Soak banked fascia lata early so as not to delay the surgical procedure.
- Palpate the supratrochlear notch before marking to be aware of neurovascular bundle.
- Always keep the fascial needle tip up as you pass to make sure you are in preaponeurotic fat pad and do not damage the globe during passes.
- Form a pocket in the temporalis for a sling knot prior to passing the sling. Reposit the knot into frontalis prior to finalizing lid height, because thicker-browed individuals

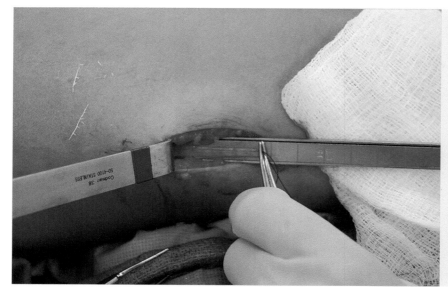

Fig. 14.5 Fascia strip is held on tension during harvest.

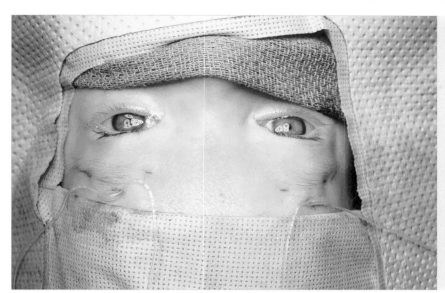

Fig. 14.6 Ends of silicone, passed in opposite directions away from center of the brow incision.

may exhibit more loss in lid height when knot is reposited.

- Close lid margin incisions prior to tightening sling material, otherwise these incisions may be difficult to access.
- Silicone ends should be passed through Watzke sleeve in opposite directions so that no silicone tips are left projecting toward the wound. This will help prevent extrusion (► Fig. 14.6).
- Placing a shield and elastic adhesive bandage (such as Elastoplast) postoperatively creates a moisture chamber and protects the cornea from trauma while local anesthetic wears off and orbicularis tone returns. Do not use an eye patch, which could cause a corneal abrasion.
- Keep an eye shield on the eye for 24 hours postoperatively. This reminds the patient and others to take it easy on day 1. Also, in bilateral cases, shielding one eye means that there is only one eye that the parents have to lubricate on the first night, which is less daunting in a resistant child.
- Compliance with postoperative lubrication in pediatric cases can be more challenging than in adults. This challenge can be obviated in at least one eye by placing a reverse frost suture and eye shield with elastic adhesive bandage over the operated eye for the first 24 hours, to be removed in the office on postoperative day 1. In bilateral cases, only cover one of the eyes to not overly alarm the patient.
- Overcorrections usually resolve. Except in cases of abrasion or lid malposition causing either eversion or inversion, defer revision for at least 6 months.
- An initially straight postoperative lid margin will become a graceful and physiologic curve around 1 month postoperatively.

14.10 What to Avoid

- Possibility of suture granuloma at fascia knot or silicone sleeve reinforcement can be limited or avoided by using vicryl rather than permanent material such as mersilene, which can extrude.

- Over-tightening can result in lid distraction from globe. Avoid this by carefully inspecting the relationship of lid margin on globe prior to finalizing the knot.
- Extrusion likelihood is decreased by delicate handling of incision. The use of skin hooks rather than forceps when repositing the sling will decrease trauma to this critical skin, especially in infant skin. In addition, once the sleeve is reposited, direct the ends of the silicone sling in opposite directions, away from the wound.

14.11 Complications/Bailout/ Salvage

- **Infection with or without extrusion:** When using silicone, the infected sling and sleeve should be removed and allowed to heal while the patient is placed on oral antibiotics. Schedule sling replacement at least one month after resolution of infection. Frequently, the effects of the sling persist due to the fibrous tract that formed around the infected sling. In these cases, the sling may not need to be replaced for years. Banked and autogenous fascia-related infections can often be successfully managed with oral or IV antibiotics. If part of the knot extrudes, the extruding tip can be excised, unextruded part of the knot reposited, and skin closed (in office or OR, depending on the age of the patient). The fascia sling is left in place and often completely responds to the antibiotic treatment. In such a case, revision is not always necessary.
- **Exposure and abrasion:** Exposure keratopathy and corneal abrasion are the main complications of this procedure. When encountered early in the postoperative period, it is often sufficient to simply increase lubrication. Consider bandage contact lenses if there is severe lagophthalmos or place a frost suture in the OR for a couple of days (► Fig. 14.7). Rarely, early sling revision is required in cases of postoperative lid margin malrotation causing entropion or ectropion.

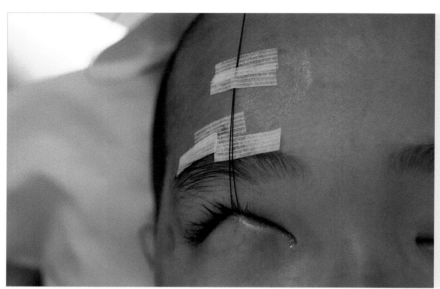

Fig. 14.7 Frost suture, placed under dressing to ensure no abrasion occurs during first 24-hour postoperative period. Removed in office on postoperative day 1.

- **Lagophthalmos and/or overcorrection:** Overcorrection causing lagophthalmos often relaxes in the first 6 postoperative months, during which time revision should be avoided. If necessary, revision (via lid margin incision or lid crease approach, where sling is undermined to relax its attachment to underlying tarsal connections) can salvage the sling rather than removing entirely.

14.12 Postoperative Care

Apply antibiotic ointment to skin incisions three times/day for 5 days. Lubricate the eye multiple times daily for the first 24 hours. Remove dressing and frost suture on postoperative day 1. After that day, it is usually sufficient to apply lubricating ointment during nighttime sleep and naps. This may be required for days, months, or indefinitely depending on lag. Older patients with fascia lata may also benefit from artificial tears four to six times/day indefinitely.

References

[1] Lee MJ, Oh JY, Choung HK, Kim NJ, Sung MS, Khwarg SI. Frontalis sling operation using silicone rod compared with preserved fascia lata for congenital ptosis a three-year follow-up study. Ophthalmology. 2009; 116(1):123–129

[2] Kim CY, Yoon JS, Bae JM, Lee SY. Prediction of postoperative eyelid height after frontalis suspension using autogenous fascia lata for pediatric congenital ptosis. Am J Ophthalmol. 2012; 153(2):334–342.e2

[3] Kersten RC, Bernardini FP, Khouri L, Moin M, Roumeliotis AA, Kulwin DR. Unilateral frontalis sling for the surgical correction of unilateral poor-function ptosis. Ophthal Plast Reconstr Surg. 2005; 21(6):412–416, discussion 416–417

[4] Anderson RL, Dixon RS. The role of Whitnall's ligament in ptosis surgery. Arch Ophthalmol. 1979; 97(4):705–707

[5] Antoszyk JH, Tucker N, Ling C, Codere F. Interlocking Crawford triangles in frontalis suspension. Arch Ophthalmol. 1993; 111(6):875–878

15 Repair of Upper Eyelid Retraction (Internal and External)

Natalie Homer and N. Grace Lee

Summary

Retraction of the upper eyelid may lead to significant ocular surface vulnerability and discomfort. This most commonly occurs in the setting of thyroid eye disease, but can also be seen in congenital eyelid malformation, or following surgery or trauma. The proper eyelid height can be restored by an external or internal approach, with external levator recession providing the maximal eyelid recession. These procedures can be further augmented with use of fixed or adjustable sutures for additional eyelid contour enhancement. Intraoperative eyelid height assessment is essential. Obtaining reliable results can be particularly challenging in patients with thyroid eye disease. Serious postoperative complications are rare.

Keywords: eyelid retraction, scleral show, thyroid eye disease, exposure keratopathy, eyelid recession, blepharotomy

15.1 Goals

- Ocular surface protection.
- Restoration of eyelid height, contour and symmetry.

15.2 Advantages

- The external approach to upper eyelid retraction repair allows for complete levator complex access and maximal upper eyelid recession via full thickness blepharotomy. The internal approach avoids a visible scar, but permits a more limited eyelid recession.

15.3 Expectations

- Patients should expect a lowered upper eyelid height, with improved ocular protection and comfort. Patients should be warned about the frequent need for reoperation to achieve and maintain an ideal eyelid height and contour, particularly those patients with thyroid eye disease.[1]

15.4 Key Principles

- An external approach through an eyelid crease incision can be utilized for recession of the levator muscle, the levator aponeurosis, and Müller muscle (often in combination) to achieve a desired amount of eyelid lowering.[2]
- An internal approach through the superior palpebral conjunctiva provides access to Müller muscle and levator aponeurosis for smaller scale eyelid recessions.
- Eyelid retraction repair can be performed with and without the use of sutures, which can be placed in a fixed or adjustable fashion.[3]
- Some recession techniques utilize spacer grafts derived of sclera, deep temporal fascia,[4] and Müller-conjunctivo-tarsal

tissue from the contralateral eyelid.[5] These techniques will not be outlined in this chapter.

15.5 Indications

- Upper eyelid retraction is defined as an upper eyelid position elevated beyond the ideal 1 to 2 mm below the superior limbal border. Etiologies of upper eyelid retraction include thyroid eye disease, congenital causes (including congenital fibrosis syndrome), iatrogenic or overcorrected ptosis following ptosis or blepharoplasty surgery, and trauma. Pseudoretraction can be seen in cases of proptosis. In few cases, upper eyelid retraction can be seen after glaucoma filtering and scleral buckle surgeries.[6]
- Upper eyelid retraction may induce lagophthalmos and significant corneal exposure, leading to globe-threatening keratopathy and discomfort, as well as an undesirable ocular appearance and exacerbated disfigurement from the often-concomitant proptosis.
- Upper eyelid retraction repair is undertaken to provide corneal protection, relieve ocular discomfort, and promote cosmetic rehabilitation.

15.6 Contraindications

- Eyelid retraction repair should not be performed in cases of active thyroid disease, particularly those requiring orbital decompression or strabismus surgery. Most recommend that a patient be biochemically and symptomatically euthyroid for at least 6 months prior to surgical recession.[7] The height of the eyelid should also be stable for approximately 6 months. Alternatives to surgery must also be considered in patients who are unable to stop blood thinners. As this surgery involves postseptal tissue, risk of retrobulbar hematoma is greater than preseptal surgery.

15.7 Preoperative Preparation

Preoperative evaluation should include bilateral eyelid contour assessment and measurement of marginal reflex distance, eyelid excursion, and lagophthalmos. A detailed slit-lamp examination should be performed to assess for consequential corneal pathology, including keratopathy and corneal thinning. In addition, external photography should document preoperative eyelid position. If the patient is on blood thinners, these should be held for an appropriate period of time to avoid postseptal hemorrhage. The patient should be made aware that their cooperation is necessary during surgery and that surgical eyelid recession should be performed under conscious sedation anesthesia to allow for patient participation in intraoperative eyelid height assessment. During surgery, very low–volume local anesthetic (< 1 mL) should be used, with careful measures taken not to infiltrate and paralyze the levator complex.

15.8 Operative Technique

15.8.1 External

Proximal Levator Muscle Recession

- Indicated in severe bilateral upper eyelid retraction.
- Recommended anesthesia: general anesthesia (due to patient discomfort with muscle belly manipulation, often thickened from fibrosis, with inability to locally anesthetize the muscle belly to allow for its functional intraoperative assessment).
- An upper eyelid crease incision is made through skin and orbicularis. The orbital septum is opened and preaponeurotic fat is carefully retracted to expose the levator aponeurosis. Dissection is proceeded to expose the levator muscle proximal to Whitnall ligament. A muscle hook is passed under the muscle belly from medial to lateral, and the entire levator muscle is transected. A mattress suture using 6–0 monofilament polypropylene is placed first through transected distal levator muscle and then through the proximal cut end of the muscle, after which both needle ends are externalized through the anterior upper eyelid edge and secured with rubber bolsters. Using this technique, fine adjustments can be made over the first 2 postoperative weeks by augmenting suture tension.
- Advantages to recessing the levator muscle belly include maximizing recession by completely devitalizing the muscle, addressing the area of primary thyroid orbitopathy pathology in the muscle belly and preserving the distal tarsus insertion for maintenance of good eyelid contour. The Müller muscle and levator aponeurosis complex are also left intact for future refinement of eyelid position, if necessary.

Full-Thickness Blepharotomy

- Indicated in severe unilateral or bilateral eyelid retraction due to thyroid eye disease (▶ Fig. 15.1).
- Recommended anesthesia: conscious sedation.

- An upper eyelid crease incision is made through skin and orbicularis (▶ Fig. 15.2). Dissection is performed to the superior border of the tarsus (▶ Fig. 15.3), from which the levator aponeurosis is disinserted. With a corneal protective shield in place, an incision is made through Müller muscle and conjunctiva across the entire extent of the upper eyelid. An option to place a 6–0 prolene suture along the medial 1/3rd versus leaving a strand of conjunctiva connected at this point will aid in the contour and prevent awkward sloping of the peak of the eyelid (▶ Fig. 15.4). The eyelid crease incision is then closed with a running 6–0 gut or prolene suture.

Levator Aponeurosis Recession

- Indicated in mild-to-moderate upper eyelid retraction, often due to overcorrected ptosis, moderate thyroid eye disease, or trauma.
- Recommended anesthesia: conscious sedation.
- An upper eyelid crease incision is made through skin and orbicularis. The orbital septum is opened and preaponeurotic fat is carefully retracted to expose the levator aponeurosis. The levator aponeurosis is dissected away from the underlying Müller muscle using an electrocautery needle, with the proximal arcade vessels marking the anterior surface of Müller muscle. The levator aponeurosis is isolated laterally, and the "horn" seen bisecting the lacrimal gland is identified and transected. A 6–0 polypropylene double-armed suture is threaded through cut edge of levator aponeurosis, externalized through orbicularis and skin, tied over rubber bolster and taped to forehead for future adjustments.
- If fixed sutures are preferred, the transected levator aponeurosis can instead be reapposed to the superior edge of the tarsus using two to three interrupted vicryl sutures, loosely tied in a "hang-back" technique. The patient should be periodically brought to a sitting position to assess eyelid height, prior to permanent tying of the sutures. The eyelid crease orbicularis and skin can be closed using a running 6–0 gut suture.[1]

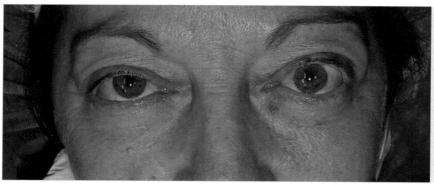

Fig. 15.1 Preoperative photo showing significant left upper eyelid retraction in a patient with thyroid eye disease.

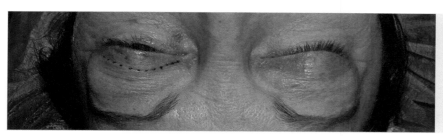

Fig. 15.2 The left upper eyelid crease is marked in preparation for incision (surgeon's view).

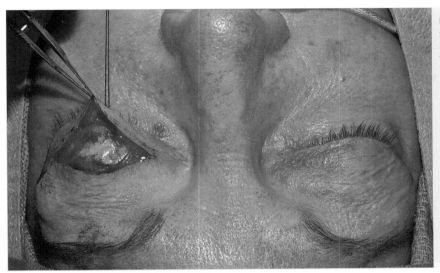

Fig. 15.3 Following entry into the postseptal space, dissection is carried down to reveal the levator aponeurosis and superior border of the tarsus.

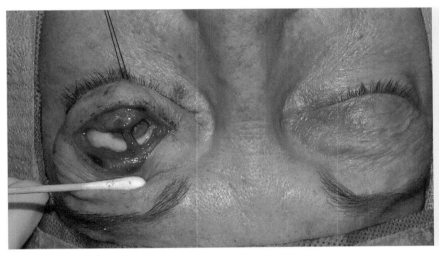

Fig. 15.4 A small strip of conjunctiva is preserved to aid in final eyelid contour.

15.8.2 Internal

- Indicated in mild (1–2 mm) upper eyelid retraction, and in cases where rapid, bilateral retraction repair is indicated.
- Recommended anesthesia: conscious sedation or local anesthesia only.
- A corneal protective shield is placed over the eye for globe protection. A 4–0 silk traction suture through edge of lid margin and the upper eyelid is everted over a Desmarres retractor. The conjunctiva is grasped with toothed forceps just over the superior tarsal border and incised using Westcott scissors or high temp cautery. Dissection is undertaken layer by layer through Müller muscle and the levator aponeurosis, with frequent checking of eyelid position until adequate recession has taken place. Eyelid position can be further augmented by completely disinserting the levator aponeurosis from its tarsal attachment, or by vertically stripping the levator aponeurosis. The patient is asked to look upward to determine the amount of induced ptosis, and the aponeurosis is directly re-fixated to the tarsus using interrupted 6–0 chromic sutures. The eyelid crease

orbicularis and skin are then closed using a running 6–0 gut suture.

15.9 Tips and Pearls

- The patient should be brought to a sitting position at various times throughout the procedure to assess lid height and symmetry.
- Overcorrection can be addressed intraoperatively by reattaching severed muscles to their original attachments.
- The surgeon may assess for significant inferior rectus muscle restriction contributing to upper eyelid retraction by noting a significant reduction in upper eyelid retraction in downgaze. If present, an inferior rectus recession should precede eyelid surgery.[8] One can also perform forced-duction testing.[1]
- Removing prolapsed preaponeurotic fat, as well as prominent postorbicularis fat pad, in Graves patients, reduces the fullness of the upper lid and brow.[9] However, avoid excessive preaponeurotic fat removal as this can lead to formation of a second, higher eyelid crease.[8]

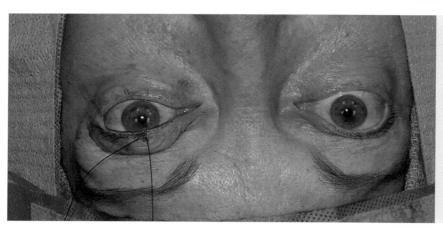

Fig. 15.5 Slight overcorrection of the left upper eyelid retraction can be seen immediately postoperatively.

- Hang-back sutures can be used in external levator muscle recession, with suture length estimated to be double the distance of desired eyelid recession.[8]
- Anticipate an additional 1.0 to 1.5 mm lowering of the upper eyelid after the local anesthetic has worn off.
- Some experts recommend placement of a nonabsorbable suture to prevent further spontaneous disinsertion with eyelid movement.[7]
- If the patient has simultaneous mild upper and mild-to-moderate ipsilateral lower eyelid retraction, consider harvesting a free tarsal graft from the retracted upper eyelid to place in the lower eyelid, and through the same internal incision, recess the Müller muscle of the upper eyelid.

15.10 What to Avoid

- Anticipate Hering law by placing the surgical eyelid slightly higher than that of the nonsurgical lid, with the expectation that the "normal" lid will elevate.
- Avoid flattening of the central eyelid contour and lateral eyelid flare by cutting the lateral horn of the aponeurosis and ensuring full lateral recession of the levator complex.[9]
- Take careful measures to avoid overcorrection medially by unintentional dissection of the far-medial aponeurosis and Müller muscle. If medial overcorrection occurs, the aponeurosis should be reattached to the tarsus with suture.[7]
- Avoid infiltration of the levator complex with local anesthetic.
- Avoid poor hemostasis, as perioperative hemorrhage will distort the surgical view and eyelid height assessment.

15.11 Complications/Bailout/Salvage

- Obtaining reliable results can be particularly challenging in patients with thyroid eye disease, due to physiologic variation in eyelid height, proptosis-related changes in globe position, disease progression, Hering law and need for subsequent strabismus surgery.[1]
- It is expected that the eyelid will appear ptotic in the initial postoperative period (▶ Fig. 15.5) and will gradually elevate over 1 to 4 weeks.[8,10] If the lid remains ptotic postoperatively,

elevation can be enhanced by patching the normal unoperated eyelid, which forces the patient to recruit the operative eyelid ipsilateral eyebrow, bringing the recessed tissues into closer approximating during the healing.
- If the lid retracts postoperatively, the patient should perform lid massage while elevating the eyebrow.[8,10]
- Superior relocation of the eyelid crease, due to aponeurotic fiber attachments to skin and orbicularis muscle, occurs in the majority of patients.
- Complications are uncommon, but may include minor eyelid margin numbness that typically resolves over the first 3 postoperative months.[9] Rare cases of eyelid fistulas have been reported.[9]

15.12 Postoperative Care

Postoperative care consists of ice on the operated eyelid for the first 48 hours. Rest and limitation of strenuous activity and swimming should be enforced for at least 1 week. Topical antibiotic ointment over the external incision (in external approach) or directly onto the ocular surface (in internal approach) for three times daily use is recommended for 5 to 10 days postoperatively, and female patients are asked to refrain from wearing makeup for the first 2 weeks to prevent incorporation of makeup pigment into the wound.

15.13 Acknowledgment

Thanks to Dr. Michael Yoon for providing the intraoperative patient photographs included in this chapter.

References

[1] Small RG. Surgery for upper eyelid retraction: three techniques. Trans Am Ophthalmol Soc. 1995; 93:353–365, discussion 365–369

[2] Cho IC, Kang JH, Kim KK. Correcting upper eyelid retraction by means of pretarsal levator lengthening for complications following ptosis surgery. Plast Reconstr Surg. 2012; 130(1):73–81

[3] Tucker SM, Collin R. Repair of upper eyelid retraction: a comparison between adjustable and non-adjustable sutures. Br J Ophthalmol. 1995; 79(7):658–660

[4] Schwarz GS, Spinelli HM. Correction of upper eyelid retraction using deep temporal fascia spacer grafts. Plast Reconstr Surg. 2008; 122(3):765–774

[5] Crawford JS. Correction of upper eyelid retraction using tissue removed in blepharoptosis repair. Am J Ophthalmol. 1986; 101(5):600–604

[6] Mauriello JA, Jr, Palydowycz SB. Upper eyelid retraction after retinal detachment repair. Ophthalmic Surg. 1993; 24(10):694–697

[7] Mourits MP, Sasim IV. A single technique to correct various degrees of upper lid retraction in patients with Graves' orbitopathy. Br J Ophthalmol. 1999; 83 (1):81–84

[8] McNab AA, Galbraith JEK, Friebel J, Caesar R. Pre-Whitnall levator recession with hang-back sutures in Graves orbitopathy. Ophthal Plast Reconstr Surg. 2004; 20(4):301–307

[9] Harvey JT, Corin S, Nixon D, Veloudios A. Modified levator aponeurosis recession for upper eyelid retraction in Graves' disease. Ophthalmic Surg. 1991; 22 (6):313–317

[10] Putterman AM. Surgical treatment of thyroid-related upper eyelid retraction: graded Müller's muscle excision and levator recession. Ophthalmology. 1981; 88(6):507–512

16 Upper Eyelid Gold/Platinum Weight Placement

Liza M. Cohen and Suzanne K. Freitag

Summary

Upper eyelid loading via gold or platinum weight placement is a gravity-dependent method of enhancing dynamic eyelid closure. It is used to treat exposure keratopathy due to lagophthalmos, which is commonly the result of facial nerve paralysis. Advantages of the procedure include its simplicity, reversibility, safety profile, and improved eyelid closure and cosmesis compared to other treatments for lagophthalmos. Preoperative preparation involves appropriate patient selection and weight fitting to determine the ideal implant weight. Key steps in the procedure include making an upper eyelid crease incision, dissecting a pretarsal pocket, suturing the weight to the tarsus and levator aponeurosis, and closing orbicularis oculi muscle and skin. Placement of the weight high on the tarsus and layered closure of orbicularis and skin can prevent weight migration and extrusion. Other potential complications include poor cosmesis, allergy, infection, under- or overcorrection, and astigmatism. Postoperative upper eyelid ptosis and continued need for topical lubrication are to be expected. Overall, upper eyelid gold/platinum weight placement is a straightforward and effective procedure to improve dynamic eyelid closure in patients with lagophthalmos and mitigate exposure keratopathy.

Keywords: gold weight, platinum weight, lagophthalmos, facial nerve paralysis, exposure keratopathy

16.1 Goals

- To treat lagophthalmos due to dysfunction of the orbicularis oculi muscle by improving eyelid closure upon blinking and forced closure. Orbicularis muscle dysfunction commonly occurs as a result of facial nerve paresis or paralysis.
- To provide corneal protection in cases of lagophthalmos, thereby preventing complications such as corneal ulceration and perforation.
- To establish an acceptable aesthetic appearance.

16.2 Advantages

- Upper eyelid weight placement allows for enhancement of dynamic eyelid function.
- The results are immediate and lasting.
- It is a straightforward, simple procedure to perform with rare need for readjustment.
- The procedure is reversible; the weight can be easily removed if orbicularis function returns and the weight is no longer needed.
- It is possible to simulate the predicted postoperative result prior to performing the procedure via weight fitting (see Preoperative Preparation).
- It provides a better cosmetic result compared to other surgical treatments of lagophthalmos, including medial and lateral tarsorrhaphies, lower eyelid elevation, temporalis muscle transfer, and facial nerve repair/grafting.

- The procedure is well tolerated with fewer complications compared to other techniques for dynamic eyelid reanimation, including silicone band and palpebral wire spring placement.[1]
- It reduces the need for conservative treatments for exposure keratopathy, such as topical lubricants, eyelid taping, moisture chambers, and contact lenses.
- Upper eyelid weight placement can be utilized in conjunction with procedures to correct the position of the lower eyelid such as medial/lateral tarsorrhaphies, lower eyelid elevation, or ectropion/retraction repair.

16.3 Expectations

- After upper eyelid weight placement, the lid should have improved excursion with the patient in a vertical position.
- Postoperative mild upper eyelid ptosis may occur following upper eyelid weight placement.
- The effect on eyelid closure is gravity-dependent; therefore, lubricating ointment, eyelid taping, and/or careful patching at nighttime while the patient is supine may be necessary.

16.4 Key Principles

Upper eyelid loading via placement of a gold or platinum weight is a method of treating exposure keratopathy due to lagophthalmos, which is commonly the result of facial nerve paresis (weakness) or paralysis. The weight functions in a gravity-dependent manner, assisting the eyelid to fall and thus inducing eyelid closure when the levator muscle relaxes, as in downward gaze, blinking, and forced eyelid closure (► Fig. 16.1). The weight provides improved eyelid closure without causing complete ptosis or significantly compromising cosmesis. A functioning levator muscle allows the eye to open normally, usually with minimal ptosis.

16.5 Indications

- Upper eyelid weight placement is an excellent first-line therapy for the treatment of exposure keratopathy due to facial nerve paresis or paralysis when maximal medical therapy is inadequate to maintain the health of the cornea. This applies to both acute, severe lagophthalmos and chronic cases unlikely to regain normal eyelid function.
- Secondary procedure when other surgical methods of eyelid closure have failed (i.e., extrusion or fatigue of a silicone band or palpebral spring) or have provided an unacceptable aesthetic result.

16.6 Contraindications

- Comatose or otherwise supine patients would not benefit from placement of an upper eyelid weight, given the weight's effect is gravity-dependent.

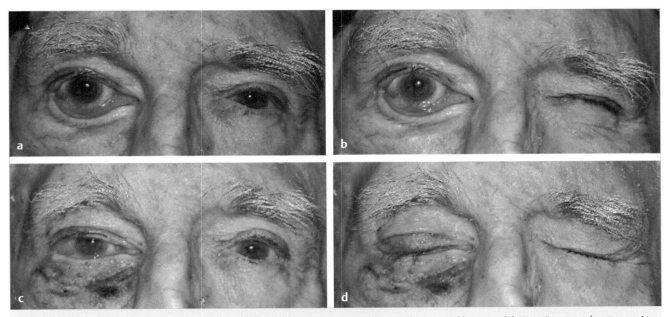

Fig. 16.1 Preoperative and postoperative photographs of a patient with lagophthalmos and upper and lower eyelid retraction secondary to scarring post-Mohs micrographic surgery resection of skin cancer. **(a)** Preoperative photograph at rest demonstrating right-upper eyelid retraction and right-lower eyelid cicatricial ectropion. **(b)** Preoperative photograph with forced eyelid closure showing complete lagophthalmos of the right eye. **(c)** Postoperative photograph at rest 1.5 weeks post-placement of a 1.6-gram right-upper eyelid platinum weight and right-lower eyelid lysis of adhesions with placement of a full-thickness skin graft. There is improvement in the upper eyelid position with a slight right-upper eyelid ptosis and in the lower eyelid position with the eyelid margin at the limbus. **(d)** Postoperative photograph with forced eyelid closure demonstrating good closure with marked improvement in lagophthalmos.

- A history of gold allergy is a contraindication to gold weight placement. Likewise, a history of allergy to platinum, iridium, or nickel is a contraindication to platinum weight placement.
- Very thin skin with an atrophic orbicularis muscle is a relative contraindication, as the color and bulk of the weight may become apparent in the eyelid.[1]

16.7 Preoperative Preparation

Elements of the history and physical examination that are important to assess prior to placing an upper eyelid weight include blink frequency and completeness, severity of facial nerve dysfunction, corneal sensation, lagophthalmos, Bell reflex, and orbicularis muscle function. Understanding the etiology and prognosis for facial nerve recovery are also important in deciding whether temporizing measures should be employed versus this more durable surgical procedure.

The next step is selecting the appropriate weight. Although gold was traditionally favored, platinum has recently gained popularity, given its smaller profile due to increased density compared to gold and lower rate of tissue reaction. Platinum weights are available as chains or segments, which provide the ability to make adjustments by adding or removing a portion of the implant rather than exchanging the entire implant.[2] Thin-profile gold and platinum weights are also available and are 0.6 mm in thickness compared to the traditional 1 mm thickness. Both gold and platinum weights range from 0.6 to 2.8 grams in 0.2-gram increments (▶ Fig. 16.2), are curved to match the curvature of the tarsus, and usually contain three holes for suture fixation.

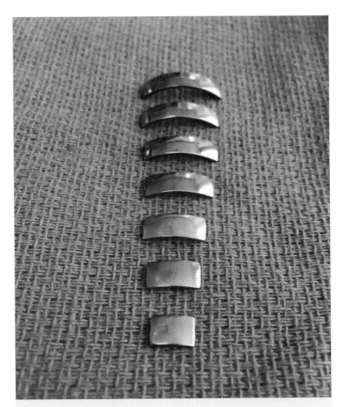

Fig. 16.2 Weight sizer trial set demonstrating the range of weights available.

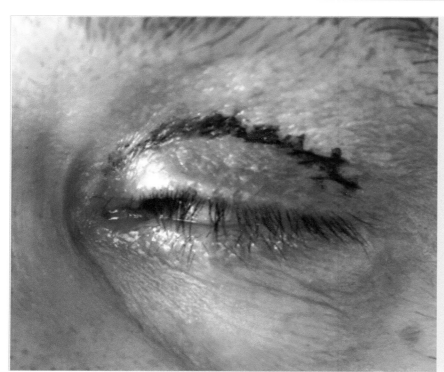

Fig. 16.3 Upper eyelid crease marking.

Weight fitting is done prior to the procedure in order to determine the desired weight of the implant. A weight is affixed to the affected upper eyelid using adhesive, with the upper border of the weight just below the upper eyelid crease. A thin strip of tape may be placed horizontally so as not to obstruct eyelid opening. The eyelid position and completeness of eyelid closure are assessed both in the sitting and supine positions. If the weight does not provide adequate eyelid closure or produces an unacceptable amount of ptosis, then it is removed and the procedure is repeated using the next heavier or lighter weight, respectively. This process is continued until the lightest weight that provides optimal closure is identified. At rest, approximately 1 mm of upper eyelid ptosis is considered ideal.[3] Many patients do well with a 1.2 or 1.4-gram weight. Given that the next heavier weight may be necessary for complete eyelid closure, it is wise to have at least two weights available for the procedure.[1]

16.8 Operative Technique

This procedure is typically performed under local anesthesia or monitored anesthesia care. The upper eyelid crease is marked (▶ Fig. 16.3). Local anesthetic consisting of a mixture of bupivacaine and lidocaine with 1:100,000 epinephrine is injected into the upper eyelid. The patient is prepped and draped in the normal sterile fashion for oculoplastic surgery. A corneal shield can be placed to protect the globe. A #15 blade is used to incise the premarked area of the skin between the medial and central thirds of the eyelid. Westcott scissors are used to dissect through the orbicularis oculi muscle down to the anterior face of the tarsus. Dissection is extended along the anterior tarsal

surface medially and laterally to accommodate the width of the implant as well as inferiorly to create a pretarsal pocket (▶ Fig. 16.4). Dissection should remain at least 2 mm superior to the upper eyelid margin, as this avoids damage to the eyelash roots and prevents the weight from migrating inferiorly to the eyelid margin.[1,3] One should also consider undermining up to 2 mm superiorly to ensure complete coverage of the implant.

The weight is then introduced into the field. The weight of the implant should be confirmed by visualizing the engraved numbers on its inner surface. The implant is placed into the pretarsal pocket on the anterior face of the superior two-thirds of the upper eyelid tarsus. The weight can be positioned slightly medially or laterally to obtain optimal eyelid contour. The superior edge of the implant should be at or slightly below the superior border of the tarsus. The orbicularis oculi muscle and skin should be pulled over the weight to ensure there is no skin tension prior to suturing the weight into place. Once in position, the inferior aspect of the weight is anchored to the tarsus using 7-0 Nylon sutures (▶ Fig. 16.5). First, a partial-thickness bite is taken through the tarsus and then through the predrilled hole in the weight from anterior to posterior, allowing for the knot to be buried. The lid is everted following each tarsal pass to ensure it is partial thickness. The upper aspect of the weight is then sutured to the extension of the levator aponeurosis on the anterior face of the tarsus via the predrilled hole in the weight.

Closure of tissue over the weight is performed in layers in order to minimize the risk of postoperative exposure or extrusion. The orbicularis oculi muscle is closed first using 6-0 Vicryl (polyglactin) in a running fashion to ensure watertight closure. Then, the skin is closed using a 6-0 plain gut suture in a running fashion. The corneal shield is removed, and antibiotic ointment is placed over the incision and on the cornea.

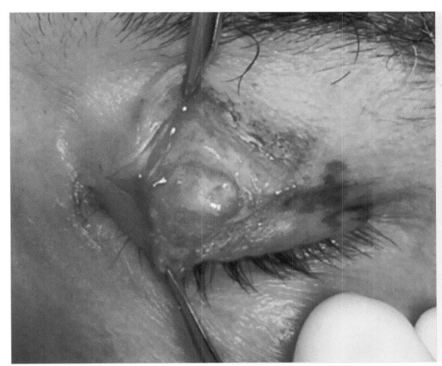

Fig. 16.4 Dissection of pretarsal pocket through orbicularis oculi muscle with exposure of the anterior face of the tarsus.

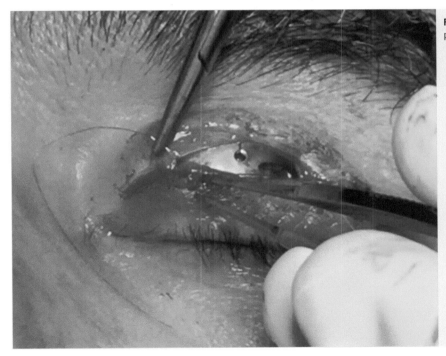

Fig. 16.5 Platinum weight being sutured into position using 7–0 nylon suture.

16.9 Tips and Pearls

- Careful dissection directly through the orbicularis oculi muscle to the tarsus followed by dissection along the anterior tarsal surface allows for a full-thickness layer of muscle to cover the weight, thus providing maximal protection from implant extrusion.
- Careful pretarsal dissection is essential in order to create the correctly sized pocket for placement of the weight. This holds the weight in position and limits the risk of migration within the pretarsal plane.[4,5,6]
- Placement of the weight high on the tarsus has advantages compared to placement low on the tarsus, including less visibility of the weight, lower chance of extrusion due to a greater thickness of tissue layers covering the weight, and creation of the eyelid crease.
- Layered closure of orbicularis muscle and skin over the weight can help prevent postoperative extrusion as compared to single-layered closure.

- Use of a platinum rather than gold weight is optimal, given the lower risk of tissue reactivity to platinum and its slightly smaller profile (higher density).[7]
- Patients with highly effective weight placement and resolution of exposure keratopathy may still have mild lagophthalmos. Consulting physicians who are non-ophthalmologists should be educated that the bottom-line goal is corneal health, which can only be assessed with slit lamp biomicroscopy.
- Patients with decreased corneal sensation (cranial nerve V dysfunction) are at higher risk for corneal breakdown than those with facial nerve dysfunction alone. More aggressive management may be required in these cases, and there should be a lower threshold for surgical management.
- Consideration should be given to placement of a small (one stitch) lateral tarsorrhaphy at the time of weight placement. It adds very little to the surgical time and postoperative recovery and provides added ocular surface coverage and some improvement in lower eyelid support and position.

16.10 What to Avoid

Placement of the implant too low on the tarsus may result in postoperative migration and eyelash compromise. Tension on the skin covering the weight should be avoided to decrease the probability of weight extrusion. This is accomplished via adequate dissection and undermining and can be evaluated prior to skin closure. Contamination of the implant can be avoided by employing sterile operative technique and introducing the implant into the surgical field at the time of insertion coupled with irrigation of the surgical bed with sterile balanced salt solution prior to closure.

16.11 Complications/Bailout/Salvage

- Poor cosmesis: Bulkiness or lumpiness at the site of the weight may be particularly noticeable in cases of gold weight placement due to the thicker profile of the weight and formation of a fibrous tissue capsule compared to platinum weights.[7,8,9] Discoloration of the skin and distortion of eyelid contour can also occur. If cosmesis is deemed unacceptable, the implant may be removed and replaced with a thinner profile or platinum weight.
- Migration of the weight: This can be avoided by placing the weight at least 2 mm above the upper eyelid margin. If the weight has migrated to a position where it is no longer functional or cosmetically acceptable, it can be removed and resutured more superiorly to the upper aspect of the anterior face of the tarsus.
- Extrusion of the weight: This is best avoided by performing layered closure of orbicularis oculi muscle and skin over the weight. If extrusion occurs, the weight should be removed and the eyelid should be allowed to heal by secondary intention. The patient is instructed to increase lubrication to protect the eye during the several weeks that a weight is absent. Then, a weight of a different material than was previously placed is inserted. The granulation tissue acts as a firm protective barrier from future extrusion.
- Infection: Infection is best prevented by placing the weight under sterile conditions and avoiding contamination of the implant or wound. Postoperative topical and oral antibiotics can also prevent this potential complication. An infected weight will become exposed and extrude, and the same management should be employed as described above.
- Allergy: Gold allergy can occur in patients undergoing gold weight placement. It may be managed by treatment with corticosteroids (either oral or a local injection), removal of the implant, and/or replacement with a platinum implant.[10] In patients with a known history of gold allergy, a platinum weight should be utilized. Although platinum allergy is a less frequent occurrence, platinum weights should be avoided in patients with a known history of allergy to platinum, iridium, or nickel.
- Undercorrection or overcorrection of upper eyelid position: This may be prevented by preoperative weight fitting. If there is insufficient eyelid closure or cosmetically unacceptable ptosis, the weight can be exchanged for a heavier or lighter one, respectively.
- Astigmatism: Refractive error related to the gravitational effect of the weight upon the cornea can occur and may warrant removal of the weight and placement of a lighter weight.

16.12 Postoperative Care

Given that the procedure may not result in complete eyelid closure, especially while lying supine, topical lubrication with drops or ointment is often still required after weight placement. Generally this need is much less than preoperatively, hence simplifying eye management for the patient.[5] Elevating the head at night can aid with nocturnal eyelid closure. Antibiotic ointment should be placed on the upper eyelid crease incision and cornea several times daily for the first week after the procedure. One should also strongly consider the use of an oral antibiotic to prevent infection of the implant. The patient is seen 1 week postoperatively, and the effect of the weight on eyelid closure and corneal exposure is assessed. Skin sutures, if nonabsorbable, can be removed at 1 week postoperatively. Close follow-up of patients who have undergone weight placement is essential in order to ensure the cornea remains protected, especially in cases of corneal hypesthesia where patients may not become aware of exposure keratopathy.

References

[1] Liu D. Gold weight lid load. In: Tse DT, Wright KW. Color Atlas of Ophthalmic Surgery: Oculoplastic Surgery. Philadelphia, PA: Lippincott Williams and Wilkins; 1992:225–230

[2] Malhotra R, Ziahosseini K, Poitelea C, Litwin A, Sagili S. Platinum segments: a new platinum chain for adjustable upper eyelid loading. Br J Ophthalmol. 2015; 99(12):1680–1685

[3] Nerad JA. Abnormal movements of the face. In: Techniques in Ophthalmic Plastic Surgery: A Personal Tutorial. Philadelphia, PA: Saunders Elsevier; 2010:252–255

[4] Seiff SR, Sullivan JH, Freeman LN, Ahn J. Pretarsal fixation of gold weights in facial nerve palsy. Ophthal Plast Reconstr Surg. 1989; 5(2):104–109

[5] Gilbard SM, Daspit CP. Reanimation of the paretic eyelid using gold weight implantation: a new approach and prospective evaluation. Ophthal Plast Reconstr Surg. 1991; 7(2):93–103

[6] Jobe RP. A technique for lid loading in the management of the lagophthalmos of facial palsy. Plast Reconstr Surg. 1974; 53(1):29–32

[7] Silver AL, Lindsay RW, Cheney ML, Hadlock TA. Thin-profile platinum eyelid weighting: a superior option in the paralyzed eye. Plast Reconstr Surg. 2009; 123(6):1697–1703

[8] Bladen JC, Norris JH, Malhotra R. Indications and outcomes for revision of gold weight implants in upper eyelid loading. Br J Ophthalmol. 2012; 96(4):485–489

[9] Townsend DJ. Eyelid reanimation for the treatment of paralytic lagophthalmos: historical perspectives and current applications of the gold weight implant. Ophthal Plast Reconstr Surg. 1992; 8(3):196–201

[10] Bair RL, Harris GJ, Lyon DB, Komorowski RA. Noninfectious inflammatory response to gold weight eyelid implants. Ophthal Plast Reconstr Surg. 1995; 11 (3):209–214

17 Upper Blepharoplasty

Michael E. Migliori

Summary

Upper lid blepharoplasty is not just about removing excess skin and fat. Achieving a satisfactory functional and aesthetic result after upper lid blepharoplasty can only be attained by understanding the anatomical changes that are responsible for the objectionable features causing symptoms, and by understanding how those features are addressed to leave a more youthful and normally functioning upper eyelid.

Keywords: dermatochalasis, ptosis, brow ptosis, margin reflex distance, lacrimal gland prolapse, browpexy

17.1 Goals

- Removal of excess skin with or without removal of prolapsed fat in the upper eyelids to improve visual function and cosmesis.

17.2 Advantages

- Removal of redundant eyelid skin and contouring of prolapsed fat as needed eliminates the physical barrier of these tissues overhanging the visual axis, allowing for improvement in visual function and an increase in the superior visual field.
- Upper eyelid blepharoplasty also improves the cosmesis of heavy, tired-appearing eyelids.

17.3 Expectations

- Patients should expect improvement in the redundancy of the upper eyelid skin with a more visible and defined eyelid crease and a decrease in visible fat prolapse. Patients should be aware that there will be a scar hidden along the upper eyelid crease. When surgery is properly performed, patients should expect to maintain normal eyelid function with complete closure of the eyelids.

17.4 Key Principles

- In youth, the upper lids are typically full. For some, very little of the tarsal platform is visible, while in others there is a larger visible area below the lid crease and above the upper eyelid lashes. With aging, the upper lid skin tends to lose elasticity and may stretch. The crease may become less defined. The preaponeurotic fat and medial orbital fat may prolapse into the lid (▶ Fig. 17.1). These fat compartments may be modified during blepharoplasty surgery. There is a trend toward being conservative in any modification to the preaponeurotic fat in an effort to not hollow out the upper lid sulcus area and instead to maintain youthful volume.[1]
- Laterally, the orbital lobe of the lacrimal gland may also prolapse anteriorly into the lid (▶ Fig. 17.2). It is important to recognize the lacrimal gland as such in order to avoid mistaking it for prolapsed fat and excising it (i.e., there is no "lateral" fat pad in the upper eyelid). The lacrimal gland may be resuspended into the bony lacrimal gland fossa via the upper blepharoplasty incision.
- In addition, there may be dehiscence or detachment of the levator aponeurosis resulting in upper lid ptosis (▶ Fig. 17.3). Removing redundant skin may be enough for some patients to regain a normal upper eyelid position, but other patients will require formal correction of eyelid ptosis (such as levator repair) to achieve their goals of improving superior field of vision or creating a more aesthetically pleasing upper eyelid configuration.
- Brow ptosis is quite common and results in additional redundancy of skin over the upper lids, especially temporally (▶ Fig. 17.4). It is important to identify brow ptosis during the preoperative clinical evaluation and make the patient aware of its contribution to excess eyelid skin, as patients often lack this insight. Concurrent correction of brow ptosis should be considered at the time of upper blepharoplasty.
- It is common to consider blepharoplasty as the removal of excess skin and fat from the upper lid. However, a better way to approach this procedure may be to focus on how much tissue is left behind rather than how much is removed. It is critical to leave adequate tissue to allow for eyelid function

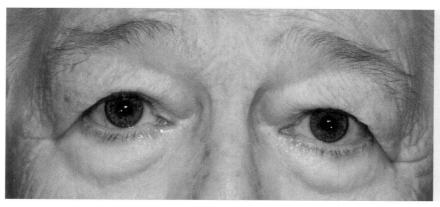

Fig. 17.1 A patient exhibiting bilateral upper eyelid dermatochalasis and prolapse of medial fat pads.

and closure. Optimizing the fine line between adequate tissue removal and safety is key to successful surgery.

- Underlying baseline asymmetry of facial anatomy is the norm, albeit to varying degrees among individuals.[2] This must be noted and discussed preoperatively. While surgical maneuvers can serve to ameliorate certain degrees of underlying preexisting asymmetry, patients should be counseled that there is a tendency for some return of asymmetry during healing and that underlying bony asymmetry, etc. is not corrected via blepharoplasty.

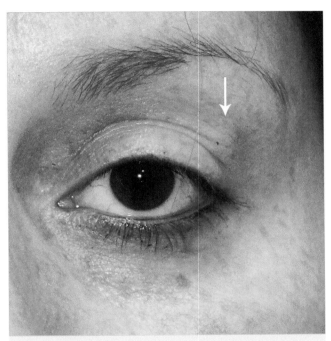

Fig. 17.2 Fullness over the lateral left upper lid crease *(arrow)* in a young woman representing a prolapsed lacrimal gland.

17.5 Indications

- Desire for cosmetic improvement of excess skin and prolapsed soft tissues of the upper eyelids.
- Desire for improved visual function by relieving the obscuration of the superior visual field caused by redundant upper lid tissues.

17.6 Contraindications

- Upper eyelid blepharoplasty should not be performed in cases of baseline severe dry eye disease that is not well-controlled or in cases of lagophthalmos. A tenet that all eyelid surgeons must remember is that the main purpose of the eyelids is to protect the eye. The lids must be able to open, close, and blink. Any surgical procedure aimed at improving either function or aesthetics must not compromise the ocular protection provided by the lids. Even a small amount of lagophthalmos or incomplete blinking may result in corneal exposure and pain (► Fig. 17.5).
- Patients who are anticoagulated for any reason, such as medications or thrombocytopenia or other disorders of clotting, should undergo blepharoplasty with caution, especially if the orbital septum is to be opened for fat debulking or levator repair, due to the risk of orbital or retrobulbar hemorrhage that may be sight-threatening if unrecognized or inadequately treated.

17.7 Preoperative Preparation

Preoperatively the surgeon should record the margin-reflex distance (MRD1), the height of the upper lid crease, the position of the upper lid skin fold, and the amount of levator excursion. Brow position should be noted as well as its contribution to excess upper lid skin. Brow position can be measured both in the alert, eyelids open position, and with the patient resting the

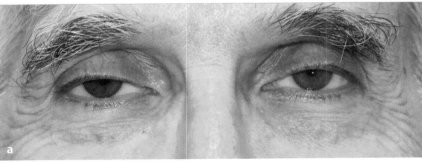

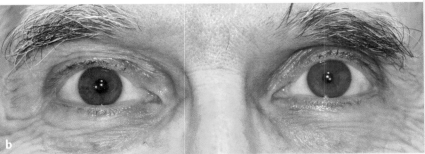

Fig. 17.3 (a) Significant bilateral upper eyelid ptosis, consistent with levator dehiscence, showing high/absent upper lid crease and superior sulcus configuration. Often when the levator is dehisced and recesses back into the orbit, it will pull the preaponeurotic fat back with it, which leads to the hollow upper sulcus appearance. (b) External levator repair alone was performed and led to normal eyelid position as well as appropriate upper sulcus configuration.

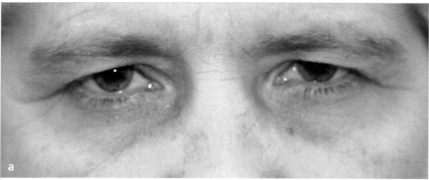

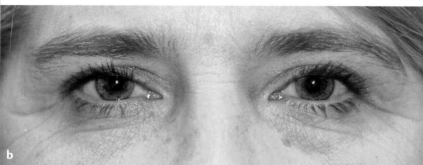

Fig. 17.4 **(a)** A 54-year-old female with severe brow ptosis and overlying dermatochalasis. **(b)** A tricophytic brow lift and concurrent blepharoplasty were performed yielding an excellent improvement in cosmesis and clearance of the visual axis.

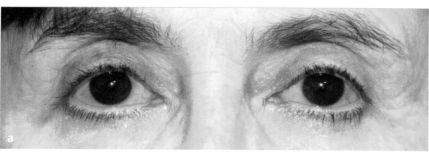

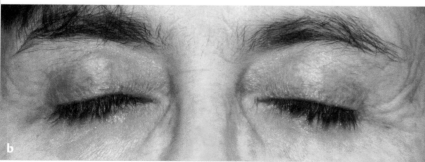

Fig. 17.5 **(a)** A 67-year-old female patient who underwent uneventful blepharoplasty and external levator repair surgery. She has normal MRD1. **(b)** Postoperatively she has trace lagophthalmos, with a small space just visible between the lashes when she closes her eyes gently (her right greater than left). This is enough to cause her significant discomfort. Great care must be taken in avoiding lagophthalmos, particularly in patients with preexisting dry eyes.

eyelids closed with the forehead relaxed; if in the relaxed position the brows fall well below the orbital rims the brows would be considered significantly ptotic. The ocular protective mechanisms including orbicularis strength, position, and horizontal laxity of the lower lid, tear film adequacy, and the presence or absence of the Bell phenomenon should also be documented. Preoperative photographs in the frontal and lateral planes should be obtained and preexisting facial asymmetry should be noted and discussed with the patient.

Equally important is to understand what the patient's goals and expectations are, and which procedures the patient may be willing to undergo (such as complex brow lift in addition to blepharoplasty versus blepharoplasty alone). Patients need to know why their lids look like they do, what can be accomplished to address this, and what to expect from surgery. Informed consent should include, among other things, the possibility of bleeding, infection, asymmetry, the possible need for additional surgery, and although rare, a significant orbital hemorrhage that could lead to blindness, as well as any risks associated with anesthesia such as sedation. If the patient is on blood thinners, it is important to weigh the risks and the benefits of suspending the blood thinners prior to surgery, especially in cases where postseptal eyelid fat removal is planned. It should be stressed that the final external appearance may not be realized for a period of many months.

17.8 Operative Technique

- The eyelid crease is delineated with a marking pen. Typically, the central crease is 8 to 10 mm from the lid margin, tapering 1 to 2 mm medially and laterally. In the Asian eyelid, the crease is lower due to the lower insertion of the orbital septum on the levator aponeurosis. The crease should not extend more medially than the upper punctum; otherwise there is risk of scarring and webbing to develop postoperatively in this region. Laterally, the crease incision should extend no further than the end of the brow but should demarcate any lateral hooding and should be relatively horizontal or up-angled lateral to the lateral canthal angle—in no way should there be a downward slope (▶ Fig. 17.6a).
- The skin to be removed is demarcated using the pinch technique. One blade of a smooth forceps is placed on the lid crease and the other blade pinches the skin above the crease at the point just inferior to where the upper lashes start to evert (▶ Fig. 17.6b). A mark is made on the skin at that point. The points are then connected in an arcuate line from the medial end to the lateral end of the lid crease incision (▶ Fig. 17.6c). It is helpful at this point to ask the patient to open the eyes to see if the demarcated area of excision is symmetric and includes any temporal hooding.
- The upper lids are infiltrated with local anesthetic. Hemostasis is better and the anesthetic affect lasts longer with anesthetics that have epinephrine, and the addition of hyaluronidase allows for easier dispersion. Anesthetic injections should be subcutaneous rather than intra- or submuscular to reduce the risk of a hematoma. The use of a ½ inch needle in the eyelid area is helpful in knowing the exact location of the needle tip in order to prevent inadvertent damage to the globe.
- Skin incision is made along the skin marker lines with a scalpel, Colorado needle, radiofrequency electrode, or CO2 laser (▶ Fig. 17.6d). The skin is dissected off from the underlying orbicularis oculi muscle and hemostasis is achieved with battery or bipolar cautery (▶ Fig. 17.6e). In patients with bulkier eyelids, the orbicularis muscle may be removed along with the skin ellipse.
- If fat is to be removed, a buttonhole is made in the orbital septum medially to access the medial and preaponeurotic fat pads and can be extended more centrally if necessary, to facilitate accessing the preaponeurotic fat (▶ Fig. 17.6f). The

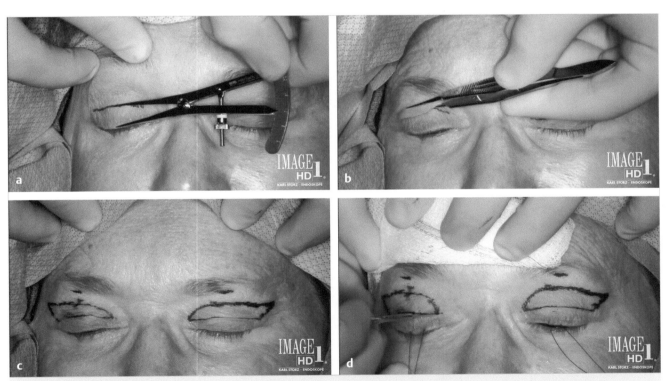

Fig. 17.6 (a) The eyelid crease is marked within the natural eyelid crease if it is normal for that patient (i.e., the crease is not abnormally elevated in association with significant eyelid ptosis, etc.). A caliper is used to confirm appropriate position and symmetry between the two eyes.
(b) A fine forceps is used to pinch excess skin while the eyelid is closed and the brow is in a resting position. This skin delineates the maximum amount of skin that may safely be removed. A caliper may further be used to confirm symmetry between the two sides for sub-brow skin symmetry. (c) The marking is completed in an elliptical fashion, generally matching the curvature of the orbit and not extending medially to the level of the lacrimal punctum. Laterally, the incision should generally not proceed past the tail of the brow. Some surgeons may bring the incision down to a lateral canthal rhytid and some surgeons may place an "upsweep" to the extension of the crease incision bringing it up to the sub-brow incision, as is depicted. (d) The incision is made with the skin on tension to improve cutting efficiency and accuracy. The incision is made through skin only. Generally, the incision is made through the eyelid crease first so that this incision is made while the skin is at maximum stability, as it is important that the crease be made very precisely. (continued)

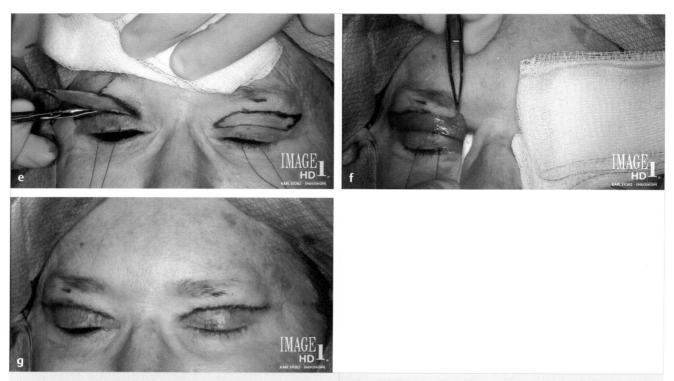

Fig. 17.6 (*continued*) **(e)** A skin flap or skin-muscle flap is excised. This is facilitated again by having the eyelid tissues on tension. **(f)** If any liposculpture is to be performed, a small "buttonhole" incision through orbital septum can be made medially with Westcott scissors to grant access to the preaponeurotic and medial fat pads. **(g)** Closure is then performed from a medial-to-lateral direction; in this way, if a standing cone or "dog-ear" is created it can be more readily dealt with laterally. Generally, the wound can be closed without this problem; however, one should be careful to "gather" the skin and account for the change in arc length of the incision (sub-brow vs. crease) as one proceeds through the closure at the outer third.

fat is meticulously removed using careful technique to maintain hemostasis and avoid orbital hemorrhage. It is important to keep in mind that excessive preaponeurotic fat removal can lead to a deep superior sulcus and loss of the upper lid convexity. Opening the orbital septum centrally and removing preaponeurotic fat also creates the potential for variability in lid crease position postoperatively if this procedure is not performed symmetrically from side to side, so great care must be taken.

- A buttonhole can be made in the septum laterally to approach a prolapsed lacrimal gland or to perform a browpexy. This incision should be close to the upper wound edge.
- A row of cautery in the orbicularis muscle along the lower wound edge will create a cicatrix that will help fortify the eyelid crease if needed in a patient with weak or multiple creases noted preoperatively.
- The incision is then closed with sutures. Most surgeons use 6–0 suture to close the lid. The choice of absorbable versus nonabsorbable suture, and interrupted versus running suture, is the surgeon's preference. Some surgeons place a few interrupted sutures to align the wound edges prior to closing with a running suture (▶ Fig. 17.6g). Patients appreciate not having to have sutures removed and may request absorbable sutures, but gut sutures lose their tensile strength quickly yet may not fully "absorb" internally for a period of months, leaving small suture cysts during this process of resolution.

17.9 Tips and Pearls

- Adjuvant procedures can be performed at the same time as blepharoplasty:
  - Concomitant ptosis is treated with standard ptosis repair techniques. Conjunctivo-Müller muscle resection is easier to perform after the lid is marked but before the skin resection is made (otherwise the lid is too "thin" to be incorporated into the clamp properly upon lid eversion). External levator ptosis repair is performed via the blepharoplasty incision.
  - A prolapsed lacrimal gland can be resuspended simultaneously with the blepharoplasty. Once the orbital rim is exposed bluntly, the orbital septum is opened directly over the prolapsed gland. Blunt dissection is then extended along the orbital roof in the lacrimal gland fossa to expose the periorbital of the orbital roof. Both arms of a double armed 5–0 polyglactin or 6–0 silk suture are passed through the lacrimal gland capsule at the anterior pole of the gland. Both arms of the suture are passed in a posterior-to-anterior direction through the periosteum just posterior to the rim within the lacrimal gland fossa. The gland is gently pushed back into the orbit and the suture is tied and cut flush to the knot.
  - One way to address a ptotic lateral brow is with internal browpexy. This should not be considered a brow-lifting

technique but rather a method of stabilizing the brow to prevent further descent. Through a lateral orbicularis buttonhole, blunt dissection is extended above the brow in line with the lateral canthal angle. Dissection continues in the pre-periosteal plane for about 2 cm. A 5–0 polypropylene suture is passed through the skin at the inferior row of cilia full thickness through the brow flap, leaving the suture end externalized. The needle is grasped under the flap and then passed through the periosteum about 1 cm above rim, in line with the lateral canthal angle. Looking under the flap, the suture from the original full-thickness pass marks the inferior row of brow cilia. The needle is then passed through the deep tissue of the flap at the exit point of the suture. The tail of the suture is then pulled through under the flap and tied. More aggressive brow lifting can be performed using standard techniques. The caveat is that a browlift should be performed prior to the upper lid blepharoplasty, to avoid excessive eyelid skin excision.

   ○ If there is lateral canthal laxity, a lateral canthopexy may be performed via the upper blepharoplasty incision.[3] The orbicularis is bluntly separated lateral to the lateral orbital rim just above the lower skin edge. The lateral orbital rim and tendon are bluntly exposed. Both arms of a 5–0 polyglactin suture are passed through the lateral end of the lower tarsus/lateral canthal tendon through this buttonhole. The sutures are then passed through the lateral rim periosteum in a posterior-to-anterior direction and tied where the lateral canthal angle is in its appropriate position. The orbicularis does not need to be closed.

- The resectable upper lid skin is notably thinner than the skin just below the brow, and skin excision should not extend into the thicker sub-brow skin except to a small degree temporal to the lateral canthal angle if there is significant lateral hooding and the brows will not be elevated. There should be at least 15 mm between the inferior brow cilia and the superior aspect of the skin to be excised, and at least 20 mm minimal total skin between the lower brow cilia to the lashes centrally to avoid over-resection of skin and to maintain normal function and appearance of the eyelids.[4] Note that the pinch technique as previously described determines the *maximum* amount of skin that can safely be removed, not the amount of skin that ought to necessarily be removed. With time a surgeon develops a sense of appropriate skin removal to yield reliably successful outcomes that are very infrequently over- or undercorrected while yielding desirable cosmesis.

- When closing the incision, the suture bites should be very close to the wound edge, no more than 1 mm away. Long bites are more likely to leave suture marks or cause the wound edge to curl under.

- Laser or electrocautery incisions may take slightly longer to heal as a result of thermal impact to the tissue, so whichever suture is chosen, it must retain some tensile strength long enough for good wound integrity. While there is thermal injury causing micro wound edge tissue necrosis from instrumentation such as Colorado needle electrocautery, the end cosmetic result between such instrumentation and "cold steel" scalpel incisions is not significantly different.[5]

- The incision should be closed from medial to lateral, and care should be taken when starting. There is often more lax skin remaining above and medial to the medial end of the incision, especially if there is medial brow descent. To avoid having the medial skin slide down over the medial lid crease, the first four or five suture passes should also include a thin pass through the orbicularis close to the upper edge of the incision. This will support the crease and prevent the tissue from sliding inferiorly. If there is more residual lax skin than can be addressed with simple closure, a small Burow triangle may be excised from the upper edge about 4 mm from the medial end of the incision. This will effectively shorten the upper arm of the incision and advance the medial skin laterally to reduce laxity.

17.10 What to Avoid

Upper blepharoplasty seems to be a relatively straightforward and simple procedure; however, it does require care and skill to avoid significant complications. It is always possible to go back and remove additional tissue, but very difficult to put it back if too much is removed. It is important to pay special attention to achieving even tarsal platform show (as a result of skin crease and skin flap configuration), as asymmetry of the tarsal platform postoperatively is particularly noticeable and bothersome to patients.[6] With good preoperative planning and careful technique, and thinking of blepharoplasty as restoring a more youthful anatomy rather than a subtractive procedure that removes skin and fat, it should be easy to achieve excellent functional and aesthetic results that satisfy both the surgeon and more importantly the patient.

17.11 Complications/Bail-Out/ Salvage

- Temporary lagophthalmos may ensue during the first days to weeks postoperatively. It is important to reinforce the importance of lubrication with ointment on the ocular surface during the immediate postoperative period.

- Permanent lagophthalmos can be present if too much skin is excised, from aggressive levator advancement, or from incorrect wound closure. This may require an additional surgical procedure with a skin graft to allow for full excursion and closure. With careful marking and surgical technique, this should be a truly rare situation.

- Rarely a medial web can result from exuberant scar tissue formation. Early injection of steroid or wound revision via z-plasty may be warranted if the patient is bothered by the appearance. This risk can be minimized by taking care to not extend the incision too medially (i.e., generally not medial to the lacrimal punctum).

- Prompt removal of sutures will avoid suture tracks, which patients find quite bothersome on the eyelid crease. Reassurance that incision line lumpiness will improve in weeks to months after surgery is often required.

17.12 Postoperative Care

After surgery, physical activity should be limited for 1 to 2 weeks to avoid hemorrhage and edema. The patient should apply cold compresses to the eyelids during the first few days after surgery. Head-of-bed elevation helps to avoid excess eyelid edema. Makeup should be avoided around the eyes for approximately 2 weeks to avoid incorporation of the material into the wound during healing. Follow-up is usually performed 1 to 2 weeks after surgery, with nonabsorbable sutures removed at approximately 1 week.

References

[1] Zoumalan CI, Roostaeian J. Simplifying blepharoplasty. Plast Reconstr Surg. 2016; 137(1):196e–213e

[2] Perumal B, Meyer DR. Facial asymmetry: brow and ear position. Facial Plast Surg. 2018; 34(2):230–234

[3] Georgescu D. Surgical preferences for lateral canthoplasty and canthopexy. Curr Opin Ophthalmol. 2014; 25(5):449–454

[4] Flowers RS. Blepharoplasty. In: Courtiss EH, ed. Male Aesthetic Surgery. St. Louis, MO: Mosby; 1982

[5] Arat YO, Sezenoz AS, Bernardini FP, Alford MA, Tepeoglu M, Allen RC. Comparison of Colorado microdissection needle versus scalpel incision for aesthetic upper and lower eyelid blepharoplasty. Ophthal Plast Reconstr Surg. 2017; 33(6):430–433

[6] Lew H, Goldberg RA. Maximizing symmetry in upper blepharoplasty: the role of microptosis surgery. Plast Reconstr Surg. 2016; 137(2):296e–304e

18 Asian Blepharoplasty

Shu-Hong (Holly) Chang and Do Eon-Rok

Summary

Asian blepharoplasty, commonly known as "double eyelid surgery," refers to surgery designed to create or define an upper eyelid crease. In this chapter, the authors review the relevant eyelid anatomy and provide detailed step-by-step explanations as well as diagrams for both non-incisional and incisional Asian blepharoplasty techniques. Surgical pearls and advice for avoiding complications, such as redundant crease formation, crease disappearance over time, prolonged edema, and iatrogenic ptosis, are also presented.

Keywords: Asian blepharoplasty, double eyelid surgery

18.1 Goals

Asian blepharoplasty, commonly known as "double eyelid surgery," or "ssangkkeopul" surgery in South Korea where the practice has been popularized, refers to surgery designed to create or define an upper eyelid crease. Due to the unique anatomic characteristics of the Asian eyelid as well as specific functional and aesthetic expectations from patients, Asian blepharoplasty surgery has been the topic of entire textbooks and a large body of research. In this chapter, we will distill this body of research and our experience into key points for performing successful Asian blepharoplasty surgery.

18.2 Advantages

Asian blepharoplasty surgery lends itself to incorporating adjunctive techniques such as excision of dermatochalasis, ptosis modification, epicanthoplasty, and palpebral fissure widening to significantly alter the anatomy and appearance of the eyelids, while at the same time improving visual functioning. Therefore, it is critical for the surgeon to understand patient expectations and clarify the goals and limitations of surgery before embarking on the surgical journey.

18.3 Expectations

We cannot overemphasize the importance of understanding patient expectations when planning Asian blepharoplasty surgery. Asians are not a homogeneous group and it can be counterproductive to make generalizations. Beauty ideals differ between the various Asian ethnicities and cultures, in addition to specific individual patient preferences. Our experience tells us, however, that nearly all patients expect short recovery time and minimal scarring. And most patients seeking Asian blepharoplasty surgery do so because they desire larger appearing eyes. It is important to clarify the following expectations before surgery:

- What is the desired crease height and tarsal platform show?
- What is the desired crease depth? Does the patient want a deep or "harsh" crease or a softer more natural crease that is less visible with the eyelids closed but has a higher risk of fading away over time?
- Is the goal of surgery to have larger appearing eyes or to change the shape of the eyes? If so, what are the patient's thoughts on adjunctive procedures like ptosis modification, epicanthoplasty, or lateral Hotz procedure to widen the palpebral fissure in multiple vectors?

18.4 Key Principles

The Asian eyelid has several key anatomic differences from the Caucasian eyelid, which are well documented in the medical literature[1,2] and succinctly summarized by Kiranantawat et al.[3]

- The Asian eyelid skin is often thicker, with pretarsal and suborbicularis oculi muscle adipose layers that are rarely present in the Caucasian eyelid.
- The inferior most extent of the preaponeurotic fat pad lies lower in the Asian eyelid. While the mechanism of this descent remains a topic of debate among anatomists, there is emerging evidence that the fusion area between the orbital septum and the distal levator aponeurosis plays a role. This area of fusion has been variably termed "septoaponeurosis junctional thickening," "septoaponeurotic vehicle," or simply "junctional thickening."[4]

The two primary methods of creating an eyelid crease are non-incisional and incisional. The non-incisional technique is less invasive and forms a more natural appearing eyelid crease with faster postoperative recovery, but carries a higher risk of long-term surgical failure. Patient selection is critical in determining which surgical method to use.

18.5 Indications

Indications for surgery include eyelid asymmetry; incomplete, redundant, or missing creases; and desire for cosmetic improvement. Patients are candidates for non-incisional (suture) crease formation if they do not require excess skin excision and have relatively thin eyelid soft tissues that can maintain a crease temporarily created by indenting the eyelid with a Q tip at the desired crease line. Patients who require skin excision to achieve the desired amount of tarsal platform show, those with thick eyelid tissues that do not maintain a temporary crease, and patients with scarring from previous blepharoplasty surgery are better suited for incisional blepharoplasty.

18.6 Contraindications

While no true contraindications exist, it is important to recognize that eyelid surgery is elective in nature, and should be balanced against the patient's general medical health as well as psychological wellbeing. Caution should be exercised and appropriate medical consultations obtained when recommending sedation for patients in poor health. Similarly, patients who exhibit signs of body dysmorphic disorder should be dissuaded from surgery and/or referred for counseling. The principle of "first do no harm" is especially important when undertaking elective surgery.

18.7 Preoperative Preparation

The preoperative surgical design process is critical. This dynamic maneuver should be performed with the patient seated upright at the surgeon's eye level. With the patient looking down, a clean toothpick or surgical tool designed for this purpose is used to gently depress the eyelid skin at the level of the intended eyelid crease. In our experience, the optimal location for the Asian eyelid crease is 7 to 8 mm from the eyelid margin. An eyelid crease placed at this height is aesthetically pleasing and facilitates deeper dissection and fixation as needed. With 7 to 8 mm as a starting point, the patient is then asked to look straight ahead as the toothpick is removed while the contour and durability of the eyelid fold is assessed. This maneuver is repeated until the crease location and design is optimized, then a marking pen is used to dot along the intended eyelid crease.

The amount of skin to be excised depends on the desired pretarsal show. If a large amount of skin excision is needed, either the skin pinch or raise-and-drop methods may be used to gauge the amount of skin to be excised. Most cosmetic Asian blepharoplasty surgeries, however, require only a few millimeters, if any, of skin excision. In these cases, the amount of skin excision can be directly measured, subtracting 1 to 1.5 mm in patients with thick skin to account for the width of the tissue forming the base of the skin that drapes over the eyelid crease (▶ Fig. 18.1).

It is our practice to have patients discontinue the use of any blood thinners 7 to 10 days prior to surgery.

Surgery is generally performed under local anesthesia or light sedation such that the patient is able to open and close the eyes intraoperatively to allow the surgeon to gauge symmetry and crease formation. In our experience, oral diazepam or intravenous ketamine, in conjunction with intravenous or intramuscular midazolam, creates the optimal level of sedation while maintaining the patient's ability to cooperate with eye opening and closure. Intravenous propofol can render the patient less cooperative.

After instillation of proparacaine or tetracaine anesthetic eye drops, local anesthetic consisting of 2% lidocaine with epinephrine 1:100,000 is injected subcutaneously across the entire surgical area, using a 30-gauge needle, administered in 0.2 to 0.3 mL aliquots. Injecting above the orbicularis oculi muscle plane avoids hematoma formation, which could cause difficulties gauging symmetry during surgery. Surgeons have the option of adding hyaluronidase (to facilitate anesthetic diffusion) and/or sodium bicarbonate (to buffer the pH and decrease pain with injection) to the local anesthetic mixture. We recommend avoiding longer-acting anesthetics such as bupivacaine in case of unintended spread to the levator muscle causing prolonged intraoperative ptosis that render it difficult for patients to open and close the eyes during surgery. One should always have local anesthesia available on the sterile field for intraoperative administration as needed. The entire face is prepped with dilute betadine solution.

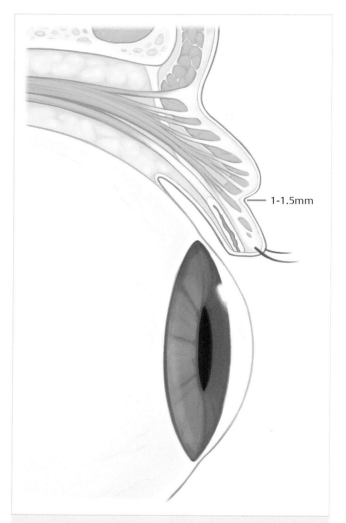

1-1.5mm

Fig. 18.1 When determining the amount of skin to be excised during blepharoplasty surgery, it is important to subtract 1 to 1.5 mm in patients with thick skin to account for the width of the tissue forming the base of the skin that drapes over the eyelid crease.

18.8 Operative Technique

For non-incisional eyelid crease formation, we prefer a continuous buried suture method.[5,6] Compared with interrupted suture techniques, the continuous suture method more evenly distributes tension and offers a natural appearing eyelid crease. Following design of the eyelid crease line, six entry points are marked loosely corresponding to the medial limbus, mid-pupillary line, and lateral limbus with the eye in primary position (▶ Fig. 18.2, ▶ Fig. 18.3). At each of the six points, a No. 11 blade is used to create a 1-mm stab incision extending from the skin to the orbicularis oculi muscle. The fifth stab incision is made deeper into the muscle layer, facilitating removal of a small amount of the orbicularis oculi muscle to create a pocket in which to bury the suture knot. A 20-mm tapered 3/8 circle needle on a 7–0 clear nylon suture is passed through entry point #5, entering skin and exiting the conjunctiva 1 mm above the superior tarsal border. The needle reenters the adjacent

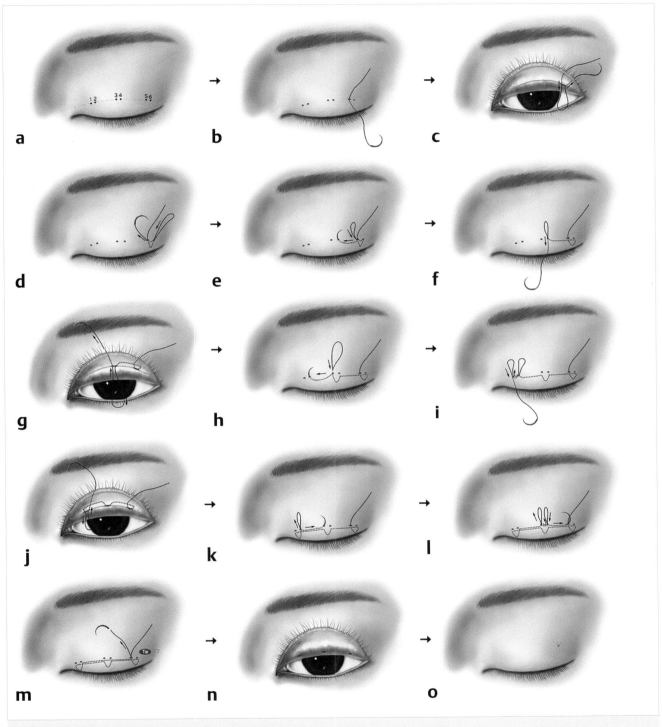

Fig. 18.2 (a-o) Non-incisional eyelid crease formation technique.

conjunctiva to exit skin at stab incision #6, thereby creating a small loop with minimal exposed suture on the conjunctival surface. Although we have not encountered corneal abrasions caused by the short segment of exposed conjunctival surface suture in our practice, this risk can be further minimized by entering the conjunctiva at the exit point then traversing the subconjunctival space before completing the pass in the same

manner as described. After exiting the skin at stab incision #6, the needle reenters incision #6 and is advanced medially in the subcutaneous plane until it exits stab incision #4. Then the needle reenters #4, exiting on the conjunctival surface 1 mm above the superior tarsal border, reentering the adjacent conjunctiva to exit at stab incision #3. The needle passes in the transverse subcutaneous plane from #3 to #1. A third conjunctival pass is

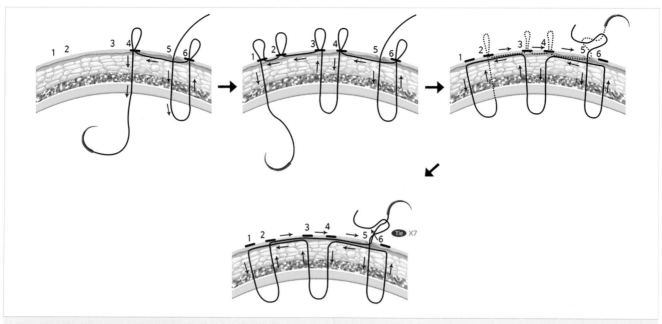

Fig. 18.3 Non-incisional eyelid crease formation technique.

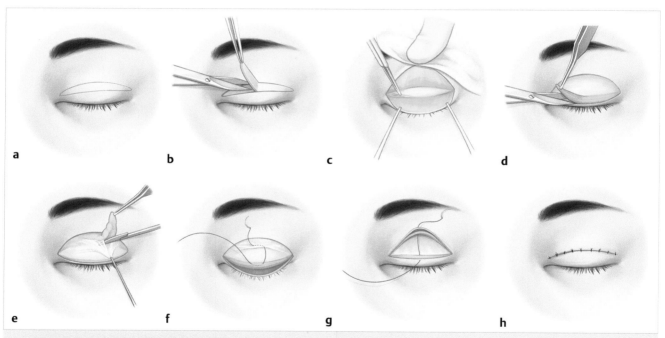

Fig. 18.4 (a–h) Incisional blepharoplasty technique.

made in similar fashion, entering stab incision #1 and exiting at #2. The needle reenters stab incision #2 and travels through the subcutaneous plane, alternately exiting and reentering at #3 and #4 to incision #5. Prior to exiting incision #5, the needle dives deep under the orbicularis oculi muscle such that the knot can be tied and buried deep into the dissection pocket. The suture is tied with controlled tension (a minimum of six single throws) and buried. The skin at stab incision #5 is closed with residual 7–0 nylon suture.

The incisional technique begins with excision of the previously determined skin flap using a No. 15 blade and curved Stevens tenotomy scissors (▶Fig. 18.4). With the assistant retracting the inferior lip of the incision using two single-prong skin hooks, a monopolar cautery on cutting mode or radiofrequency surgical device is used to incise the orbicularis oculi muscle at the level of the eyelid crease and undermine toward the eyelid margin in the pretarsal plane. The extent of undermining depends on the patient's degree of pretarsal fullness,

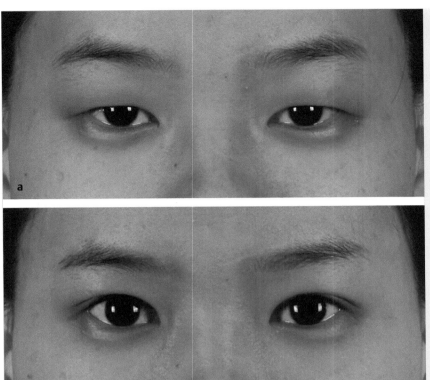

Fig. 18.5 (a) Before and (b) 14-month follow-up result after incisional Asian blepharoplasty.

but generally includes the superior half of the tarsus. With undermining complete, scissors are used to excise a 2 to 3 mm strip of orbicularis oculi muscle and pretarsal soft tissues along the inferior lip of the incision. More aggressive pretarsal tissue excision may be required for severely puffy eyelids, but can cause prolonged postoperative edema. If needed, additional muscle excision can be performed along the superior lip of the incision to expose the orbital septum overlying the preaponeurotic fat pad. The septum is incised across the eyelid and, in the case of a puffy eyelid, the preaponeurotic fat can be judiciously debulked. In most patients, we prefer to preserve the fat because overly aggressive fat debulking can cause contour irregularities and formation of redundant folds. The inferior lip of the now opened orbital septum, as it inserts onto the anterior tarsal face, has been shown to divide into an anterior layer that fuses with tarsus and a posterior layer that blends into the levator aponeurosis. This is the aforementioned septoaponeurotic junction (SAJ), which some anatomists believe retains elasticity with normal eyelid opening and closure, and that the eyelid crease should be fixated to this junction to create a dynamic eyelid crease that naturally softens with lid closure but maintains its efficacy. Residual septal stump is trimmed, preserving the SAJ. Crease fixation is performed using multiple 7–0 nylon sutures placed in buried fashion to anchor the orbicularis muscle at the inferior lip of the incision to the SAJ. Again, the number and locations of the fixation sutures vary depending on crease design, but we generally place five to six such sutures, taking special care to fixate the medial eyelid crease because this area is prone to crease disappearance over time. Skin closure is performed with 7–0 silk or nylon sutures, starting with three guiding sutures placed along the midpupillary, medial limbus, and lateral limbus lines. These guiding sutures enter skin at the inferior lip of the incision, incorporate orbicularis at the inferior aspect of the wound, then incorporate the suborbicularis fascia in addition to muscle tissue at the superior lip of the wound, and exit skin superiorly. Orbicularis closure in this manner helps to prevent formation of redundant creases. Finally, skin is closed with multiple interrupted or 7–0 silk or nylon sutures, incorporating pretarsal soft tissue as needed for reinforcement of the crease. ▶ Fig. 18.5 and ▶ Fig. 18.6 respectively demonstrate results of incisional and non-incisional Asian blepharoplasty surgery.

18.9 Tips and Pearls

- It is useful to have high resolution photographs of the patient to refer to intraoperatively.
- Lighting is an important consideration in Asian blepharoplasty surgery, because the patient is repeatedly asked to open and close the eyes for the surgeon to gauge crease contour and symmetry. The vast majority of patients are unable to fully open their eyes with the overhead surgical lights shining in their eyes. To avoid wasting time in repeatedly moving the overhead surgical lights, we recommend either a foot pedal control for the overhead lights or the surgeon to wear a headlight so that he or she can quickly move the light away from the patient's eyes when asking the patient to open/close his or her eyes.
- Fat removal is seldom performed except in cases of truly puffy eyelids. If fat is removed, do not discard the fat. Rather, keep the excised fat on a telfa or gauze pad so as to compare

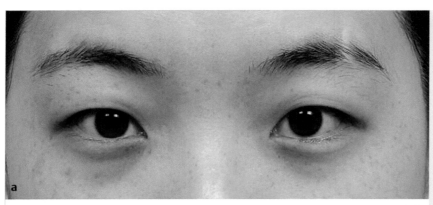

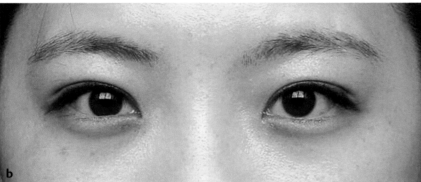

Fig. 18.6 **(a)** Before and **(b)** 2-year follow-up result after non-incisional Asian blepharoplasty.

the amount excised between the two eyelids to ensure comparable fat excision.

- In many surgeries, suture closure of the incision is a task left to the junior assistants because the senior surgeon has performed the "important" parts of the surgery. In Asian blepharoplasty, incision closure is arguably the most important part of the surgery because this is when the crease is defined and symmetry is of utmost importance. This task should not be left to an inexperienced surgeon.
- In a patient who is able to maintain a crease well but desires more tarsal platform show, we occasionally combine continuous suture crease formation with skin-only excision blepharoplasty to provide the benefits of a more natural crease without the prolonged edema anticipated with full blepharoplasty suture.[7] In this technique, it is important to incorporate the crease formation suture in the skin closure to avoid multiple creases.

18.10 What to Avoid

- Aggressive pretarsal tissue removal may lead to iatrogenic ptosis due to levator aponeurosis dehiscence. If this is suspected, a prophylactic suture can be placed to stabilize the levator aponeurosis to the tarsus.
- Care should be taken to avoid causing a hematoma that can distort the tissue anatomy and, even worse, mechanical ptosis. Anesthetic injection in the subcutaneous plane (rather than suborbicularis plane) and meticulous intraoperative hemostasis are two ways to avoid hematoma formation.

18.11 Complications/Bailout/ Salvage

Asian blepharoplasty is subject to complications that can be seen with any type of blepharoplasty surgery, including hemorrhage, infection, asymmetry, worsening dry eyes, and lagophthalmos. In the body of this chapter, we have provided tips to avoid specific complications such as redundant crease formation, crease disappearance over time, prolonged edema, and iatrogenic ptosis. Nonetheless, reoperations are not uncommon in Asian blepharoplasty patients with unmet expectations, continued age-related eyelid changes, or those who experience surgical complications.[8]

Reoperations are often the most challenging surgeries due to scar formation and distortion of anatomic tissue planes. Reoperations always start with excision of the skin scar. The preaponeurotic fat is a useful landmark to help identify the levator aponeurosis. If the eyelid planes simply cannot be identified or are scarred together, we recommend initiating the dissection laterally where the levator aponeurosis condenses into the lateral horn that dives deep, so there is a relative zone of safety for exploration that carries less risk of transecting the levator aponeurosis.

18.12 Postoperative Care

At the conclusion of surgery, ophthalmic antibiotic ointment is applied on the incisions and icing is started immediately upon arrival to the recovery room. Oral antibiotics are administered for

5 to 7 days, ophthalmic antibiotic ointment is used three times daily for 1 week, and icing is continued for the first 48 hours.

We recommend suture removal 5 days after surgery to minimize scarring while allowing for adequate wound healing. To remove the fine 7–0 silk sutures, it is easier to use a #11 blade, occasionally with loupes or stand magnification.

References

[1] Doxanas MT, Anderson RL. Oriental eyelids: an anatomic study. Arch Ophthalmol. 1984; 102(8):1232–1235

[2] Chen WPD. Asian Blepharoplasty and the Eyelid Crease, with DVD, 2nd ed. Philadelphia: Butterworth Heinemann; 2006

[3] Kiranantawat K, Suhk JH, Nguyen AH. The Asian eyelid: relevant anatomy. Semin Plast Surg. 2015; 29(3):158–164

[4] Kim HS, Hwang K, Kim CK, Kim KK. Double-eyelid surgery using septoaponeurosis junctional thickening results in dynamic fold in Asians. Plast Reconstr Surg Glob Open. 2013; 1(2):1–9

[5] Baek SM, Kim SS, Tokunaga S, Bindiger A. Oriental blepharoplasty: single-stitch, nonincision technique. Plast Reconstr Surg. 1989; 83(2):236–242

[6] Fan J, Low DW. A two-way continuous buried-suture approach to the creation of the long-lasting double eyelid: surgical technique and long-term follow-up in 51 patients. Aesthetic Plast Surg. 2009; 33(3):421–425

[7] Cho BC, Byun JS. New technique combined with suture and incision method for creating a more physiologically natural double-eyelid. Plast Reconstr Surg. 2010; 125(1):324–331

[8] Weng CJ, Noordhoff MS. Complications of Oriental blepharoplasty. Plast Reconstr Surg. 1989; 83(4):622–628

19 Floppy Eyelid Syndrome (FES) Repair

Blair K. Armstrong and Vy Nguyen

Summary

Floppy eyelid syndrome is characterized by excess horizontal eyelid laxity allowing for spontaneous eversion and mechanical irritation. Patients present with chronic papillary conjunctivitis and nonspecific irritation. Though conservative measures can be tried, these are usually not effective and surgery is necessary. The upper and lower eyelid lateral tarsal strip procedure allows for horizontal tightening of the eyelid to limit eversion, irritation, and patient complaints.

Keywords: floppy eyelid syndrome, lateral tarsal trip, obstructive sleep apnea, papillary conjunctivitis, eyelash ptosis

19.1 Goals

Floppy eyelid syndrome (FES) consists of excessively elastic and rubbery upper eyelids that are easily everted with minimal effort (▶ Fig. 19.1a). The condition is often asymmetric and the worse side corresponds to the side the patient most often sleeps on. Presumably, nocturnal eversion of the eyelid allows for exposed palpebral conjunctiva and mechanical trauma. This results in a chronic papillary conjunctivitis (▶ Fig. 19.1b).[1] Associated ocular findings can also include punctate epitheliopathy, keratoconus, dermatochalasis, blepharoptosis, eyelash ptosis, and blepharitis.[1]

The goal of surgery is to improve patient symptoms through limitation of nocturnal exposure and mechanical irritation. This can be achieved primarily through an upper and lower eyelid lateral tarsal strip (LTS) procedure. While initially described as a lower eyelid procedure, the LTS can also be used in the upper eyelid with excellent results. Associated periocular morbidities such as eyelash ptosis, blepharoptosis, dermatochalasis, upper eyelid entropion, or lower eyelid ectropion can be addressed concurrently.

19.2 Advantages

There are various surgical techniques described to treat FES. These include pentagonal full-thickness wedge resection (FTWR), upper eyelid medial canthal/lateral canthal tendon plication, and upper eyelid medial canthal strip. The upper eyelid LTS procedure offers the advantage of preservation of eyelid structures, namely the central tarsal plate that contributes to the structural integrity of the eyelid. Higher recurrence of FES is seen with FTWR alone. To achieve adequate tightness of the eyelid, FTWR necessitates resection of a large percentage of tarsal plate. Histopathologic studies reveal a decrease in tarsal stromal elastin fibers and increased matrix metalloproteinase activity.[2] Aggressive resection and manipulation of the attenuated tarsus may further degrade the abnormal tarsal plate and predispose a patient to recurrence of FES.[3]

The upper and lower LTS procedure produces an aesthetic scar within the horizontal relaxed skin tension lines of the eyelid and lateral canthus. The classic pentagonal FTWR creates incisions perpendicular to the relaxed skin tension lines of the eyelid and has the potential for noticeable scarring. Variations on the classic pentagonal FTWR have been described to enhance cosmesis of scars.[4]

In contrast to plication of the medial canthal or lateral canthal tendons, the LTS serves to create a new scar plane between the fashioned tarsal strip and the lateral orbital rim. The created tarsal strip is wider than the tendon and is fixated to the lateral orbital rim at two points with a double-armed suture. This forms a broad-based scar plane that may better anchor the lid laterally, thus limiting rotation around this axis and spontaneous eversion of the eyelid.[3]

19.3 Expectations

The expectation of the upper and lower LTS procedure is to reduce horizontal eyelid laxity and to create a broader pivot point at the lateral canthus, thereby limiting spontaneous eyelid eversion. In the upper eyelid, this is accompanied by resection of the upper limb of the lateral canthal tendon which is approximately 10 mm in length. This achieves horizontal tightening and maximal preservation of the tarsus.

19.4 Key Principles

- In general, patients with FES benefit from LTS procedure on both upper and lower eyelids.
- Maximal resection of the lateral canthal tendon should precede any tarsal shortening, though some lateral tarsal shortening may be necessary to optimize eyelid tone.
- Permanent suture should be used to fixate the tarsal strip to the periosteum of the inner orbital rim at Whitnall tubercle.
- Optimal fixation can be achieved by using the horizontal mattress technique. A double armed suture can facilitate this.
- Upper and lower LTS can be combined with other procedures to address associated periocular morbidities.

19.5 Indications

Surgeons must maintain a high index of suspicion for FES. While initially described in obese, middle-aged males,[5] it can also affect women, non-obese patients, and even children.[1,6] Patients typically present with chronic ocular irritation, redness, and mucous discharge.[1] FES has systemic associations, most notably obstructive sleep apnea (OSA) and all patients must undergo a sleep study.[1,7] Patients diagnosed with OSA are often treated with nocturnal positive airway pressure machines that can exacerbate mechanical eyelid irritation and exposure keratoconjunctivitis through airflow leakage. Nonsurgical measures may initially be tried, including refitting of the positive airway pressure mask, nighttime eyelid taping and patching, eyelid hygiene, ocular surface lubrication, ocular steroids, and punctal plugs.[1,8] When conservative measures fail, surgical intervention is indicated.

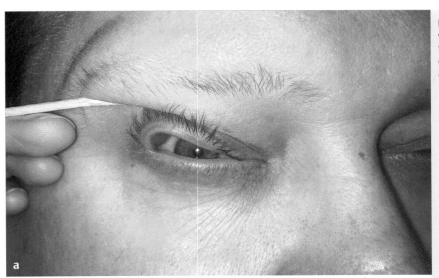

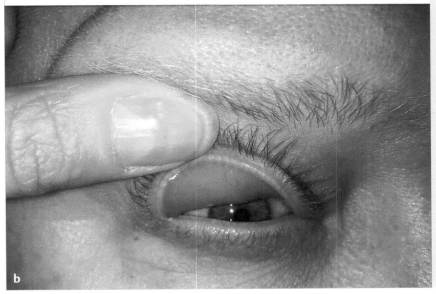

Fig. 19.1 **(a)** The upper eyelid is easily everted when gentle pressure is applied with a cotton tipped applicator. **(b)** On eversion of the upper eyelid, a papillary conjunctivitis can be appreciated on the palpebral conjunctiva.

19.6 Contraindications

Patients who are poor surgical candidates or who do not desire surgical intervention can be treated with conservative measures to minimize and treat irritation. Patients with FES who are asymptomatic or who improve with nonsurgical measures can also be observed. In some eyelids, eyelash ptosis may be noted to be associated with an area of attenuated tarsus; these patients may be better served by pentagonal FTWR of the affected tarsus (refer to section II-4 for repair of the eyelid margin). As with any eyelid surgery, every effort should be made to safely discontinue anticoagulant and antiplatelet medications perioperatively. If discontinuation is not possible, then the patients symptoms should be weighed against the increased risk of bleeding related complications including retrobulbar hemorrhage.

19.7 Preoperative Preparation

- A slit-lamp examination of the eyelids, conjunctiva, and cornea is performed with careful documentation of superficial punctate keratopathy, papillary conjunctival reaction, and eyelash ptosis.
- Eyelid measurements such as marginal reflex distance (MRD), interpalpebral fissure height (IPF), and levator function (LF) can be measured and documented to detect any associated eyelid morbidities and for postoperative comparison.
- We recommend preoperative photography.
- The upper eyelid skin crease is marked with a marking pen as are the horizontal, lateral canthal rhytides created by the orbital orbicularis or "crow's feet."

- The upper eyelid laxity is assessed and the amount of tarsus to be shortened is determined. This is delineated as a perpendicular line from the lid margin with a marking pen.
- The lateral canthal angle and lateral skin of the upper and lower eyelid are infiltrated with 3 to 5 mL of 1% lidocaine with 1:100,000 epinephrine and adequate time is allowed for hemostasis and anesthesia.

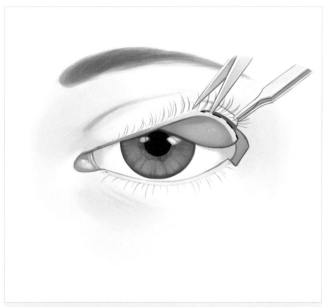

Fig. 19.2 The anterior lamella (skin and orbicularis) is separated from the posterior lamella (tarsus and conjunctiva) by sharp dissection using tenotomy scissors. This is facilitated by holding the eyelid on lateral stretch to provide counter traction.

19.8 Operative Technique

- The patient is prepped and draped in standard, sterile ophthalmic fashion.
- The lateral orbital rim is located by digital palpation and a lateral canthotomy incision is created with a #15 bard-parker blade extending approximately 5 mm from the lateral commissure.
- The upper eyelid is grasped with toothed forceps and elevated away from the face. The superior limb of the lateral canthal tendon is strummed with Stevens scissors and incised.

19.8.1 Upper Eyelid

- Following successful cantholysis, the periosteum of the lateral orbital wall is exposed and the lateral tarsus of the upper eyelid is freely mobilized.
- The eyelid is grasped laterally to provide horizontal tension and dissection proceeds between the anterior lamella (skin and orbicularis) and posterior lamella (tarsus and conjunctiva) with Stevens tenotomy scissors Fig. 19.2.
- The mucocutaneous junction, including the pilosebaceous units, is excised using Westcott scissors.
- The lateral canthal tendon is shortened to desired length. If significant laxity is present, it may also be necessary to shorten tarsus. The lateral edge of the tarsal plate is grasped with toothed forceps and stretched to identify amount of tarsal excision required to achieve desired eyelid tone. The excess tarsus is excised with Westcott scissors. Shortening should correspond to the perpendicular line marked preoperatively (▶ Fig. 19.3).
- A 4–0 double-armed permanent suture on a half-circle needle is then passed through the created strip posterior to anterior. One arm of the suture is then passed intraorbitally in the region of Whitnall tubercle incorporating a purchase

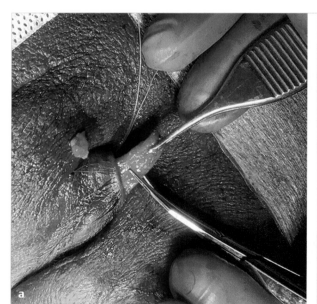
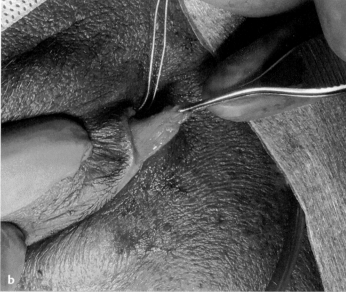

Fig. 19.3 (a,b) After excision of redundant lateral canthal tendon, it is often necessary to shorten the tarsus to achieve desired eyelid tone and reduced spontaneous eversion. The eyelid is placed on lateral stretch to provide counter traction and the desired amount of tarsus is excised with surgical scissors. This should correspond to the preoperative markings.

of periosteum as the needle leaves the orbit and then exiting at the lateral canthotomy site. The second arm of the double-armed suture is passed through the identical structures in a slightly inferior pathway to complete the mattress suture. The suture is left loose at this point.

19.8.2 Lower Eyelid

- The lateral lower eyelid is grasped with toothed forceps and elevated vertically away from the face. Closed tenotomy scissoris are directed infero-temporally in the inferior limb of the lateral canthal tendon identified by a strumming technique. The scissors are then opened to straddle and cut the inferior tendon.
- A lower LTS fashioned by dissecting between anterior and posterior lamella. This dissection should extend to include the lateral tarsus to be resected. The mucocutaneous junction is excised. The resultant robust LTS is shortened to desired, predetermined length using Westcott scissors. In FES, this is often significant and may extend for one-third to one-half of the eyelid.
- The lower eyelid tarsal strip is engaged with a 4–0 double-armed polyester fiber suture on a half-circle needle posterior to anterior. The sutures are then passed intraorbitally incorporating periosteum adjacent to the upper eyelid sutures.

19.8.3 Concluding the Procedure

- The upper eyelid sutures are tied and cut. This results in improved tightening of the upper eyelid. The lower eyelid sutures are similarly tied and cut.
- The unshortened anterior lamella can create a "dog ear of skin." The lateral edge is grasped with toothed forceps and stretched horizontally. The redundant skin and orbicularis can be excised. Where possible, this incision can be created to coincide with the eyelid crease to produce a more aesthetic scar (▶ Fig. 19.4).
- The anterior lamella of the upper and lower eyelid at the canthotomy site can then be sutured together with a 6–0 plain gut absorbable suture.

19.9 Tips and Pearls

- Take into consideration any eyelid abnormalities that might be encountered ahead of time in order to plan for successful surgical correction.
- The addition of hyaluronidase to the local anesthesia mixture can enhance tissue infiltration and minimize distortion of patient anatomy.
- Recall that the lateral canthal tendon naturally lies 2 to 3 mm above the medial canthal. This anatomic relationship should be preserved. When both the upper and lower lids have been released from the lateral orbital rim, extra care must be taken to preserve the patient's natural lateral canthal angle position, as one lid attachment does not remain as a landmark for the other.
- Horizontal eyelid tightening through LTS or other surgical approaches can improve eyelid height and increase the upper marginal reflex distance-1 (MRD1). This may obviate the need for concurrent blepharoptosis repair in mild cases.[9]

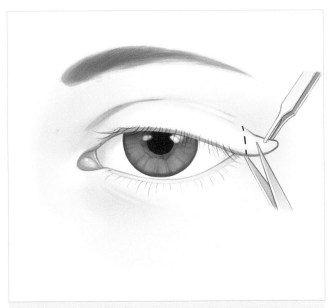

Fig. 19.4 To prevent a dog ear, it is often necessary to excise redundant anterior lamella (skin and orbicularis). Where possible, this should be constructed so that the postoperative scar is hidden in the relaxed skin tension lines of the lateral canthus.

19.10 What to Avoid

- The lacrimal gland and its ductules are located 5 mm superior to the lateral most edge of tarsus in the upper eyelid. The lacrimal gland should be carefully avoided to limit injury to the gland, incorporation of the gland into suturing, damage to ductules and associated dry eye or subsequent dacryops formation, etc.
- The lateral canthal tendon should be fully resected. If additional horizontal tightening is indicated, the lateral portion of the tarsus can be resected. Care should be taken to avoid excessive resection or overcorrection that can lead to lagophthalmos or ectropion.
- The mucocutaneous junction and redundant anterior lamella of the upper eyelid should be resected to avoid epidermal inclusion cysts or lash incorporation into closure and subsequent trichiasis.
- Avoid periocular and retrobulbar hemorrhage with meticulous hemocauterization.

19.11 Complications/Bailout/ Salvage

Complications include ectropion, lateral canthal deformity, failure to achieve symptomatic relief, or recurrence of FES. In the event of overzealous shortening of the tarsus of the upper or lower eyelid, the tissue may be under too much tension to close primarily. If this occurs, an orbital-based periosteal flap can be created by vertically incising the periosteum along the anterior aspect of the lateral orbital rim for approximately 6 mm length. A Freer elevator is used to elevate the periosteum 2 to 3 mm inside the lateral orbital wall. The tarsal strip of the upper or lower eyelid can then be fixated to the periosteal flap approximating the location of Whitnall tubercle.[10]

19.12 Postoperative Care

The surgical site can be left open to air; no patching is necessary and the patient should keep the area clean and dry. Antibiotic ointment can be applied to the wounds and to the conjunctival surface three times a day for 7 days postoperatively. The patient should be instructed to aggressively ice the surgical area, especially for the first 2 postoperative days. Ideally, this will be for a minimum of 10 minutes every hour and can reduce postoperative edema, ecchymoses, and pruritus. The patient should be counseled to avoid excessive eyelid rubbing to protect the surgical site and to minimize additional mechanical trauma to the palpebral conjunctiva. Nocturnal shielding with a plastic or aluminum fenestrated shield can be beneficial. The patient should be evaluated 1 week postoperatively for healing, signs of infection, or wound dehiscence.

References

[1] Pham TT, Perry JD. Floppy eyelid syndrome. Curr Opin Ophthalmol. 2007; 18 (5):430–433

[2] Schlotzerschrehardt U. Stojkovic M, Hofmannrummelt C, Cursiefen C, Kruse F, Holbach L. The pathogenesis of floppy eyelid syndrome: involvement of matrix metalloproteinases in elastic fiber degradation. Ophthalmology. 2005; 112(4):694–704

[3] Ezra DG, Beaconsfield M, Sira M, et al. Long-term outcomes of surgical approaches to the treatment of floppy eyelid syndrome. Ophthalmology. 2010; 117(4):839–846

[4] Valenzuela AA, Sullivan TJ. Medial upper eyelid shortening to correct medial eyelid laxity in floppy eyelid syndrome: a new surgical approach. Ophthal Plast Reconstr Surg. 2005; 21(4):259–263

[5] Culbertson WW, Ostler HB. The floppy eyelid syndrome. Am J Ophthalmol. 1981; 92(4):568–575

[6] Rao LG, Bhandary SV, Devi AR, Gangadharan S. Floppy eyelid syndrome in an infant. Indian J Ophthalmol. 2006; 54(3):217–218

[7] Karger RA, White WA, Park WC, et al. Prevalence of floppy eyelid syndrome in obstructive sleep apnea-hypopnea syndrome. Ophthalmology. 2006; 113 (9):1669–1674

[8] Viana GAP, Sant'Anna AE, Righetti F, Osaki M. Floppy eyelid syndrome. Plast Reconstr Surg. 2008; 121(5):333e–334e

[9] Mills DM, Meyer DR, Harrison AR. Floppy eyelid syndrome: quantifying the effect of horizontal tightening on upper eyelid position. Ophthalmology. 2007; 114(10):1932–1936

[10] Burkat CN, Lemke BN. Acquired lax eyelid syndrome: an unrecognized cause of the chronically irritated eye. Ophthal Plast Reconstr Surg. 2005; 21(1):52–58

Part V

Eye Brow

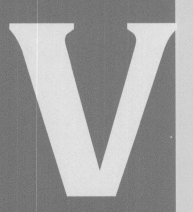

20 Direct Brow Lift

Natalie Wolkow and Suzanne K. Freitag

Summary

The direct brow lift is a highly effective, durable, and predictable procedure that can be performed expeditiously under local anesthesia, and which does not require special equipment. The procedure is best suited for functional brow elevation. Its major drawback is the potential for scar. Patients seeking cosmetic brow elevation should be offered alternative approaches. This chapter discusses preoperative considerations, operative technique, postoperative care, possible complications of the procedure, and ways to avoid them.

Keywords: direct brow lift, brow ptosis, browplasty, functional brow lift, rhytides, scar, local anesthesia, complications

20.1 Goals

The direct brow lift is one of many options available to surgically correct ptotic eyebrows. It may be performed under local anesthesia or with sedation and may be combined with other procedures, such as blepharoplasty. In particular, a direct browplasty is useful for correcting temporal brow ptosis in patients who have preexisting rhytides and present mainly with functional rather than cosmetic complaints.

20.2 Advantages

A main advantage of the direct browplasty is that it does not require special equipment, such as endoscopes, screws, or tacks, and can be performed with readily available sutures. The surgical skills required to perform this procedure are basic and it does not require endoscopic surgical competence. In addition, it is not a time-consuming procedure and can be performed under local anesthesia or with minimal sedation in an office or operative setting. The surgical results are very predictable, as it is possible to carefully control the amount of brow elevation, even in cases of significant brow asymmetry, because the lift is a direct result of tissue excision. Furthermore, the surgical results are lasting, and are not expected to diminish over time. This is in contrast to other methods such as endoscopic brow lifting where the brow is suspended and at risk of falling as suspension materials stretch or give way.

20.3 Expectations

Surgical expectations should be discussed with patients to ensure that they are appropriate candidates for the procedure. Patients should be forewarned that they almost certainly will have a visible scar postoperatively and that they will have numbness surrounding the incisions, which will improve over time. They should know that the vertical distance of the forehead between the brows and the hairline will decrease in size. This may be desirable in those with a high hairline, but may be a concern in those with a short distance between hairline and brow. Men, in particular, should know that the procedure will elevate and often arch the brow, which may have an undesirable feminizing effect. Efforts should be made to minimize this arched configuration in male patients through careful incision design. Patients should be warned that in rare instances, damage to the temporal branch of the frontal nerve may occur, leading to paralysis of the frontalis muscle; also, in rare instances, damage may occur to the supraorbital nerve, leading to permanent numbness of the ipsilateral forehead and part of the scalp. The surgeon should stress that the purpose of a direct browplasty is to improve the functional rather than the cosmetic aspects of brow ptosis, and that if a patient is more concerned with cosmetic outcomes, an alternative brow-lifting procedure may be more appropriate, where the incision is created at or behind the hairline.

20.4 Key Principles

A key principle in successfully performing a direct browplasty is to carefully select appropriate surgical candidates, who will be happy with the functional improvements in vision and will not be bothered by a potential scar. The surgeon should remember to avoid branches of the frontal and supraorbital nerves to minimize the risks of numbness and paralysis. In addition, the surgeon should be attentive to where preoperative surgical marks are placed and how much tissue will be removed in order to create a pleasantly arched eyebrow in women and avoid feminizing effects in men.

20.5 Indications

A direct browplasty is an excellent option in patients who do not want general anesthesia, in older men and women with skin of lighter pigmentation who do not mind a faint scar postoperatively, in patients with significant temporal brow ptosis, in patients with a long forehead who could benefit in moving the brows closer to the hairline, and in patients who do not mind an arched eyebrow or a smoothed contour of the upper eyebrow hairs. Patients with scarring of the tissue in or around the brow may benefit more from this powerful procedure than one involving a more remote incision placement. This procedure is also highly effective in patients with facial nerve paralysis resulting in a nonmobile brow.

20.6 Contraindications

This procedure should not be performed in younger individuals or in patients who insist upon an excellent cosmetic outcome without a scar. It should also be avoided in patients who form keloids or hypertrophic scars, and patients with darker skin who may have depigmented scars for a prolonged time period. Caution should be exercised in patients who have underlying dry eye or lagophthalmos, as overaggressive brow elevation can result in lagophthalmos. The procedure should not be performed in patients with a vertically short forehead, as removal of additional skin between the eyebrows and hairline will only worsen this feature. Men who do not want to risk a feminizing effect, either from arching of the eyebrow or from loss of the rough, feathered appearance of eyebrow hairs at the superior border of the brow should be advised not to undergo this procedure.

20.7 Preoperative Preparation

Preoperatively the patient should refrain from taking anticoagulant medications for an appropriate time prior to surgery, as determined by consensus of the surgeon and the prescribing physician. The surgeon and patient should discuss whether the direct browplasty will be performed in isolation or will be combined with a blepharoplasty or other procedure, such as ptosis repair or mid-face lift. If a blepharoplasty will be performed in conjunction, the direct browplasty should be performed first as it may alter the amount of skin that will be removed during the blepharoplasty. In addition, the surgeon should decide whether the browplasty will involve only the temporal portion of the brow or a more extensive segment.

The necessary preoperative materials should be obtained, including a signed informed consent and appropriate patient identification, a ruler, marking pen, 5% povidone iodine, topical anesthetic drops, local anesthetic (typically a 1:1 mixture of 2% lidocaine with 0.75% marcaine and 1:100,000 epinephrine), a #15 blade, forceps, Stevens scissors, cautery, 4–0 or 5–0 polyglactin 910 or poliglecaprone 25 sutures for deep closure and 5–0 polypropylene or nylon for cutaneous closure.

20.8 Operative Technique

1. After a time-out has been performed, the surgical sites should be marked. The surgeon may want to identify the supraorbital notch and mark its location so that the supraorbital nerve and vascular structures may be avoided. In situations where a supraorbital notch cannot be palpated, a line drawn vertically up from the caruncle closely approximates the location of the supraorbital foramen (▶ Fig. 20.1).[1] Similarly, the surgeon may want to identify the area where the temporal branch of the facial nerve likely enters the frontalis muscle (▶ Fig. 20.2).[2,3] With the patient in an upright vertical position, the incision lines are carefully drawn with a surgical marking pen. This step is an extremely important part of the procedure. The lower aspect of the ellipse of tissue to be removed is drawn at the superior margin of the brow cilia (▶ Fig. 20.3, ▶ Fig. 20.4).

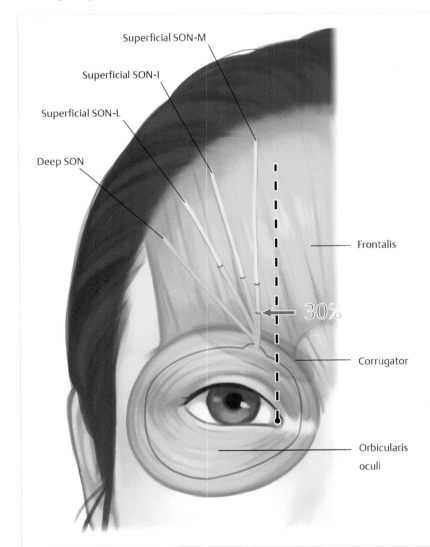

Superficial SON-M

Superficial SON-I

Superficial SON-L

Deep SON

Frontalis

30%

Corrugator

Orbicularis oculi

Fig. 20.1 Surgical anatomy of the supraorbital nerve. The supraorbital nerve is a sensory nerve, which is a branch of the frontal nerve. The location of the supraorbital nerve may be identified by palpating the supraorbital notch and marking the overlying skin. If the patient has a supraorbital foramen or a supraorbital notch that cannot be palpated, a vertical line may be traced from the caruncle to the superior orbital rim to approximate the location of the supraorbital foramen or notch (dotted line). The supraorbital nerve branches into a deep supraorbital nerve (deep SON) and three superficial branches, lateral (SONs-L), intermediate (SONs-I), and medial (SONs-M). The superficial branches initially course underneath the corrugator and frontalis muscles, and then pierce the frontalis muscle and continue on its superficial aspect. The medial branch becomes superficial closest to the superior edge of the brow. In up to 30% of individuals, the medial branch may pierce the corrugator and frontalis muscles prematurely, and may be at risk for injury during a direct browplasty.

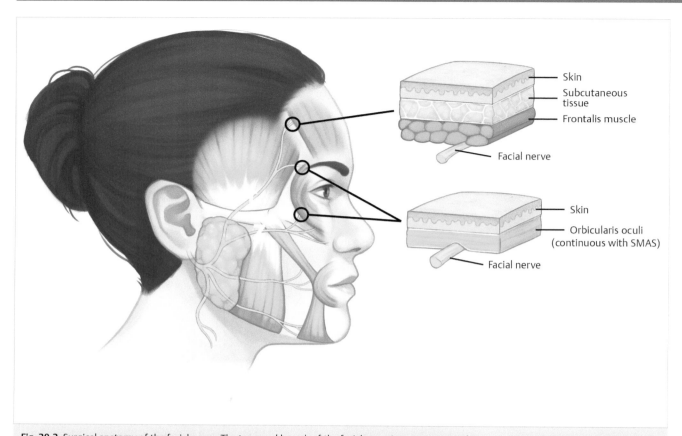

Fig. 20.2 Surgical anatomy of the facial nerve. The temporal branch of the facial nerve is a motor nerve that courses over the zygomatic arch and over the temporalis muscle to innervate the frontalis and orbicularis oculi muscles. While the frontalis muscle is innervated only by the temporal branch, the orbicularis oculi is innervated by both the temporal and zygomatic branches. Throughout its course, the temporal branch of the facial nerve is located underneath or within the inferior portion of the superficial musculoaponeurotic system (SMAS). Thus, the nerve should be protected if dissection does not disturb the SMAS during a direct browplasty.

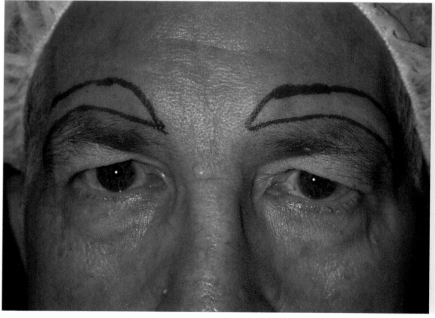

Fig. 20.3 Surgical markings for direct browplasty, anterior view. The inferior border of the markings is just above the brow hairs, while the superior border is flattened so as to avoid a feminine postoperative contour.

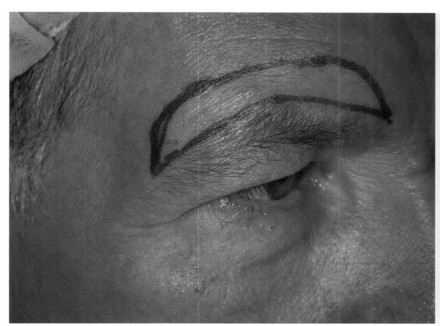

Fig. 20.4 Surgical markings for direct browplasty, lateral view. The lateral aspect of the surgical markings does not extend far beyond the lateral border of the frontalis muscle in order to avoid areas where the temporal branch of the frontal nerve is not as well protected.

Alternatively, the lower incision line can be drawn in a low-lying horizontal forehead furrow. Next, the brow is manually elevated to the desired position and the number of millimeters of desired elevation should be determined for the horizontal extent of the brow. This desired distance plus 2 mm should be marked above the previously drawn line demarcating the lower aspect of the ellipse (▶ Fig. 20.3, ▶ Fig. 20.4). It is important in male patients to make the upper marking as flat as possible without an arch, in order to prevent a high-arched brow as the surgical outcome.

2. Topical anesthetic drops are instilled in the eyes and local anesthetic containing epinephrine is injected along the skin markings. The surgical site is prepped and draped in a sterile fashion. Protective scleral shells are placed over the eyes.

3. An incision is first made along the superior aspect of the brow with a #15 blade. The blade should be beveled so that it is parallel to the insertion of the hair follicles to avoid damaging them and causing permanent hair loss. The incision should be shallow near the area of the supraorbital nerve. The superior portion of the ellipse is then incised.

4. Stevens scissors are used to excise the tissue ellipse, including within it skin and subcutaneous fat, and taking care to stay superficial near the area of the supraorbital nerve.

5. Hemostasis is achieved with judicious cautery and manual pressure.

6. Deep closure is performed with 4–0 or 5–0 polyglactin 910 or poliglecaprone 25 buried interrupted sutures. These sutures should approximate the wound edges so that subsequent skin closure does not have any tension, and risks of scarring are minimized. It is important to cut these suture ends short so that they stay buried and do not stick out of the wound causing poor healing. For patients with facial nerve paralysis, these deep sutures may incorporate a small bite of periosteum in order to fixate the brow at the desired height. The height is determined by examining the dynamic range of movement of the contralateral non-paretic brow and selecting a height in the middle of this range.

7. The skin is closed with 5–0 polypropylene or nylon suture to minimize scarring. Many surgeons advise interrupted using vertical mattress sutures or running horizontal mattress for skin closure to maximally evert the skin edges for optimal prevention of scar depression, as this is a big risk of this procedure.

8. Antibiotic ointment is applied to the incision sites and eyes, and the patient is instructed to apply ice compresses for the first 48 hours to minimize swelling and bruising. Consideration should be given to prescribing oral antibiotics. Cutaneous sutures are removed after 1 week.

20.9 Tips and Pearls

- Patient selection for this procedure is critical. Direct browplasty is a highly effective, durable, and predictable procedure. However, the presence of a visible scar above the brow is a huge negative for many cosmetically oriented patients (▶ Fig. 20.5, ▶ Fig. 20.6, ▶ Fig. 20.7, ▶ Fig. 20.8).[4,5,6,7]

- To avoid periorbital nerve damage, the surgeon should be aware of the locations of the supraorbital nerve and the temporal branch of the facial nerve, and it may be useful to mark their locations while marking the incision lines in the skin (▶ Fig. 20.1, ▶ Fig. 20.2). The superficial branches of the supraorbital nerve initially course under the corrugator and frontalis muscles, then pierce the frontalis and run superficially. In as many as 30% of individuals, the medial branch of the superficial supraorbital nerve pierces the corrugator and frontalis muscles prematurely, exposing it to injury if dissection is not kept superficial in the area. Fibers of the temporal branch of the facial nerve run within or below the superficial musculoaponeurotic system (SMAS) and enter the posterior surfaces of the frontalis and orbicularis oculi muscles; thus, as long as the surgical dissections remain superficial to these tissues (i.e., within the subcutaneous plane only), these nerve fibers should be protected from injury. Intraoperatively, the nerve fibers may be identified as small white strands coursing through the tissue.

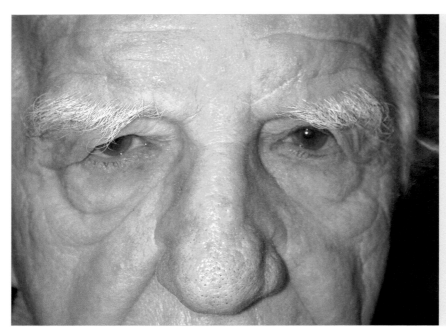

Fig. 20.5 Preoperative appearance of a patient who was a suitable candidate for a direct browplasty. Note the significant brow ptosis, which is contributing to visual obstruction, as well as numerous preexisting forehead rhytides and a preexisting scar over the left eyebrow.

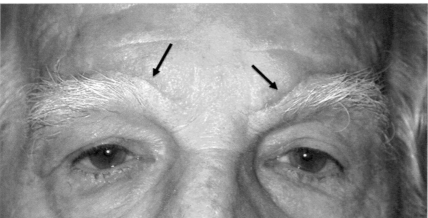

Fig. 20.6 Postoperative scarring. Postoperative photograph of the patient in ▶ Fig. 20.5. Although the postoperative brow contour is acceptable, and the visual axis is now clear, a significant degree of scarring remains at this 6-week follow-up visit *(arrows)*. This is expected to fade significantly over the next months.

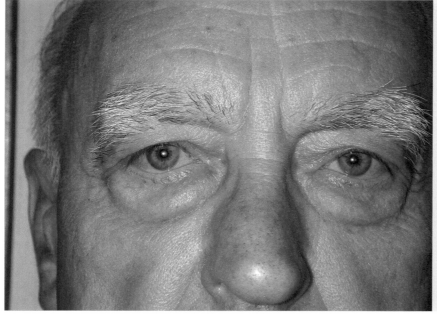

Fig. 20.7 Preoperative appearance. A man with brow ptosis, dermatochalasis, and lower eyelid steatoblepharon.

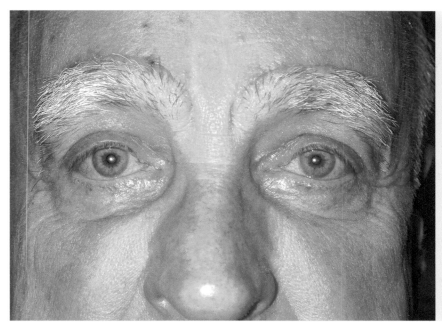

Fig. 20.8 Postoperative surprised appearance. Postoperative photograph of the patient in ▸ Fig. 20.7. In the early postoperative period, scarring is still quite apparent but expected to fade. The brow contour is more arched than preoperatively, which some would consider undesirably feminizing. Note that the patient also underwent a bilateral lower eyelid blepharoplasty.

- The most important surgical step in this procedure is careful drawing of the incision lines, taking care to elevate the brow by the desired amount, as well as making sure the upper incision line is flat in male patients to avoid creation of a high-arched feminine brow or surprised appearance (▸ Fig. 20.7, ▸ Fig. 20.8).
- To minimize postoperative scarring, the deep sutures of the wound should bear the tension of the closure and should bring the wound edges together, while the skin sutures should be stress-free. A vertical mattress or running horizontal mattress suture may be used for skin closure to maximally evert wound edges of this thick skin.

20.10 What to Avoid

- Avoid damaging the supraorbital nerve and its associated vascular structures in order to prevent long-lasting forehead and scalp numbness.
- Avoid extending the lateral aspects of the excisions too far or deep to avoid injury to branches of the facial nerve resulting in frontalis paralysis.
- Avoid feminizing male brows by excising too much tissue or by overly arching the brow centrally.
- Avoid causing eyebrow hair loss by keeping incisions parallel to hair follicles.

20.11 Complications/Bailout/Salvage

- A potential complication is worsening of dry eye and lagophthalmos. To avoid this, the inexperienced surgeon should be conservative in skin excision, as additional skin can always be removed if the initial excision was inadequate.
- Meticulous attention should be paid to hemostasis prior to placing deep sutures, and the supraorbital vascular structures should be avoided to minimize bleeding.

- Infection is rare after this procedure, particularly if oral and topical antibiotics are prescribed.
- Most complications of this procedure, such as injury to neural structures or patient dissatisfaction with postoperative appearance, can be avoided if appropriate care is taken during preoperative planning.

20.12 Postoperative Care

Minimal postoperative care is required. Antibiotic ointment is applied to the incision lines several times per day, and sutures are removed at the 1-week postoperative visit. Consideration should be given to prescribing oral antibiotics. It is not necessary to bandage or cover the incisions. Scars and numbness related to the procedure may take 6 months or more to improve.

References

[1] Gil YC, Shin KJ, Lee SH, Song WC, Koh KS, Shin HJ. Topography of the supraorbital nerve with reference to the lacrimal caruncle: danger zone for direct browplasty. Br J Ophthalmol. 2017; 101(7):940–945

[2] Agarwal CA, Mendenhall SD, III, Foreman KB, Owsley JQ. The course of the frontal branch of the facial nerve in relation to fascial planes: an anatomic study. Plast Reconstr Surg. 2010; 125(2):532–537

[3] Liebman EP, Webster RC, Berger AS, DellaVecchia M. The frontal nerve in the temporal brow lift. Arch Otolaryngol. 1982; 108(4):232–235

[4] Dutton JJ. Direct brow elevation. In: Dutton, JJ, ed. Atlas of Oculoplastic and Orbital Surgery. Philadelphia: Lippincott Williams & Wilkins, a Wolters Kluwer business; 2013: 72–73

[5] Korn BS, Kikkawa DO. Direct browplasty. In: Korn, BS and Kikkawa, DO, eds. Video Atlas of Oculofacial Plastic and Reconstructive Surgery. China: Elsevier; 2017: 138–142

[6] Nerad JA. Involutional periobital changes: dermatochalasis and brow ptosis. In: Nerad, JA, ed. Techniques in Ophthalmic Plastic Surgery: A Personal Tutorial. China: Saunders Elsevier; 2010: 129–156

[7] Tyers AG, Collin JRO. Direct brow lift. In: Tyers, AG and Collin, JRO, eds. Colour Atlas of Ophthalmic Plastic Surgery. China: Butterworth Heinemann Elsevier; 2001: 243–245

21 Endoscopic Brow Lift

Anne Barmettler, Michael Tseng, and Javier Servat

Summary

The endoscopic brow lift is a minimally invasive technique that allows for elevation of the entire brow and glabellar area, while utilizing a well-hidden, post hairline approach. Other methods, like a direct brow surgery, do not address glabellar ptosis and have visible scars or, in the case of pretrichial and coronal approaches, have much larger surgical incisions and have the potential for more postoperative scalp numbness and scalp alopecia.[1] These aspects are unappealing for most patients. The minimally invasive approach of endoscopic brow lifts also decreases postoperative healing time and morbidities compared to the conventional coronal or pretrichial incision.[1]

Using an endoscopic approach and fixation devices, the glabellar area is addressed, visible scars are avoided, and a long-lasting, natural appearing result can be achieved. Instrumentation is inserted through a 4- to 5-cm elliptical incision over the temple posterior to the hairline, staying deep to the deep temporalis fascia. Superiorly, one to three incisions are made posterior to the hair line. Once periosteal attachments, as well as procerus and corrugator muscle attachments, to the orbital rim are released, the fixation device holes are drilled into the cranium and the fixation device placed. The brow is then lifted and secured to the fixation devices to give the appropriate height and contour. In the temporal incisions, the deep temporal fascia is closed with 2–0 PDS suture and the scalp incisions are closed with skin staples. This safe and effective mode for addressing brow ptosis leads to excellent results with no visible scars.

Keywords: endoscopic, endobrow, eyebrow, glabella, forehead, lift, elevation, Endotine, brow ptosis, fixation device

21.1 Goals

An endoscopic brow lift encompasses three goals. First, it lifts and reshapes the brow, glabella, and temporal skin without a visible scar. Second, the surgery decreases transverse forehead rhytides and vertical glabellar rhytides, improves lateral canthal hooding, and thins the nose at the level of the nasofrontal angle (▶ Fig. 21.1). Finally, it achieves a long-lasting result with less morbidity and a shorter postoperative recovery time.

21.2 Advantages

- Excellent, long-lasting elevation of eyebrows and glabella (direct brow lifts do not address the glabellar area).
- Ability to decrease function of procerus and corrugator muscles, which decreases dynamic wrinkling.
- Ability to avoid visible scars (direct brow and pretrichial approaches have incisions in more easily apparent areas, ▶ Fig. 21.2a,b).
- Ability to be used in patients who wear their hair pulled back or have minimal to moderate receding hairlines, which are typical contraindications for the pretrichial approach (▶ Fig. 21.2c).
- Shorter operative times, shorter postoperative recovery period (smaller incisions than coronal approach, ▶ Fig. 21.2a,b).[1]

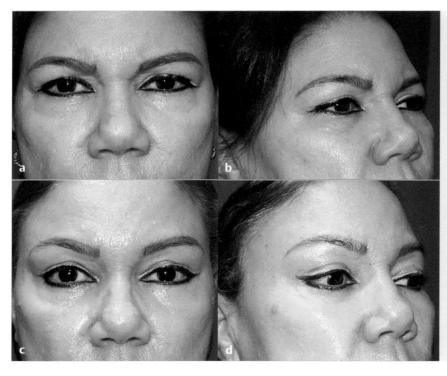

Fig. 21.1 The endoscopic forehead lift addresses more than just the eyebrow position. It also improves transverse forehead rhytides, vertical glabellar rhytides, lateral canthal hooding, and thins the nose at the level of the nasofrontal angle. Preoperative (**a**) En face, (**b**) Three quarters. Postoperative (**c**) En Face, (**d**) Three quarters.

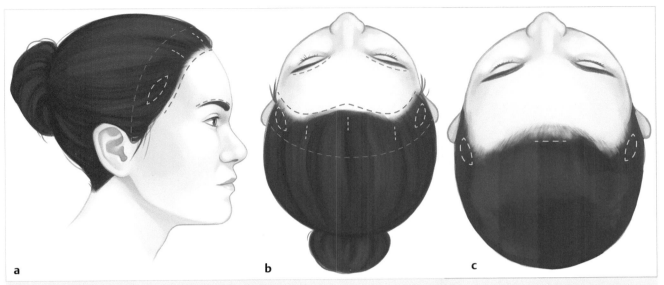

Fig. 21.2 Brow lift incision sites for four types of approaches: coronal, endoscopic, pretrichial, and direct. **(a)** Profile view. **(b)** Bird's-eye view. **(c)** Alternative approach for receding hairlines Birds eye view.

21.3 Expectations

The expectation of endoscopic brow lift is to achieve an elevation of the entirety of the brow, as well as the glabellar area. Endoscopic brow lift is intended to be performed in conjunction with fixation, typically via two Endotines (Microaire Aesthetics, Inc, Charlottesville, VA).

21.4 Key Principles

- Excessive corrugator activity and brow ptosis can create an unintended appearance of being angry, upset, or tired (▶ Fig. 21.1a,b).
- Endoscopic brow lifts allow for elevation and shaping of the entire brow and glabellar area, whereas direct brow lifts cannot lift the glabellar area and result in surgical scars in visible locations.
- Minimally invasive endoscopic approaches have been shown to be associated with less blood loss, reduced operating room time, and reduced recovery time when compared to the conventional open approaches.[2]

21.5 Indications

Poor brow position can be inherited or acquired, whether via age, paralysis, or trauma. Descent of the eyebrow can occur in the head, the body, or the tail, with the tail being the most frequent in involutional brow ptosis. Brow ptosis should be on the differential for any patient with redundant upper eyelid skin. Significant overhanging skin in the upper lid, especially medially next to the nose and laterally in the "crow's feet" area, is unlikely to improve with eyelid surgery alone and therefore raising the brow should be considered.

The role of brow ptosis can easily be underestimated, by both surgeons and patients. Both can be mistaken into believing a blepharoplasty will resolve the "upper lid" redundancy, but post-

operative disappointment awaits the misinformed. For this reason, understanding normal anatomy is important. In women, the eyebrow typically is arched, resting superior to the orbital rim. In men, the brow is typically more flat and is positioned on the orbital rim.[3] Measuring brow ptosis in all droopy upper eyelid complaints aids in establishing patient expectations, in addition to obtaining a great surgical outcome and happy patient.

21.6 Contraindications

- Evaluate cosmetic surgery patients for unrealistic expectations or psychological instability.
- Defer or avoid brow surgery in patients with lagophthalmos or exposure keratopathy until these have been addressed, as brow elevation can exacerbate these conditions.
- Patients who have an eyebrow tattoo placed superiorly to the anatomic location can be poor endoscopic brow lift candidates. In certain cases, a brow lift will result in the tattooed brow being elevated into an overly high and unnatural looking position.
- Consider the increased surgical complexity in patients with a high or receding hairline and possible increased visibility of surgical scars. Similarly, in patients with very short hair, receding hairline, or balding, the surgical scar will be visible, although less so than any other brow lift approach.

21.7 Preoperative Preparation

21.7.1 Patient Discussion

- With the patient looking into a mirror, ask the patient to describe their goals. Oftentimes, a patient will point to the brow or lift the brow to indicate their desired outcome and this is a cue to evaluate the eyebrow in addition to the rest of the eyelid.[3]

- Discuss any asymmetries with the patient and potential outcomes.
- Explain typical postoperative course, including postoperative scalp numbness, alopecia, and the palpability of the fixation devices for up to a year.

21.7.2 Examination

- Measure eyelid positioning and upper lid skin to determine the presence of concurrent blepharoptosis, dermatochalasis, or a low lid crease. Eyebrow elevation alone will not address these issues.
- Assess for lagophthalmos or exposure keratopathy, as eyebrow elevation may worsen this.
- Examine the patient's hairline and hairstyle for the following: receding hairline, amount of balding, very short hair. A patient, who has balding or wears their hair very short, needs to be aware that the surgical scar will still be visible on examination of their scalp. While this is still less noticeable than the incisions from a direct brow or a pretrichial incision, it will still be visible. A high hairline will make surgery more technically difficult, and endoscopic brow surgery may make the hairline appear even higher.

21.8 Operative Technique

21.8.1 Marking

The right and left temporal crescent, where the conjoined tendon fuses the periosteum, deep temporal fascia, and superficial temporal fascia, is palpated and marked. Posterior to the hairline, this is marked in an ellipse, which measures approximately 4 to 5 cm in length and 1 to 2 cm in width. The superior incisions consist of a central vertical incision and two paramedial vertical incisions in most patients (▶ Fig. 21.2a,b). The central incision begins about 1 cm behind the hairline and measures about 2 cm in length. Similarly, the paramedian incisions are created about 4 to 5 cm laterally to the central incision. In those with a hair temporal hairline or the beginning of a receding hairline, a single incision in the horizontal direction can be used (▶ Fig. 21.2c). Mark the site of the Endotines at the anterior aspect of the paracentral incisions. These are typically more medial and closer together in men to create the straighter appearance of a male brow. In women, the Endotines are typically placed more laterally and further apart in order to create the more feminine brow arch.

Mark the supraorbital notch and a safety zone of about 1 to 2 cm around this to protect the supraorbital and supratrochlear nerves. Approximately 50% of skulls have bilateral supraorbital notches, 25% have bilateral supraorbital foramina, and 25% have a foramen on one side and a notch on the other.[3] The safety zone allows the surgeon to increase caution when entering the area to dissect the periosteum while paying careful attention for the aforementioned nerves.

In order to increase visibility and decrease interference of hair during the surgery, the hair can be pulled back into rubber bands (colorful ones are easier to find postoperatively).

21.8.2 Anesthesia

Local anesthesia with sedation or general anesthesia can be used. Local anesthesia is made of 2% lidocaine with 1:100,000 epinephrine in a 50/50 mixture with 0.5% bupivacaine with 1:100,000 epinephrine. This is placed along the superior and lateral orbital rims, the incision sites and throughout the forehead and temple.

21.8.3 Surgery

A #15 blade is used to incise the temporal skin along the elliptical markings. The depth of the incision is deep to the superficial temporalis fascia to avoid facial nerve damage. Remove the ellipse of skin, muscle, and fascia. When obtaining hemostasis, cauterize scalp edges gently as this decreases postoperative alopecia. With an optical dissector on the endoscope and a 10-mL syringe attached filled with saline, you will have an excellent view and can use the saline as needed to clear blood or debris from your field of view. At the plane deep to the superficial temporalis fascia and superficial to the deep temporalis fascia, dissect with a straight, spatulated raspatory to the orbital rim. The inferior extent of the dissection is the sentinel vein, which is found 1 cm lateral to the lateral canthal angle.

Turn to the central and paracentral incisions (or the single horizontal incision, see section Marking to decide). Use the #15 blade to incise the skin all the way down to the bone along the markings. Use the spatulated raspatory dissector in the plane deep to the periosteum. Dissect to the outer limits of the safety zone and free periosteal attachments to the orbital rim lateral to the zone. If the forehead is very high or curved, a curved spatulated raspatory dissector may help you obtain the necessary angle. Medial to the safety zone, dissect the corrugators and procerus muscles off of the nasal bone. Within the safety zone of the supraorbital and supratrochlear nerves, use a blunt tipped scissors to carefully dissect this area until the neurovascular bundle is visualized. Do not cut with the scissors! The scissors are being used to stretch and dissect the tissue gently, doing their work in being opened (not closed).

Ensure that all periosteal attachments are completely freed from the orbital rim.

There are quite a number of methods to fixate the forehead into the desired position, including resorbable screws,[4] adhesives,[5] cortical tunnels,[6] and other fixation devices.[7,8] The fixation device, Endotine, is biodegradable, easy to place, and its multiple fixation points provide a diffuse area of lift to prevent peaking. Typically, a 3.0-mm device is used in women and 3.5-mm in men.

At the conclusion of the case, a simple, but thoughtful addition is to use shampoo and a comb to clean the blood and debris from the patient's hair prior to a compression dressing.

Duration of surgery typically lasts about 1 to 2 hours.

21.9 Tips and Pearls

- Placement of the incisions and fixation device is one of the most important steps. Take the necessary time to measure and determine fixation placements.

- When dissecting from the temporal incision, ensure that the dissection is superficial to the temporalis muscle and deep to the superficial temporalis fascia. This will keep the dissection in a safe plane, deep to the facial nerve.
- Thorough dissection of the periosteal attachments to the eyebrow rim allows for the most lift. While doing so, use caution in the supraorbital nerve region to avoid postoperative paresthesia. The most common reason for failure is inadequate release of periosteum and depressor muscles.[9]
- When determining shape and height of the eyebrows, gender and patient desires are important factors. The ideal female eyebrow tends to be more arched with the brow peak typically being above the lateral canthus. The ideal male eyebrow tends to be flatter, so the fixation devices typically need to be placed more medially in men than in women.[3,10] Stand at the head of the bed to assess for symmetry when elevating and fixating the brow to the fixation devices.
- Examine the scalp for any deformities, such as osteomas, which may be in the way of placing a fixation device. The etiology of these abnormalities should be determined, as well as the possible need for different fixation placement.
- Have more than the necessary number of fixation devices available than needed, just in case one is deformed or otherwise mishandled.

21.10 What to Avoid

- Ensure that patients have gotten medical clearance, as this is an elective procedure and may not be a good fit for the debilitated. Patients should be off of blood thinners for the appropriate amounts of time prior to the procedure.
- Avoid large movements in the temporal pocket to prevent indirect damage to the facial nerve.
- Make sure your patient understands possible surgical outcomes in terms of appearance as well as the postoperative healing period. This includes understanding that most rhytides discussed will improve but will not completely disappear.

21.11 Complications/Bailout/Salvage

Bleeding and nerve damage are the biggest sources of complication.
- In the event of temporal artery bleeding, have your assistant retract, while you visualize with suction in one hand and the hemostat in another. Use a hemostat to grasp the bleeding vessel and tie with 4–0 silk suture. The temporal artery is unlikely to stop bleeding with pressure alone.
- Sentinal vein bleeding looks alarming while visualized with the endoscope but stops quickly with the application of pressure.

- Supraorbital artery bleeding is worrisome as it means you have damaged the tissue adjacent to the supraorbital nerve. The bleeding will stop with pressure (but avoid cautery in this area to prevent further damage to the nerve). Postoperatively, there is a high likelihood of paresthesia, which will likely improve in the following 3 months.
- When in the temporal incisions, stay in the space just superficial to the temporalis muscle to avoid damage to the facial nerve. When in doubt, dissect deeper until the muscle is visualized, then return to the proper plane, just superficial to the muscle.

Fixation device troubles can also complicate your surgery.
- Should the Endotine not fixate properly, retry drilling in the same hole, making sure to keep the drill at 90 degrees to the skull. If this should fail, drill another hole, ensuring proper and equal pressure on the drill.

21.12 Postoperative Care

- A firm dressing of two folded abdominal pads over the forehead is secured via a roll of Kerlix to reduce postoperative swelling and is left in place, typically until the next morning.
- Antibiotics and analgesic and anti-inflammatory medication may be provided at the surgeon's discretion. A typical regimen would be cephalexin 500 mg by mouth four times daily for a week, acetaminophen with codeine, and a methylprednisolone dose pack.
- Patients can usually return to work in 1 week.
- Staples are removed in the office 7 to 10 days postoperatively.

References

[1] Ramirez OM. Why I prefer the endoscopic forehead lift. Plast Reconstr Surg. 1997; 100(4):1033–1039, discussion 1043–1046

[2] Thompson DR, Zurakowski D, Haberkern CM, Stricker PA, Meier PM. Endoscopic versus open repair for craniosynostosis in infants using propensity score matching to compare outcomes: a multicenter study from the Pediatric Craniofacial Collaborative Group. Anesth Analg. 2017

[3] Black EHNF, Gladstone G, Calvano CJ, Levine MR. Smith and Nesi's Ophthalmic Plastic and Reconstructive Surgery. New York, NY: Springer; 2012

[4] Eppley BLCJ, Coleman JJ, III, Sood R, Ha RY, Sadove AM. Resorbable screw fixation technique for endoscopic brow and midfacial lifts. Plast Reconstr Surg. 1998; 102(1):241–243

[5] Mixter RC. Endoscopic forehead fixation with histoacryl. Plast Reconstr Surg. 1998; 101(7):2006–2007

[6] Hoenig JF. Rigid anchoring of the forehead to the frontal bone in endoscopic facelifting: a new technique. Aesthetic Plast Surg. 1996; 20(3):213–215

[7] Servat JJ, Black EH. A comparison of surgical outcomes with the use of 2 different biodegradable multipoint fixation devices for endoscopic forehead elevation. Ophthal Plast Reconstr Surg. 2012; 28(6):401–404

[8] Landecker A, Buck JB, Grotting JC. A new resorbable tack fixation technique for endoscopic brow lifts. Plast Reconstr Surg. 2003; 111(2):880–886, discussion 887–890

[9] Isse NG. Endoscopic forehead lift: evolution and update. Clin Plast Surg. 1995; 22(4):661–673

[10] Griffin GR, Kim JC. Ideal female brow aesthetics. Clin Plast Surg. 2013; 40(1):147–155

22 Pretrichial Brow Lift

Senmiao Zhan and Kian Eftekhari

Summary

Pretrichial brow lift is a powerful surgical procedure to restore harmony between the upper and lower face in the properly selected patient. This technique can be used in the context of functional or aesthetic surgery to elevate the brow. Understanding the anatomic layers and relationship between the facial mimetic musculature is important to achieve the goals of the procedure. To avoid complications, knowledge of motor and sensory nerves is key. The pretrichial lift has distinct advantages. It allows direct mechanical elevation of tissue and does not require special instrumentation. In addition, pretrichial brow lift can shorten the forehead, which is useful in select patients. The key disadvantage of this procedure is the postoperative scar. Patient selection is critical. There is risk of injury to the facial nerve and sensory nerves and understanding these nuances is important before performing the pretrichial brow lift.

Keywords: brow lift, forehead, pretrichial, brow ptosis, temporal branch of facial nerve

22.1 Goals

Anatomically and functionally, there is an intimate relationship between the forehead, the brow, and the upper eyelids. Understanding this relationship is key to avoiding pitfalls of upper eyelid surgery in which the eyelids are raised without considering descent of the forehead and brow.[1] Many different procedures exist to address the brow region, from foreheadplasty surgeries such as the coronal or endoscopic forehead lift to more direct procedures addressing the brow region via a direct or transblepharoplasty approach.[2] The purpose of the current chapter is to discuss the pretrichial brow-lift procedure.

The goal of the procedure is to accomplish elevation of the brow in patients in which brow ptosis is contributing to the aesthetic appearance of looking "tired" or the functional consequence of interference with the visual field. Descent of the brow can exacerbate limitation of the superior visual field in patients with preexisting dermatochalasis. This is especially pronounced laterally, and indeed the main goal of the procedure in the modern era is to accomplish lateral elevation and reshaping of the brow. During the advent and growth period of endoscopic brow elevation in the mid-1990s, many advocates of this procedure had focused on medial and lateral brow elevation as an important goal of the procedure.[3] But as long-term results have been evaluated, this is an area that—if raised significantly relative to the lateral elevation—can induce a facial expression of surprise that can be aesthetically displeasing. In addition, extirpation of the corrugator or procerus muscles can increase the risk of intraoperative and postoperative bleeding as well as dysesthesia. The goal of any brow procedure in the modern era is lateral more than medial elevation, especially in the female population where the arch of the brow is more pronounced.[4] In select patients with an elongated forehead, however, the goal

may be intentional forehead shortening, best accomplished with a pretrichial or coronal lift over other techniques.[5]

It is important to understand the anatomy of the frontalis muscle and its relationship to the orbicularis oculi and brow depressors (▶ Fig. 22.1). The lateral portion of the upper eyelid orbicularis extends past the insertion of the frontalis muscle into the temple region, and the contraction of the orbicularis unopposed can lead to lateral brow ptosis. During patient evaluation, it is also helpful to consider the concept of "facial thirds" (▶ Fig. 22.2), and the pretrichial lift is the most direct option to restore the upper third of the face that can elongate with aging (▶ Fig. 22.3).[6]

22.2 Advantages

The advantage of the pretrichial brow lift over other techniques is the significant amount of mechanical elevation and skin excision that can be safely accomplished, as well as the open surgical exposure compared to the endoscopic approach. In patients who style their hair with bangs or have sufficient follicles at the anterior hairline, the incision from this approach can be concealed. In addition, patients with an elongated forehead may be able to achieve better symmetry between the upper, middle, and lower thirds of the face with a forehead shortening procedure via this approach.[5] The other practical advantage of the pretrichial brow lift is that it does not require any special instrumentation in contrast to the endoscopic approach. Lastly, although many different procedures have been proposed to address the ptotic brow, the coronal and pretrichial approaches have stood the test of time as reliable procedures to raise the brow, despite the larger incision.[7]

22.3 Expectations

Setting expectations is important during the preoperative planning and evaluation of any aesthetic patient, but especially in the case of the pretrichial brow lift, given the longer incision and postoperative swelling that can occur. It's important to have a frank conversation about the postoperative scar and—where possible—to advise the patient to consider styling their hair appropriately to conceal the scar for the first few months after surgery until healing has taken place. Patients should be advised that despite the best techniques to address brow ptosis, given the gravitational effects of aging there is a possibility of recurrence and descent after surgery.

22.4 Key Principles

The main principle of open brow-lift surgery is that it will involve a postoperative scar and require time for healing, and that point should be driven home to the patient during the preoperative evaluation. If patients are willing to accept this fact, the results from the surgery can be extremely satisfying. Patients best suited for this procedure include individuals with

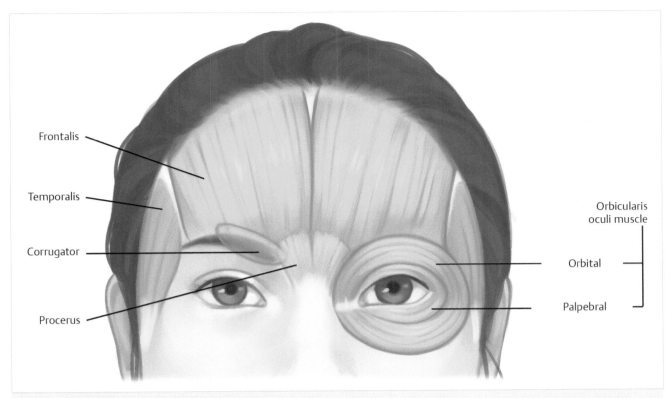

Fig. 22.1 Muscles of the forehead and periorbital region.

long foreheads. The key advantages of the procedure are its time-tested effectiveness, the ability to perform the procedure without special instrumentation, and the open exposure with the ability to mechanically and directly elevate the brow.

22.5 Indications

Indications for the surgery include descent of the brow. Some authors have suggested that a pretrichial lift should be considered especially in cases where a high forehead exists, defined as greater than 6 cm from the anterior hairline to a line drawn across the top of the brow cilia.[7]

22.6 Contraindications

There are relative contraindications to pretrichial brow-lift surgery. Patients with vertically short foreheads or low anterior hairlines may not be the best candidates for this approach, given that the surgery may further shorten the forehead. Patients with thin hairs in the anterior hairline or with balding may not be good candidates for the procedure, given the visibility of the scar.

22.7 Preoperative Preparation

Evaluation of the patient's goals is of paramount importance in the preoperative preparation. There are many different options to elevate the brow, including the coronal, pretrichial, endoscopic, mid-forehead, direct supraciliary approach, and transblepharoplasty approach. If a patient desires a durable method

to lift the brow and is willing to accept the healing period associated with the incision, they may be a good candidate for a pretrichial approach. It goes without saying that it is also important to evaluate the presence of dermatochalasis and ptosis of the eyelid preoperatively.

It is also important to preoperatively evaluate medical conditions that may affect the choice of brow surgery. Patients who are at higher risk from an anesthesia standpoint may be better suited for direct or transblepharoplasty brow elevation procedures that can be done under purely local anesthesia. In addition, given the extensive vascular supply of the forehead during the pretrichial incision and dissection, patients who are on blood thinners may be at higher risk for postoperative hematoma or seroma formation.

22.8 Operative Technique

There are several variations of the incision for the pretrichial lift that can be considered. The authors prefer an irregular pattern at the anterior hairline, and it is helpful to make a central "V" in the central forehead to assist with alignment at the time of closure (► Fig. 22.4). A lateral subcutaneous variant of the surgery can also be considered with two shorter incisions (► Fig. 22.5).[8]

A mixture of lidocaine with epinephrine and bupivacaine may be used for local anesthesia under the incision. Many authors also prefer to infiltrate the central forehead and glabella, as well as the arcus marginalis, with tumescent anesthesia to create a "vascular tourniquet."[7]

The incision may be made with a 15 or a 10 blade, and the authors prefer the latter, given its larger belly to cut through the thicker forehead skin. Beveling the incision from posterior

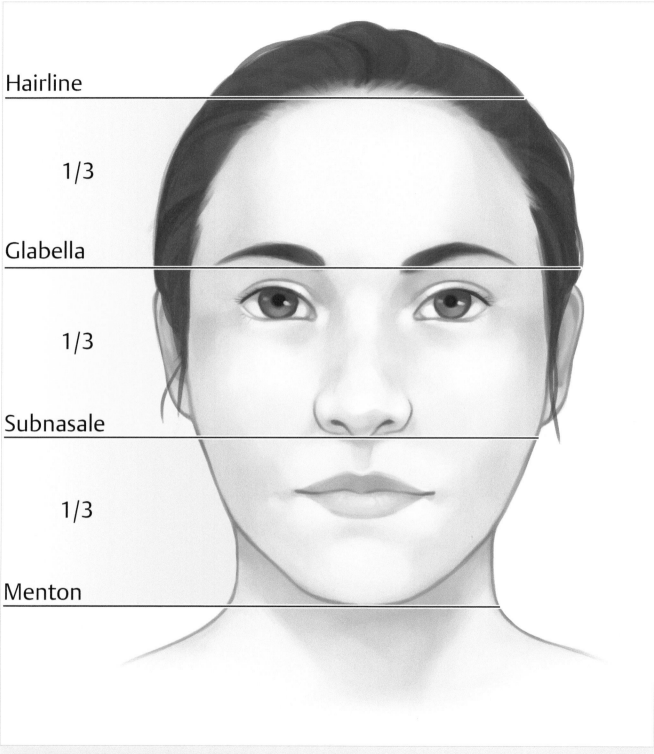

Fig. 22.2 The concept of facial thirds in the idealized face.

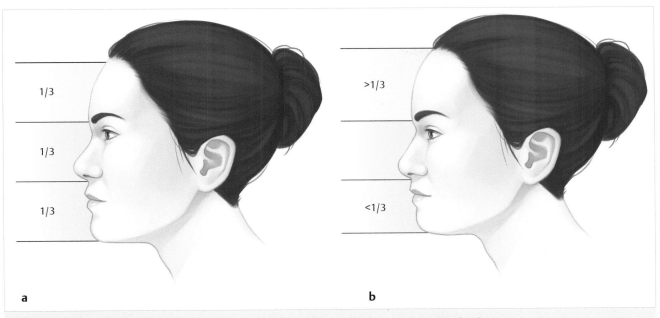

Fig. 22.3 Facial thirds in profile **(a)** in the idealized face and **(b)** showing the elongation of the forehead with aging.

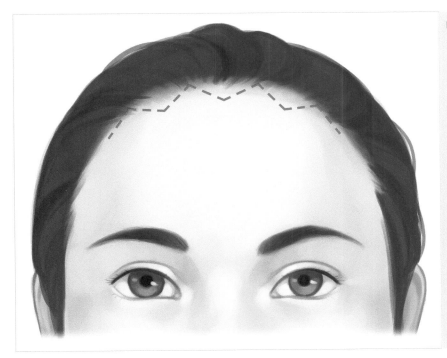

Fig. 22.4 Traditional pretrichial brow-lift incision.

to anterior may be helpful in preserving hair follicles and preventing postoperative alopecia at the incision. It is helpful to minimize cautery in the dermis at the site of the incision for this reason as well, although several vessels will be encountered in the subdermal layer.[9]

The level of the dissection depends on the type of procedure chosen. For a more extensive lift or, if the goal of surgery is to lower the forehead, then subperiosteal dissection may be necessary to try to advance the posterior scalp forward. The authors' preferred approach is along the posterior galea anterior to the periosteum, which provides a smooth dissection plane down to the arcus marginalis. If dissection is kept at the deep portion of the galea, the surgeon will avoid injury to the deep branch of the supraorbital nerve as it crosses the temporal line of fusion.[1] A third variant for the dissection is a subcutaneous approach on top of the frontalis muscle. This may be appropriate in select patients and does not present as much risk to neurovascular structures. Through the galeal approach, the central forehead muscles may be released as well as the arcus marginalis, taking care not to disturb the supraorbital

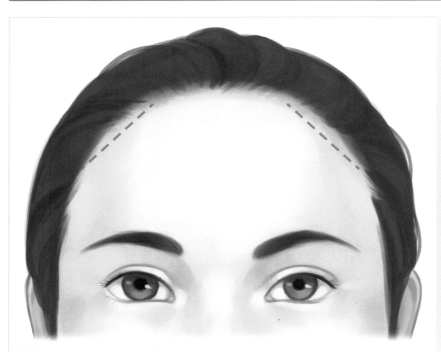

Fig. 22.5 Lateral pretrichial brow-lift incision.

neurovascular bundle. Finger dissection can also be used to release down to the lateral canthal area.[8]

After dissection is complete, the flap is mobilized upward to determine the amount of skin resection. It is helpful for an assistant to provide countertraction on the scalp at the posterior edge of the incision to determine the amount of resection. A heavy marker is used to delineate the resection amount, being careful to follow the shape of the original incision with a slight taper as it approaches the lateral edge. A #10 blade or monopolar cautery on the coagulation setting may be used to resect the excess skin. The authors prefer buried, interrupted 4–0 polygalactin suture for deep closure and running, locking 5–0 polypropylene for the skin. A postoperative head wrap in the central forehead may be useful but is not necessary, as this may exacerbate swelling in the periorbital area.

22.9 Tips and Pearls

With any aesthetic or functional procedure, the goal is often to achieve the most benefit at the least amount of risk. For the pretrichial brow lift, this downside risk includes the scar and healing period, as well as risk of motor or sensory nerve damage during the procedure. The temporal branch of the facial nerve is adjacent to the inferior portion of the dissection in the region of the arcus marginalis, and can be avoided by staying on the deep temporal fascia without dissecting into the superficial temporal fascia. This is uncommonly at risk during pretrichial brow-lift surgery, and yet must be kept in mind. The more likely nerve affected by pretrichial approaches is the deep branch of the supraorbital nerve, which travels obliquely from the supraorbital notch superotemporally to the hairline under the frontalis muscle. Damage to this nerve can cause sensory dysesthesias. The nerve is best avoided by dissecting along the deep galea, or subperiosteally, taking care to release the

temporal line of fusion from lateral to medial to avoid damage to this nerve.[1]

22.10 What to Avoid

Patient selection is key for the pretrichial brow lift. Patients with male-pattern baldness or significant thinning in the anterior hairline may not be the best candidates for the procedure. It is important also to have a discussion with patients before surgery about expected outcomes such as postoperative swelling and scar remodeling, as well as possible complications including dysesthesias of the forehead. These can occur from any type of brow lift, but are most likely in procedures that affect the supraorbital nerve, especially the deep branch. The dysesthesia can cause debilitating pruritus and sensory disturbance. It is best to take all measures to avoid this complication rather than having to treat one afterward.

22.11 Complications/Bailout/Salvage

For the pretrichial lift, the most common complication that can occur is alopecia at the site of the incision. It is best to warn patients about this possibility ahead of time. Making a beveled incision, minimizing cautery to the dermis and follicles during dissection, and avoiding excessive tension on the wound can avoid widening of the scar band and minimize alopecia.

Motor or sensory nerve damage is a potential complication of any forehead lift. For the temporal branch of the facial nerve, stretch injury can occur from tension on the flap during dissection. This injury can result in a temporary palsy of the nerve. Transection of the nerve is rare but usually permanent. Sensory dysesthesia from damage to the supraorbital nerve has been discussed. If a patient develops this complication, it may resolve after 3 to 6 months or be more permanent. Several measures can be tried. For one, it is important to instruct the patient to be careful using hot compresses in this area. Patients can get burns of the forehead and be unaware as a result of dysesthesia.[10] Distracting measures can be tried such as encouraging the patient to wear a headband or tight-fitting hat, which will stimulate the damaged sensory nerve into habituation and may relieve the symptoms. In rare cases, gabapentin or pregabalin can be tried as well.

22.12 Postoperative Care

Patients should be instructed to use ointment along the incision line for 10 to 14 days. Permanent sutures can be removed at 10 days. Some surgeons apply a wrap to the forehead after surgery with a Kerlex followed by Coban, but this is surgeon preference. The wrap may "squeegee" the postoperative edema into the periorbital area rather than prevent it from forming entirely. Hematoma is certainly a potential complication of the surgery, and patients should be checked shortly after surgery. A drain can be used if the concern for hematoma is high.

References

[1] Knize DM. Anatomic concepts for brow lift procedures. Plast Reconstr Surg. 2009; 124(6):2118–2126

[2] Georgescu D, Anderson RL, McCann JD. Brow ptosis correction: a comparison of five techniques. Facial Plast Surg. 2010; 26(3):186–192

[3] Jones BM, Grover R. Endoscopic brow lift: a personal review of 538 patients and comparison of fixation techniques. Plast Reconstr Surg. 2004; 113(4): 1242–1250, discussion 1251–1252

[4] Lee H, Quatela VC. Endoscopic Browplasty. Facial Plast Surg 2018; 34:139-144

[5] Marten TJ. Hairline lowering during foreheadplasty. Plast Reconstr Surg. 1999; 103(1):224–236

[6] Powell N, Humphreys B. Proportions of the Aesthetic Face. New York: Thieme-Stratton; 1984

[7] Walrath JD, McCord CD. The open brow lift. Clin Plast Surg. 2013; 40(1):117–124

[8] Mahmood U, Baker JL, Jr. Lateral subcutaneous brow lift: Updated technique. Aesthet Surg J. 2015; 35(5):621–624

[9] Fattahi T. Open brow lift surgery for facial rejuvenation. Atlas Oral Maxillofac Surg Clin North Am. 2016; 24(2):161–164

[10] Jones YJ, Georgescu D, McCann JD, Anderson RL. Microwave warm compress burns. Ophthal Plast Reconstr Surg. 2010; 26(3):219

Part VI

Eyelid Reconstruction

VI

23 Tenzel Semicircular Flap

Lucas Bonafede and Joseph Giacometti

Summary

The Tenzel semicircular flap was first described in 1975 by Dr. Richard Tenzel and consists of an advancement-rotational musculocutaneous flap used for direct closure of moderate-sized lower or upper eyelid defects. The procedure involves creating a semicircular skin-muscle flap rotated either upward or downward from the lateral canthal angle with selective cantholysis and advancement of the flap for direct closure. Drs. Levin and Buckman modified the procedure in 1986 to include the release of the lower eyelid retractors and inferior orbital septum to allow for more laxity and the closure of larger defects. The semicircular flap is a particularly useful technique with successful cosmetic and functional outcomes that is performed in a single stage and avoids the need for grafting of other tissues. There are several potential complications, including ectropion, lid retraction, lateral canthal webbing or dystopia, and notching of the lid margin. These may be avoided with appropriate surgical planning and technique.

Keywords: Richard Tenzel, semicircular flap, eyelid reconstruction, lower eyelid reconstruction, upper eyelid reconstruction, facial reconstruction, rotational flap, advancement flap

23.1 Goals

The goals of the semicircular flap are anatomical, functional, and cosmetic reconstruction of lower or upper eyelid defects of moderate size.[1] As with any eyelid reconstruction, it is important to create an anatomically stable and cosmetically acceptable eyelid and margin and to restore the functional ability of the eyelid to protect and lubricate the eye.

23.2 Advantages

There are several advantages to the Tenzel semicircular flap. The semicircular design of the flap generates more lateral movement of the graft than a straight-line design would permit.[1,2,3,4] The procedure is performed in a single stage and does not require temporary closure of the eyelids. This is in contrast to a tarsoconjunctival flap from the upper eyelid. Furthermore, the semicircular flap does not require grafting or manipulation of other nonadjacent tissues. It utilizes the adjacent lateral eyelid margin tissue with natural lashes for direct closure, which promotes a more favorable cosmetic appearance compared to utilizing grafted tissue without lashes. In the semicircular flap, the medially mobilized periorbital tissue that does not contain lashes is limited to the lateral eyelid.

23.3 Expectations

The semicircular flap is a reliable procedure and the surgeon can expect a reasonable cosmetic outcome with good functionality of the reconstructed eyelid. There are several minor complications that have been reported, many of which may be avoided with the appropriate preoperative planning and surgical techniques.[5]

23.4 Key Principles

The semicircular flap is an advancement-rotational musculocutaneous flap used for direct closure of moderate-sized lower or upper eyelid defects.[1,2,3,4] It should be considered when the size of the defect would not permit direct closure alone. The technique recruits the adjacent lateral remaining eyelid and periorbital tissue. It was first described in 1975 by Dr. Richard Tenzel.[2,3] The original technique was modified by Drs. Levine and Buckman to promote further mobilization by freeing the attachments of the inferior orbital septum and the lower eyelid retractors.[4] The approach to the semicircular flap varies on an individual basis, depending on the size and location of the defect, the degree of tissue laxity, and the personal preferences of the surgeon.

23.5 Indications

The Tenzel semicircular flap can be used for closure of moderate-sized upper or lower eyelid defects, which have been described as defects involving 1/3 to 1/2 of the eyelid margin. The degree of lid laxity should be considered when determining its use.[1,2,3,4,5,6] Several reports of this technique are being used to successfully repair defects involving up to 80% of the eyelid.[4,5] This procedure is best for repair of central eyelid defect with at least 2 mm of remaining tarsus on the lateral and medial wound, but has also been utilized in cases where there is minimal tarsus laterally or medially.[3] The semicircular flap is typically used for reconstruction following surgical excision of tumors or other eyelid lesions, but it may also be used for repair of traumatic defects if there is sufficient remaining tissue.

23.6 Contraindications

The Tenzel semicircular flap should not be utilized for large upper or lower eyelid defects where there is not sufficient tissue mobilization for adequate closure. Large defects are defined as involving over 50% of the upper or lower eyelid margin. While there are many reports of the semicircular flap technique being used for defects involving up to 75 to 80% of the margin, other techniques, including the Hughes flap and the Cutler-Beard procedure, may be recommended for eyelid margin defects greater than 50%.[1,4,5,6,7] Lack of tarsal remnant on the lateral or medial wound edge may limit the ability to utilize the Tenzel semicircular flap by decreasing lid stability of the final reconstruction, thereby increasing the risk for postoperative lid malposition.[3]

23.7 Preoperative Preparation

The procedure is typically performed in an ambulatory surgery center under conscious sedation. Standard instrumentation for ophthalmic plastic surgery should be available. Sutures vary depending on the specifics of the case and the personal preference of the surgeon.

23.8 Operative Technique

The key procedural steps are as follows (▶ Fig. 23.1, ▶ Fig. 23.2) [1,2,3,4]:

1. Drape and prepare the patient in the standard ophthalmic fashion.
2. Design the semicircular flap starting from the lateral canthal angle, moving superiorly and laterally and curving inferiorly for lower eyelid defects, or moving inferiorly and laterally and curving superiorly for upper eyelid defects.
3. Place topical ophthalmic anesthetic eyedrops and perform subcutaneous infiltration of local anesthetic into the operative eyelid and surrounding periocular tissue.
4. Create a curved canthotomy and skin-muscle incision following the planned semicircular flap outline.

5. Perform a selective cantholysis of the inferior or superior canthal tendon for inferior and superior defects, respectively.
6. Dissect the flap at the level of the orbicularis muscle to the lateral orbital rim.
7. Mobilize the flap medially to visualize if direct closure of the wound is possible.
8. If further mobility is necessary, the lateral attachments of the orbital septum may be severed.
9. If even further advancement is required for direct closure for lower eyelid defect, release the attachments of the inferior orbital septum from the orbital rim and the inferior retractors and conjunctiva from the inferior tarsus.
10. Advance the flap medially and perform primary closure of tarsus, eyelid margin, and overlying skin. Let's have it state: Interrupted 5-0 polyglactin (Vicryl) sutures with buried knots are used for deep fixation of the advanced tissue. The eyelid margin is sutured together with two interrupted 6-0 silk sutures placed at the gray-line and the lashline. A third marginal suture posterior to the gray-line may be applied, but may increase the risk of corneal abrasion. Leave the tails long and anchored away from the cornea in order to aid in removal at follow-up. The skin is then closed using 6-0 silk

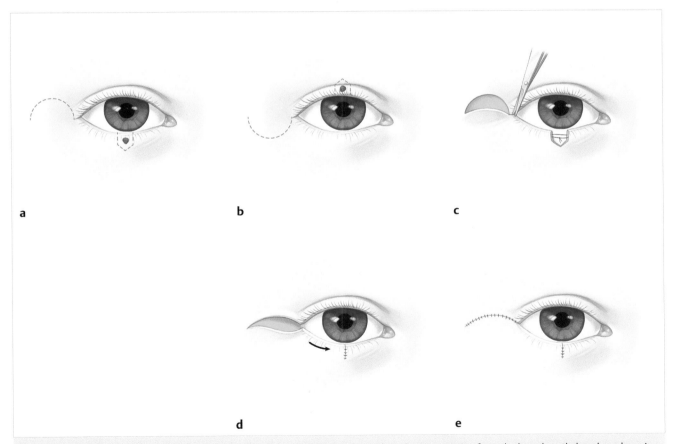

Fig. 23.1 Diagram of key steps in the Tenzel semicircular flap. **(a, b)** Create a curved canthotomy starting from the lateral canthal angle and curving superiorly or inferiorly depending on the location of the eyelid defect. **(c)** Perform a cantholysis and then dissect the flap to the lateral orbital rim. **(d)** Mobilize the flap medially and perform direct closure of the eyelid defect. **(e)** Recreate the lateral canthus and anchor the flap to the periosteum of the lateral orbital rim and close the skin wound.

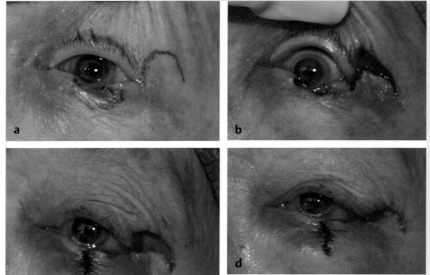

Fig. 23.2 Images of key steps in the Tenzel semicircular flap: **(a)** a lower eyelid defect centrally with a designed Tenzel semicircular flap that starts perpendicular to the lateral canthal angle and rapidly curves. **(b)** Eyelid laxity following curved canthotomy as well as inferior cantholysis and dissection of the flap at the level of the orbicularis muscle. **(c)** Direct closure of the eyelid defect. **(d)** Reconstructed lateral canthus and the closed canthotomy wound. Appropriate horizontal eyelid traction was ensured.

sutures, incorporating the tails of the lashline/gray-line sutures, in order to avoid abrasion of the ocular surface.

11. Re-create the lateral canthal angle and re-establish the stability of the lateral canthus by suturing the flap to periosteum of the lateral orbital rim. This step can be performed by using a 4–0 or 5–0 suture (polyglactin or nylon) to attach the lateral aspect of the flap to the periosteum of the lateral orbital rim at the level of Whitnall tubercle.

12. If the inferior retractors and conjunctiva were separated for further mobilization, then consider reattaching the retractors and conjunctiva following reconstruction of the lateral canthal angle.

13. Close the skin incision using either 6–0 nylon or absorbable plain gut sutures.

14. Apply antibiotic-steroid ointment to all incisions.

23.9 Tips and Pearls

- There are several variations of the specific surgical technique, depending on the size/location of defect as well as the intrinsic laxity of the patient's periocular tissue. As with any surgery, experience will help guide decision-making.
- The dimensions of the semicircular flap vary with each individual case based on the size of the defect and the amount of eyelid laxity, but the diameter of the semicircular flap is typically between 10 and 22 mm.
- In order to maintain the natural upward or downward curve of the lateral eyelid toward the lateral canthus, the curved canthotomy incision should begin at a vertical 90-degree angle from the lateral canthal angle. Failure to create this initial vertical projection of the flap could result in malposition of the flap. This vertical incision should rapidly transition to a curved canthotomy.

- Adequate vertical height of the flap must be assured to prevent vertical shortening of the reconstructed eyelid. Again, this will be determined both by the width of the defect and the laxity of the tissue.
- Once the flap has been initiated and the cantholysis has been performed, attempt to advance the tissue medially and assess the mobility and amount of tension. If additional mobility is required, further dissection should be performed. In the case of the lower lid, ensure completion of the cantholysis. Dissection in the suborbicularis/preseptal plane should be performed inferiorly to the level of the inferior orbital rim. If the lid requires further mobilization, consider releasing the orbitomalar ligament and additional dissection into the midface in a pre-periosteal plane using a periosteal elevator.
- Severing the attachments of the orbital septum and lower lid retractors as well as the deeper dissection previously described should be limited to cases that require the additional laxity for appropriate closure of the lid defect. Attempt to close the wound with the least amount of manipulation to the surrounding tissue possible. It is critical to ensure sufficient horizontal tension of the eyelid after closure.
- If there is concern for vertical shortening or entropion, the surgeon may opt not to reattach the inferior retractors and conjunctiva when closing the semicircular flap if they had been resected during the procedure.
- Appropriate re-establishment of the lateral canthus is also of critical importance for lid stability and cosmesis. This can be accomplished with optimal placement of the periosteal suture at the level of Whitnall tubercle. This suture should be placed at the medial aspect of the lateral orbital rim, approximately 1 to 2 mm superior to the medial canthal angle. Placing this suture too anteriorly (i.e., not deep enough) or too inferiorly may result in postoperative ectropion or retraction, respectively.

- Consider using 6–0 plain gut or other absorbable sutures, rather than silk sutures, in patients who may have difficulty with follow-up.

23.10 What to Avoid

- Place special attention on avoiding the lacrimal gland and its vasculature when performing a superior cantholysis, and also take care not to inadvertently suture lacrimal gland tissue into the periosteal sutures of the canthoplasty.
- Avoid excess horizontal eyelid laxity when closing the wound and reconstructing the canthus in order to prevent lid ectropion or retraction.
- Avoid integrating the septum in the sutures during eyelid reconstruction, which could also lead to retraction.
- Re-approximating the lateral canthus without accomplishing good fixation to the lateral orbital rim periosteum may lead to webbing of the newly created canthus.

23.11 Complications/Bailout/ Salvage

Several minor complications have been reported for the semicircular flap procedure; however, they can often be avoided with proper surgical planning and technique.[1,3,4,5]

- Ectropion can occur when there is excessive horizontal laxity following the closure of the defect. This problem may be exacerbated when the orbital septum and inferior lid retractors are severed and excessive dissection is performed. Ensuring adequate tension and anchoring the flap helps to prevent ectropion formation.
- Webbing of the lateral canthal angle can occur when the flap design is improperly constructed with an excessive vertical component. Proper flap dimensions and curvature help to prevent this complication.
- Symblepharon formation has been reported following reconstruction with a semicircular flap. A triangular conjunctival graft from the wound may be placed on the posterior flap surface to help minimize symblepharon formation.
- Notching of the lid margin may occur if sufficient tension is not applied to the direct lid closure. The proper placement and tension of tarsal and marginal sutures during the repair of the eyelid wound and the appropriate vertical alignment of the tarsus can minimize lid notching. Hypertrophic scarring may also lead to a poor cosmetic result.
- Protrusion of orbital fat may occur if the septum is severed during the operation.
- Eyelid malposition and fullness of the lateral canthus may occur in cases of lateral defects with minimal residual lateral tarsus that requires attachment of the tarsus to the lateral canthus. Careful selection of the correct operative techniques can help minimize complications.

- Intra- or postoperative hemorrhage and wound infections are other possible complications in patients undergoing eyelid repair.

There are several alternatives that can be utilized if the semicircular flap is not chosen for reconstruction[1,6,7,8,9]:
- A Hughes tarsoconjunctival flap from the upper eyelid may be used for large lower eyelid defects.
- A Cutler-Beard full-thickness eyelid flap may be used for reconstruction of large upper eyelid defects.
- The double lateral flap technique as described by Toribio et al.,[8] which involves a combination of a tarsoconjunctival and periosteal flap, may be an alternative to the Tenzel semicircular flap.
- Full-thickness pedicled flaps, temporal forehead transposition flaps, free transconjunctival grafts, and Mustarde rotating cheek flaps are other options for reconstruction of larger eyelid defects.

23.12 Postoperative Care

The semicircular flap tends to have favorable anatomic, functional, and cosmetic results. Following the procedure, an antibiotic-steroid ophthalmic ointment should be placed over all incisions two times per day. No patching is necessary following the surgery. Follow-up should be scheduled for 7 to 10 days after surgery for removal of marginal sutures. Follow-up can then be extended to 4 to 6 weeks and 3 months following the date of surgery.

References

[1] Shinder R, Esmaeli B. Eyelid and ocular adnexal reconstruction. In: Black EH, Nesi FA, Calvano CJ, Gladstone GJ, Levine MR, eds. Smith and Nesis Ophthalmic Plastic and Reconstructive Surgery. New York, NY: Springer; 2012: 551–569

[2] Tenzel RR. Reconstruction of the central one half of an eyelid. Arch Ophthalmol. 1975; 93(2):125–126

[3] Tenzel RR, Stewart WB. Eyelid reconstruction by the semicircle flap technique. Ophthalmology. 1978; 85(11):1164–1169

[4] Levine MR, Buckman G. Semicircular flap revisited. Arch Ophthalmol. 1986; 104(6):915–917

[5] Miller EA, Boynton JR. Complications of eyelid reconstruction using a semicircular flap. Ophthalmic Surg. 1987; 18(11):807–810

[6] Yordanov YP, Shef A. Lower eyelid reconstruction after ablation of skin malignancies: how far can we get in a single-stage procedure? J Craniofac Surg. 2017; 28(5):e477–e479

[7] Foggnolo P, Colletti G, Valassina D, Allevi F, Rossetti L. Partial and total lower lid reconstruction: our experience with 41 cases. Ophthalmologica. 2012; 228(4):239–243

[8] Álvaro Toribio J. Double lateral flap: a new technique for lower eyelid reconstruction alternative to the Tenzel procedure. Aesthetic Plast Surg. 2015; 39 (6):935–941

[9] Marcet MM, Lau IHW, Chow SSW. Avoiding the Hughes flap in lower eyelid reconstruction. Curr Opin Ophthalmol. 2017; 28(5):493–498

24 Hughes Tarsoconjunctival Flap

Sonul Mehta

Summary

The Hughes tarsoconjunctival flap is a two-stage eyelid-sharing flap that can be used for full-thickness lower eyelid defects that involve greater than 50% of the lower eyelid margin.

Keywords: lower eyelid defect, tarsoconjunctival flap, lid-sharing flap, Hughes flap

24.1 Goals

- To reconstruct large lower eyelid defects that involve greater than 50% of the horizontal lower eyelid margin.[1,2]

24.2 Advantages

- This approach offers reconstruction of wide defects of the lower eyelid with satisfactory cosmetic results and low morbidity at the donor site, and rebuilds the eyelid with its own tissue allowing restoration of normal anatomy and function.[1,2]

24.3 Expectations/Key Principles

- Two-stage eyelid-sharing reconstructive technique: First stage involves (a) advancement of a tarsoconjunctival flap (Hughes flap) from the upper to the lower eyelid defect to reconstruct the posterior lamella (tarsus and conjunctiva) and (b) reconstruction of the anterior musculocutaneous lamella with a local flap, free full-thickness skin graft, or an advancement flap. During the first stage, the eye remains covered with the pedicle flap connecting the upper lid to the lower lid. This type of flap allows for new vasculature to form within and around the graft. The second stage is performed approximately 4 to 6 weeks later and involves severing the flap pedicle and re-creating the new lower lid margin.[1,2]

24.4 Indications

- This technique is indicated in patients with posterior lamellar defects (i.e., secondary to tumor excision or trauma) of the lower lid margin encompassing greater than 50% of the horizontal lid margin.

24.5 Contraindications

- This procedure requires preservation of at least 4 mm of tarsal plate height in the upper lid (to prevent postoperative upper lid entropion, etc.) and is contraindicated in a patient with insufficient tarsus (i.e., in a patient who has had a prior surgery involving the tarsus).
- Because this procedure requires the eye to be covered for several weeks before the second stage is performed, this surgery is contraindicated in patients requiring surgery in their only-seeing eye, or in children at risk for occlusion amblyopia.

24.6 Preoperative Preparation

- Several factors should be evaluated prior to surgery: age of the patient; age of the wound; potential compromise to the vascular supply, such as active cigarette smoker or previous radiation treatment to the area, etc. Clinically, the size and orientation of the defect should be evaluated. Also, the upper lid should be everted to ensure that there is normal tarsal anatomy and no evidence of previous surgery involving the tarsus.

24.7 Operative Technique

- Flap size is determined by gently bringing together the edges of the lower lid defect. The size of the flap should roughly be the size of the residual defect.
- Local anesthetic (1% lidocaine with epinephrine 1:100000) is injected into the upper lid. Some surgeons may perform a frontal nerve block.
- A 4–0 silk traction suture is placed at the central upper lid margin.
- The 4–0 silk traction suture is then used to evert the upper lid onto a Desmarres retractor and the 4–0 silk traction suture is secured to the head drape (▶ Fig. 24.1a,b).
- With preservation of at least 4 mm of tarsus from the lid margin, a horizontal incision parallel to the lid margin and slightly shorter than the length of the defect is made to the depth of the pretarsal space with a #15 blade (▶ Fig. 24.1a,b).
- Using the same #15 blade, a vertical cut is made at each end of the horizontal incision toward the superior aspect of the tarsal plate.
- With Westcott scissors, the tarsus and conjunctiva are separated from the Müller muscle and the upper lid retractors.
- After the flap is created, it is brought down into the lower lid defect (▶ Fig. 24.1c).
- Medially and laterally, the flap is secured into place with 6–0 vicryl suture to the native, remaining, lower lid tarsal tissues and conjunctiva or lower lid retractors to complete the repair of the posterior lamella defect (▶ Fig. 24.1d).
- To replace the anterior lamellar defect, one can suture in a full-thickness skin graft (from the contralateral upper lid or retroauricular) or a myocutaneous cheek flap that is rotated in from the side. A myocutaneous flap is not recommended in patients with nonelastic, tight skin, as this can cause a cicatricial ectropion to form when it heals (▶ Fig. 24.1e,f).
- After an adequate blood supply has been established and the flap has healed (usually 4–6 weeks later), the second stage of the Hughes procedure is performed.
- Local anesthetic of 1% lidocaine is injected into the upper lid and lower lid.

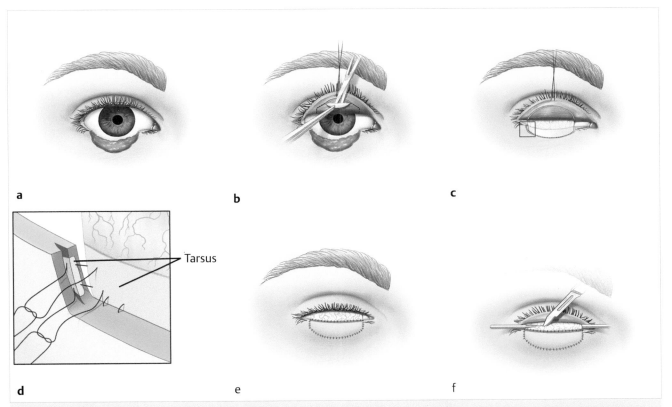

Tarsus

Fig. 24.1 **(a,b)** A 4–0 silk traction suture everting upper lid onto a Desmarres retractor, preservation of 4 mm of upper lid tarsus, and horizontal incision parallel to the lid margin with a #15 blade. **(c)** Advancement of the tarsoconjunctival flap into the lower lid defect. **(d)** Securing the tarsiconjunctival flap into the lower lid defect with suture and the flap covering the eye. **(e, f)** Reconstruction of the anterior lamella with a full-thickness skin graft. (From Codner M, McCord C. Eyelid & Periorbital Surgery. 2nd ed. New York: Thieme Medical Publishers; 2016.)

- With a grooved director under the flap, the flap is severed at the new lower lid margin with Westcott scissors, angled so that the edge of the conjunctiva is slightly higher than the anterior edge (▶ Fig. 24.2).
- The extra conjunctiva of the new lower lid margin is draped forward and secured with suture in a buried fashion to reform the lid margin. Alternatively, the neo-margin may be cut flush and allowed to heal secondarily without additional suturing.
- If tarsoconjunctival flap remains at the tarsal plate of the upper lid, this can be excised. Gentle cautery may be needed to stop bleeding.

24.8 Tips and Pearls

- The initial horizontal incision should be placed 4 to 5 mm back from the upper lid margin. Less than this will cause instability of the upper lid and entropion of the upper lid may result.
- It is important to completely release the Müller muscle from the conjunctiva during flap construction; if this is not performed adequately, then Müller muscle will effectively be advanced with the flap and will heal in this advanced position to the overlying upper lid tarsus. Upon separation of the flap subsequently, an upper lid retraction may result.

- Remember to avoid the myocutaneous cheek flap to replace the anterior lamellar defect in patients with tight, nonelastic skin, as this can result in a cicatricial ectropion.
- Patients who are cigarette smokers should be counseled to stop smoking and refrain from smoking during the healing process. Smoking can interfere with the healing process and prevent formation of an adequate vascular supply to the flap.

24.9 Complications

Complication rate following Hughes flap is relatively low. The largest reported study of 122 cases showed a low complication rate of 14% with revision required in 4%. Potential complications include lagophthalmos, eyelid retraction, lid margin hyperemia, flap dehiscence, and ectropion or entropion.[3] In order to avoid flap dehiscence, the flap should be secured with multiple 6–0 vicryl sutures with native residual tarsal bed. Close follow-up can help monitor the progress. If flap dehiscence occurs early on after repair, the wound can be freshened under local anesthesia, and additional sutures can be placed. Lid margin instability, whether ectropion and entropion, is another potential complication. To avoid an entropion, it's essential to leave at least 4 mm of tarsus in the upper lid. If this occurs postoperatively, surgical correction would be required depending on the amount of laxity in the lid and the amount of residual tarsus

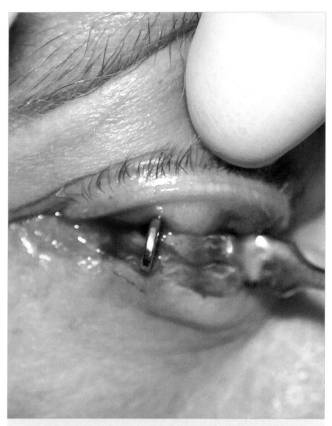

Fig. 24.2 The second stage of the Hughes procedure. A grooved director is placed under the flap, and the new lower lid margin is created by severing the tarsoconjunctival flap. (From Codner M, McCord C. Eyelid & Periorbital Surgery. 2nd ed. New York: Thieme Medical Publishers; 2016.)

remaining. Lid margin hyperemia can be avoided by trimming the conjunctival pedicle flush with the eyelid margin as opposed to advancing the conjunctiva over the lid margin as originally described.[4] Flap necrosis is very rare, given that the eyelid and periocular tissues are extremely vascular.

24.10 Postoperative Care

- Topical antibiotic ophthalmic ointment on all wounds.
- If a full-thickness skin graft was used, warm compresses to the graft.

References

[1] Maloof A, Ng S, Leatherbarrow B. The maximal Hughes procedure. Ophthal Plast Reconstr Surg. 2001; 17(2):96–102

[2] Hawes MJ, Grove AS, Jr, Hink EM. Comparison of free tarsoconjunctival grafts and Hughes tarsoconjunctival grafts for lower eyelid reconstruction. Ophthal Plast Reconstr Surg. 2011; 27(3):219–223

[3] McKelvie J, Ferguson R, Ng SGJ. Eyelid reconstruction using the "Hughes" tarsoconjunctival advancement flap: long-term outcomes in 122 consecutive cases over a 13-year period. Orbit. 2017; 36(4):228–233

[4] Bartley GB, Putterman AM. A minor modification of the Hughes' operation for lower eyelid reconstruction. Am J Ophthalmol. 1995; 119(1):96–97

25 Cutler-Beard Flap

Arpine Barsegian and Roman Shinder

Summary

Reconstruction of large full-thickness upper eyelid defects poses a challenge to oculofacial surgeons. Successful repair will maintain the function of the upper eyelid while providing an adequate cosmetic result. The Cutler-Beard flap is a lid-sharing, staged procedure to reconstruct such defects that has stood the test of time. This chapter will detail the key principles of the procedure preferred by the senior author (RS), potential complications, and alternative surgical approaches.

Keywords: Cutler-Beard flap, tarsoconjunctival flap, lid-sharing procedure, upper eyelid defect

25.1 Goals

The repair of a large full-thickness upper eyelid defect typically created after the excision of an eyelid malignancy is a surgical challenge (▶ Fig. 25.1). Cutler and Beard in 1955 described a two-stage, eyelid-sharing procedure to reconstruct such defects involving greater than 50% of the upper lid width.[1] The procedure encompasses advancing a composite full-thickness lower eyelid flap into the upper eyelid defect by passing it posterior to the remaining lower eyelid margin. The second stage of the procedure involves lysis of the flap and takes place 6 to 8 weeks after the first stage. The surgical goals are to reestablish the lid anatomy, as well as to attempt to retain function and cosmesis.

25.2 Advantages

The key advantage of this flap is that it is usable in nearly all large upper lid full-thickness defects. The flap has a good vascular supply that aids in its ultimate success. The lower lid donor tissue offers a suitable match in texture, quality, and appearance to the sacrificed upper lid. Lastly, the final outcome is often functionally and cosmetically acceptable to the patient.

25.3 Expectations

While this procedure does have its merits, the patient should be counseled that the surgery is challenging and complex and the final result will never act nor look like a completely normal upper lid, and in certain cases touch-up procedures may be warranted. The reconstructed lid tends to be relatively thick and immobile. Placement of a tarsoconjunctival graft from the contralateral upper eyelid to reconstruct the posterior lamella can improve upper eyelid stability.[2,3,4,5,6] Other possible complications include upper eyelid retraction or entropion, lower eyelid laxity or ectropion due to induced lid denervation, vascular compromise, lagophthalmos, lymphedema, keratopathy, and blepharoptosis.[2]

25.4 Key Principles

- To bring a full-thickness lower eyelid flap, harvested at least 4 mm beneath the lower eyelid margin, underneath the remaining lower lid margin "bridge" of tissue and over the globe to close the upper eyelid defect.
- The flap is traditionally separated 6 to 8 weeks after the first stage.
- One of this procedure's main shortcomings is its lack of stability in the newly created upper eyelid due to the absence of tarsus. Eyelid retraction and entropion are potential complications if a posterior lamellar graft is not utilized as an adjunct.
- The senior author (RS) has had success with the use of a tarsoconjunctival graft from the contralateral upper eyelid to reconstruct the posterior lamella in a modified Cutler-Beard procedure.

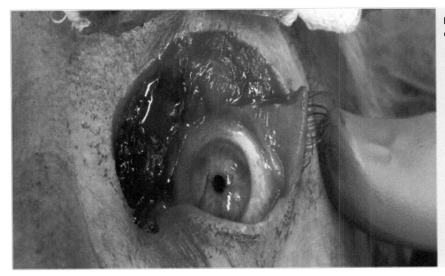

Fig. 25.1 A large full-thickness upper eyelid defect after tumor excision.

25.5 Indications

To reconstruct full-thickness defects of the upper eyelid that involve more than 50% of the eyelid width, judged to be too large for more conservative surgical strategies such as a modified Tenzel flap.

25.6 Contraindications

This surgery requires occlusion of the eye for a period of several weeks. Thus, it should be avoided in the better seeing eye of monocular patients and young children in whom occlusion amblyopia may develop.

25.7 Preoperative Preparation

Blood thinning medications are stopped for several days if possible with the help of the prescribing physician. The patient is brought to the operating room, placed in supine position, and given intravenous sedation. Alternative options for anesthesia include local anesthesia or general anesthesia in select patients. Tetracaine eye drops are delivered onto both ocular surfaces and the patient is prepped and draped in typical sterile fashion for ophthalmic surgery.

25.8 Operative Technique

- Local anesthesia consisting of 50:50 mixture of 1% lidocaine with epinephrine 1:100,000 and 0.5% bupivacaine with epinephrine 1:200,000 (with added hyaluronidase) is injected subcutaneously to the medial, lateral, and superior remnants of the ipsilateral upper lid, the entire ipsilateral lower eyelid, and contralateral upper eyelid.
- The medial and lateral upper lid remnants are pulled toward one another with forceps and the residual defect is measured horizontally with a caliper giving the "surgical width."
- The contralateral upper lid is then everted over a Desmarres retractor and the tarsal conjunctiva is marked, with the desired surgical width being 4 mm from the lid margin.
- A tarsoconjunctival graft is then harvested using a Beaver 6700 mini-blade for initial incision through the conjunctiva and tarsus, and Westcott scissors finalize the graft excision. Hemostasis is achieved with direct pressure and the donor site is allowed to heal via secondary intention. The graft is placed in a moist gauze.
- Using a caliper, a line parallel to the ipsilateral lower lid margin, and 5 mm below it to avoid the marginal arcade, is marked for the surgical width.
- After a Jaeger lid plate is placed to protect the globe, a #15 Bard-Parker blade creates a cutaneous incision at the surgical mark and Westcott scissors finalize a full-thickness blepharotomy incision through the lower lid. Two relaxing incisions are then made in similar fashion medially and laterally in an inferior direction to the inferior fornix of the posterior lamella and orbital rim of the anterior lamella (► Fig. 25.2).
- The tarsoconjunctival graft is then positioned with the conjunctival surface facing the globe and secured to the residual medial and lateral tarsal plate of the upper lid with two partial-thickness lamellar bites of 6–0 polyglactin sutures ensuring the host and graft tarsal margins are well aligned. The superior border of the graft is then secured to the cut

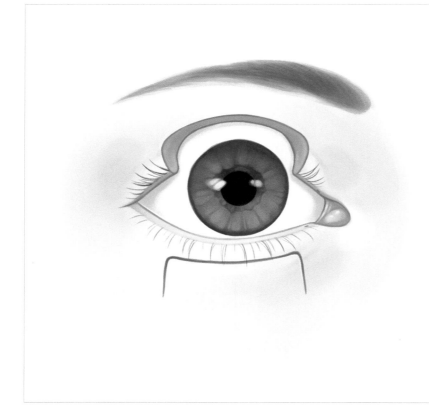

Fig. 25.2 Appearance of flap after two inferior relaxing incisions are made medially and laterally down to the inferior orbital rim.

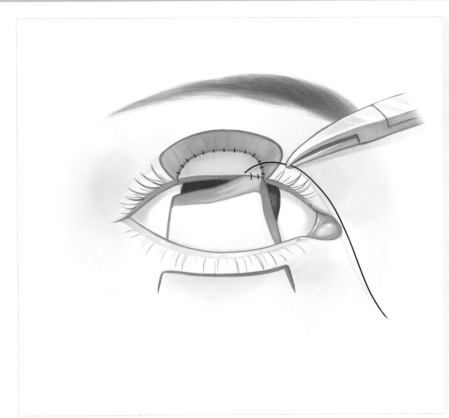

Fig. 25.3 The conjunctiva of the flap is brought up deep to the bridge and sutured to the inferior border of the tarsoconjunctival graft.

edge of the upper lid conjunctiva with a running 6–0 polyglactin suture in lamellar fashion. All conjunctival sutures placed during this and subsequent steps should be done with care, ensuring all knots face anteriorly to minimize the possibility of posterior suture exposure toward the globe and suture keratopathy.

- The flap is then secured into the upper lid defect in three layers. The conjunctiva is carefully dissected free from the lower lid retractor complex in the flap with Westcott scissors, and is brought superiorly underneath the bridge of remaining lower lid tissue, and reapproximated to the tarsoconjunctival graft inferior border with lamellar bites of running 6–0 polyglactin suture (layer 1, ▶ Fig. 25.3).
- The lower eyelid retractors and orbicularis complex in the flap are then secured to the cut edge of the levator aponeurosis with running 6–0 polyglactin suture (layer 2, ▶ Fig. 25.4). The levator will often need to initially be dissected free of adjacent attachments in the upper lid for proper exposure. This closure will lead to the eventual formation of the upper lid crease and allow for upper lid excursion. If the aponeurosis has been excised completely, then the sutures should instead secure the levator palpebrae superioris muscle.
- The skin of the flap is then secured to the upper lid skin with interrupted and running 6–0 silk suture (layer 3).
- The cut edge of the lower lid bridge tissue is left to heal via granulation.
- A healthy pink appearance to the lower lid bridge and flap skin signifies that the lower lid marginal arcade and vasculature of the flap have been preserved and the bridge, flap, and tarsoconjunctival graft should survive.

- Antibiotic ophthalmic ointment is given to all surgical sites and a pressure patch is applied to the ipsilateral eye.
- The second stage of the surgery is lysis of the flap and is usually carried out 6 to 8 weeks after the first stage.
- Under intravenous sedation, the same local anesthesia mixture is injected subcutaneously to the lower eyelid bridge and flap.
- A grooved director is placed deep to the flap through the medial and lateral palpebral fissures for globe protection.
- The flap skin is cut with a #15 Bard-Parker blade, and Westcott scissors finalize lysis at a level of 1 to 2 mm below the desired height of the new upper lid margin, angling the scissor cut so that the conjunctiva is longer than the skin (▶ Fig. 25.5). This 1 to 2 mm segment helps to prevent potential postoperative eyelid retraction and keratopathy.
- The upper lid conjunctiva is advanced anteriorly onto the newly created upper lid margin for about 2 mm with running 6–0 plain gut suture to create an anteriorly located mucocutaneous junction. This is to decrease the chance of keratinized skin or fine lanugo hair from the new upper lid margin causing keratopathy. If the flap is judged to have stretched since the first stage, excess superior flap tissue is carefully excised so that it could be secured to the lower lid bridge without laxity.
- The granulation tissue of the lower lid bridge is then denuded using a #15 Bard-Parker blade and the superior edge of the flap is attached to the bridge in two layers with interrupted 6–0 polyglactin orbicularis oculi closure and running 6–0 plain gut suture skin closure. Antibiotic ophthalmic ointment is given to all surgical sites. ▶ Fig. 25.6 shows a patient after the second stage of the Cutler-Beard flap.

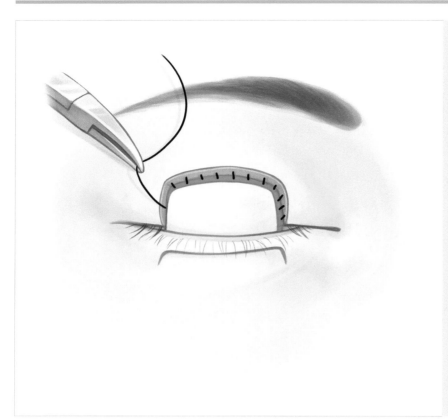

Fig. 25.4 The lower lid retractor/orbicularis complex of the flap is sutured to the cut edge of the levator aponeurosis.

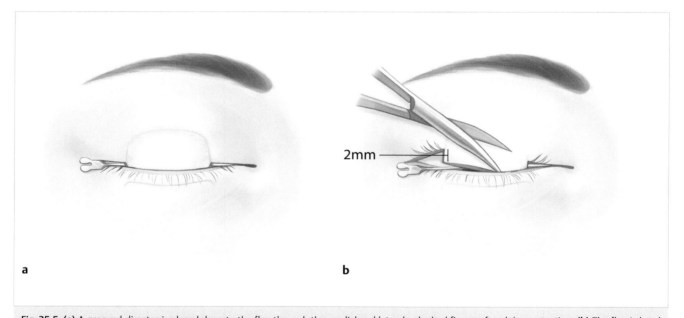

a

b

2mm

Fig. 25.5 (a) A grooved director is placed deep to the flap through the medial and lateral palpebral fissures for globe protection. **(b)** The flap is lysed with Westcott scissors 2 mm inferior to the desired height of the upper lid margin, angling the scissor so that the conjunctiva is longer than the skin.

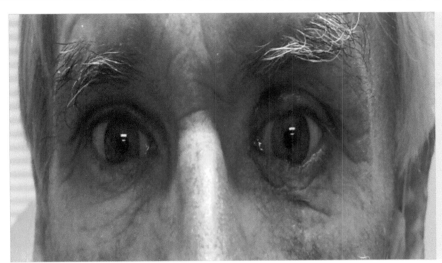

Fig. 25.6 Patient in Fig. 25.1 shown 2 weeks after second stage of the Cutler-Beard flap.

25.9 Tips and Pearls

- The flap of tissue from the lower eyelid must be approximately the same width as the upper eyelid defect. However, given the inherent laxity in the upper lid remnants, the flap may be narrower than the visible defect size because the upper eyelid remnants can be stretched to some extent to decrease the size of the defect ("surgical width").
- When forming the bridge during the first stage of the procedure, the marginal arterial arcade must be preserved by creating an incision at least 4 to 5 mm below the lid margin. If this vascular supply is sacrificed, necrosis of the bridge in the lower eyelid may occur.
- In younger patients with elastic tissue, the flap may seem contracted so that the horizontal dimension is shorter than necessary; however, if it has been measured properly initially, this will eventually stretch for an adequate result.
- The risk of postoperative upper lid entropion is decreased with the use of a tarsoconjunctival graft from the contralateral upper eyelid to re-create the upper lid posterior lamella.[2,3,4,5,6]
- It is necessary to suture the conjunctival layer of the flap to the inferior border of the tarsoconjunctival graft (layer 1) so that when the flap is opened during the second stage, this conjunctiva is available to advance over the reconstructed upper lid margin to avoid keratopathy that can result from skin lanugo hair if the mucocutaneous junction is too posterior.

25.10 What to Avoid

- The reconstructed upper eyelid bears no cilia. It is not recommended to attempt hair-bearing grafts in this location as the hair in the grafted area do not resemble normal eyelashes, and any cilia that were to take would be prone to malalignment and trichiasis/keratopathy.
- Attempt should be made to limit postoperative upper eyelid retraction. In addition to the use of a tarsoconjunctival graft from the contralateral upper eyelid, this complication can be decreased by bisecting the flap approximately 2 mm below

the level of the desired upper eyelid margin, and waiting at least 6 to 8 weeks prior to carrying out the second stage. Thus, surgeons should try to avoid the procedure without the use of a posterior lamellar substitute, lysing the flap flush with the intact upper lid margin, and attempting to do the second stage earlier than 6 weeks.

- During the second stage, the flap should be lysed with the scissor angled to leave the posterior conjunctiva 2 mm longer than the anterior skin/muscle complex. This allows the conjunctiva to be draped forward over the eyelid margin so that the lid margin will contain mucous membrane as opposed to keratinized epithelium. This helps prevent postoperative keratopathy from keratinized epithelium or fine lanugo hairs that could otherwise abrade the cornea. Surgeons should thus avoid lysing the flap in more traditional perpendicular cuts to the tissue.

25.11 Complications/Bailout/ Salvage

- A possible alternative to a Cutler-Beard procedure is placement of a free tarsoconjunctival graft from the contralateral upper eyelid for posterior lamellar repair and coverage of this graft with a myocutaneous flap for anterior lamellar repair if the amount of redundant upper eyelid tissue is sufficient. However, for deep and complex defects extending into the fornix and anterior orbit, this technique would not be adequate and the Cutler-Beard flap is more suitable.
- If the upper eyelid full-thickness defect is wide but shallow, including only a few millimeters at most past the lid margin, a tarsoconjunctival flap can be harvested from the region just superior to the defect. It can be advanced inferiorly for posterior lamellar reconstruction. This flap should be dissected well to the superior fornix. The levator aponeurosis is disinserted from its anterior tarsal attachments to prevent upper eyelid retraction during the postoperative period. The anterior lamella can be repaired with either a full-thickness skin graft or myocutaneous flap.

- In rare instances of considerable upper and lower eyelid tissue loss from trauma or tumor resection, sufficient tissue cannot be borrowed from the opposing lower eyelid to utilize the Cutler-Beard procedure. In such cases, vascular flaps must be obtained from more distant areas such as the forehead. The forehead flap can be based temporally, utilizing the superficial temporal artery as its vascular supply, or nasally using a median forehead flap. These techniques are exploited to reconstruct the upper eyelid when no other surgical options exist.

25.12 Postoperative Care

- After the first stage, a pressure patch is placed over the ipsilateral eye for 5 days to bolster the tarsoconjunctival graft to its overlying vascular flap. Antibiotic ophthalmic ointment is given three times daily to the contralateral eye for 1 week to promote healing of the tarsoconjunctival graft donor site. The patch is removed in the office and the patient begins to apply antibiotic ophthalmic ointment three times daily to the ipsilateral surgical wounds until the second stage.
- After the second stage, antibiotic ophthalmic ointment is again given three times daily to the surgical wounds for 1 week when the next follow-up is scheduled. The patient is followed thereafter every few months until adequate healing

has occurred. Lid edema/lymphedema can take up to several weeks to subside and patients are counseled to this possibility.

25.13 Acknowledgments

We would like to thank Valeriya Gershteyn for her contributions in producing the figure drawings for this chapter.

References

[1] Cutler NL, Beard C. A method for partial and total upper lid reconstruction. Am J Ophthalmol. 1955; 39(1):1–7

[2] Shinder R, Esmaeli B. Eyelid and ocular adnexal reconstruction. In: Black EH, Nesi FA, Calvano CJ, et al ed. Smith and Nesi's Ophthalmic Plastic and Reconstructive Surgery, 3rd ed. New York, NY: Springer, 2012:551–71

[3] Hsuan J, Selva D. Early division of a modified Cutler-Beard flap with a free tarsal graft. Eye (Lond). 2004; 18(7):714–717

[4] Kopecky A, Koch KR, Bucher F, Cursiefen C, Heindl LM. Results of Cutler-Beard procedure for reconstruction of extensive full thickness upper eyelid defects following tumor resection. Ophthalmology. 2016; 113(4):309–313

[5] Rajak SN, Malhotra R, Selva D. The 'over-the-top' modified Cutler-Beard procedure for complete upper eyelid defect reconstruction. Orbit. 2018; 7:1–4

[6] Yoon MK, McCulley TJ. Secondary tarsoconjunctival graft: a modification to the Cutler-Beard procedure. Ophthal Plast Reconstr Surg. 2013; 29(3):227–230

VII

26 Probing, Irrigation, and Intubation in Congenital Nasolacrimal Duct Obstruction

Jason S. Mantagos

Summary

Nasolacrimal duct probing and irrigation, as well as nasolacrimal intubation are common procedures for the management of congenital nasolacrimal duct obstruction, as well as dacryocystoceles. Both procedures have high success rates. For most patients, probe and irrigation will suffice; however, for recurrent nasolacrimal duct obstruction and complex cases the procedure of choice is nasolacrimal intubation. The salient points of each technique are reviewed, allowing ophthalmic surgeons to improve their technique and success with both procedures.

Keywords: congenital nasolacrimal duct obstruction, nasolacrimal duct obstruction, dacryocystocele, dacryocele, nasolacrimal intubation, nasolacrimal probing and irrigation, epiphora

26.1 Goals

The goal of nasolacrimal probing and irrigation (P&I), as well as of intubation is to achieve normal flow of tears within the nasolacrimal system and alleviate obstructions causing epiphora.[1] For newborns presenting with a dacryocystocele, the goal, in addition to restoring normal outflow of tears is to prevent dacryocystitis.[2] Dacryocystitis in a newborn can be life threatening because of their immature immune system.

26.2 Advantages

P&I can achieve resolution of symptoms in most children with a congenital nasolacrimal duct obstruction (CNLDO), while it can prevent dacryocystitis in children with a dacryocystocele.[1,2,3] Higher success can be achieved with nasolacrimal intubation for older children or following failed P&I.[4,5]

26.3 Expectations

Approximately 5% of infants are born with CNLDO and almost 90% of CNLDOs resolve spontaneously before the first year of life.[1,6,7] The success rate for P&I is approximately 80% for children of age groups 6 to 12 months, 12 to 24 months, and 24 to 36 months; however, the success rate declines to 56% for ages 36 to 48 months.[3] The success rate of P&I for managing a dacryocystocele is approximately 75%.[2] Nasolacrimal duct intubation has a success rate of approximately 90% for children with CNLDO less than 4 years of age.[8]

26.4 Key Principles

- 90% of CNLDO resolve prior to the first year of life without surgical management.[1,6]
- For children less than 3 years of age with persistent CNLDO, a primary P&I can be performed.[3]

- Nasolacrimal intubation should be considered as the primary procedure for children over 4 years of age with CNLDO.[4,8]
- Nasolacrimal intubation should be considered for children who have persistent epiphora following P&I.[5]
- Dacryocystocele requires urgent management, ideally while the child is still in the newborn nursery. P&I can be considered as first-line treatment.[2]
- Bilateral dacryocystocele often results in respiratory distress and requires surgical management in the operating room with assistance from an otolaryngologist.[2]

26.5 Indications

Nasolacrimal P&I is indicated for persistent symptoms of epiphora and infections in the setting of nasolacrimal duct obstruction.[1] Patients whose symptoms persist beyond the first year of life can be considered for primary P&I, as by that time the likelihood of spontaneous resolution is low and general anesthesia is safer after the first year of life.[6,7,9] P&I can be considered at earlier ages if infections require frequent use of oral antibiotics or if the symptoms prevent children from attending daycare.

P&I is indicated for patients with dacryocystocele and should be performed at the earliest opportunity if digital massage of the nasolacrimal sac fails as there is high risk of dacryocystitis if left untreated.[2]

Nasolacrimal intubation should be considered as a secondary procedure after a failed P&I, or as a primary procedure for patients over 3 years of life when a traditional P&I is more likely to fail.[3,4,5,8] In addition, nasolacrimal intubation can be considered for patients with dacryocystocele who require marsupialization of an intranasal cyst by otolaryngology.

26.6 Contraindications

- Children with acute dacryocystitis should be placed on systemic antibiotics for at least 48 hours prior to proceeding with P&I.
- While epiphora in the first year of life is most commonly caused by congenital nasolacrimal duct obstruction, it is important to rule out congenital glaucoma as a cause. In addition, lid anomalies, such as epiblepharon, and corneal disease can also present with tearing and should be ruled out prior to proceeding with P&I.
- Patients with complete punctal agenesis would require a punctal cut-down to look for elements of the punctal ampulla and canaliculus in order to enable P&I or nasolacrimal intubation; if no proximal lacrimal drainage anatomy is present, a conjunctivodacryocystorhinostomy (Jones tube) would ultimately be required.
- Patients with lacrimal fistulas require complete excision of the fistulous track at the time of surgical management.

26.7 Preoperative Preparation

- It is important to discuss the risk of recurrence with all nasolacrimal duct procedures with the family in anticipation of surgery.[3,4,5,8]
- For very young children, in-office P&I can be performed; however, it becomes increasingly difficult to perform without sedation as children get older.[9,10]
- In typical CNLDO, mask sedation can be used for P&I; however, it is important to limit irrigation as it can cause laryngospasm. If significant irrigation or nasolacrimal intubation is to be performed, then a more secure airway should be established either with a laryngeal mask airway or an endotracheal tube.
- Nasolacrimal intubation can be performed with a variety of stents, including monocanicular and bicanalicular stents utilizing the Rietleng, Crawford, or Masterka systems among others.[8,10,11,12] The type of stent to be used is the surgeon's preference.
- In newborns with dacryocystocele, P&I should ideally be performed prior to discharge from the nursery; alternatively, it can be done in the office without sedation. For these very young children, the combination of topical anesthesia with eye drops, use of a pacifier with sugar water, and swaddling them is usually enough to keep them comfortable and still for the procedure. However, patients with bilateral dacryocystocele will often experience respiratory distress as they are obligate nose breathers. Thus, early intervention in an operating room setting with assistance from an otolaryngologist is essential in order to safely and completely marsupialize the nasal aspect of the cyst.[2]

26.8 Tips and Pearls

- Occasionally, a membrane can be found covering the openings of the puncta. Either a sharp dilator or a safety pin can be used to puncture the membrane prior to proceeding with P&I.
- In choosing which punctum to dilate the nasolacrimal system from, it is felt that performing P&I through the superior punctum is more advantageous as there is less tension applied to the proximal canaliculus when the probe is rotated and passed along the nasolacrimal duct (▶ Fig. 26.1).

However, sometimes the anatomy is such that a "hard stop" cannot easily be reached through the superior punctum; in these situations, probing through the inferior punctum can be performed.

- While introducing the dilator and the probe, lateral traction should be applied to the eyelid. This maneuver stretches the canaliculus and prevents folds along its path to minimize the risk of creating a false passage (▶ Fig. 26.1).
- Starting with the smallest and sharpest dilator can minimize trauma to the proximal nasolacrimal system. Greater dilation can be achieved if one rotates the dilator along its long axis as it is being advanced forward.
- A slight bend, which matches the curvature of the eyelid, can be given to the probe; this can facilitate passage of the probe along the canaliculus.
- A 0 or 00 Bowman probe is usually the appropriate size; if significant tightness is encountered upon entering the canaliculus then a smaller caliber probe should be used.
- Once a "hard stop" has been reached, the probe should be rotated 90° and directed inferiorly toward the nose; it should glide along the nasolacrimal duct (▶ Fig. 26.2). A "soft pop" can be felt as the valve of Hasner is passed.
- If significant tightness is encountered as the probe reaches the distal end of the nasolacrimal duct, there is increased risk of failure of the P&I and one could consider placing a stent at the same time. For this reason, it is reasonable to have patients consented for P&I with possible intubation.
- Following P&I, patency of the nasolacrimal can be confirmed by irrigating the nasolacrimal system with fluorescein-stained saline. When irrigating, it is advised to place a dilator at the opposite punctum to avoid egress of saline from it. Suctioning fluorescein-stained saline through the naris or the oropharynx confirms patency. Alternatively, one can confirm patency with metal-to-metal contact, by leaving the nasolacrimal probe in place and using a second larger probe (e.g., No. 8) to enter the naris, slide under the inferior turbinate, and feeling for the distal end of the probe that is in the nasolacrimal duct (▶ Fig. 26.3).[13]
- If the space under the inferior turbinate is too tight, infracture of the turbinate toward the septum is recommended using a Freer elevator by applying steady and gentle pressure. A slight crack should be felt.

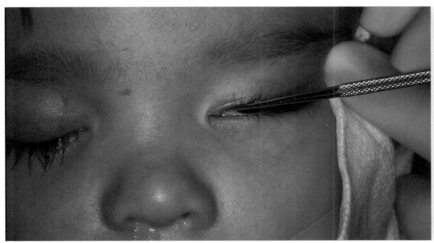

Fig. 26.1 The left upper punctum is being dilated while lateral traction is applied.

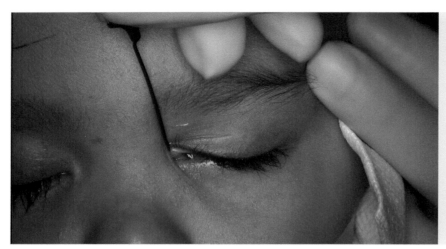

Fig. 26.2 A #0 Bowman probe has been introduced; after reaching a "hard-stop," it is rotated 90 degrees and directed inferiorly toward the nose.

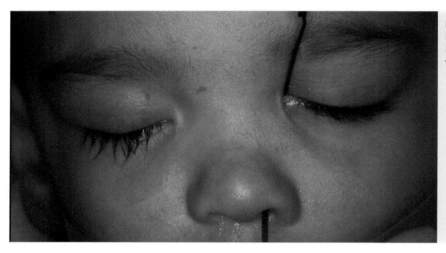

Fig. 26.3 The probe in the nasolacrimal system is left in place, while a large (# 8) Bowman probe is introduced in the nose and patency is confirmed with metal-to-metal contact.

- It can take up to 2 weeks to achieve symptom resolution following a successful P&I.
- For patients undergoing nasolacrimal intubation, a nasal vasoconstrictor, such as oxymetazoline hydrochloride 0.05%, should be administered after anesthesia has been induced. Neurosurgical patties soaked with the nasal vasoconstrictor can be placed underneath the nasal turbinate using bayonet forceps. These maneuvers constrict the nasal mucosa and decrease bleeding.
- When the Ritleng system is used for intubation (▶ Fig. 26.4), it is best to use nontoothed forceps to advance the suture within the Ritleng probe, by grasping the suture almost next to the hub of the probe and advancing the suture only a few millimeters at a time initially. This will prevent kinking of the suture. Once the suture has been advanced, it can be retrieved in the nose with a Ritleng hook (▶ Fig. 26.5).
- The author's personal preference is to use monocanalicular stents, as they are easier to place, do not require a knot in the nose, and the success rate is higher.[12] It is important to ensure that the collarette is properly seated at the punctum, of ten times it requires gentle pushing into the punctum utilizing a dilator while countertraction is provided with forceps. After the collarette has been seated, the tube is trimmed in the nose with scissors (▶ Fig. 26.6).

- If a bicanalicular stent is used then a knot has to be tied in the nose with enough tension to allow the stent to remain within the tear duct system. Pulling the portion of the silicone tube between the two puncta using a large probe or a small muscle hook allows the surgeon to ensure the appropriate tension has been placed when tying the knot in the nose. When the knot is tied, there should be enough laxity to prevent "cheese-wiring" at the proximal part of the nasolacrimal system, but it should also be tight enough to prevent extrusion of the stent.
- A bicanalicular stent that has its ends tied with two simple square knots can easily be removed by cutting the stent between the upper and lower puncta and then pulling on the residual stump from either the upper or lower punctum.
- Most pediatric ophthalmologists recommend leaving silicone tubes in place for 3 to 4 months.[10]
- For probing a dacryocystocele, swaddle the child and use a pacifier with sugar water for comfort. Dilation of the canaliculus can help decompress the dacryocystocele, making the rest of the procedure easier. The smallest probes are typically needed (0000 or 000); they should not be forced in, but rather gently advanced utilizing tactile feedback to guide the probe. Once a distal soft pop has been felt, lift the child upright as they will swallow the fluid that was filling the cyst.

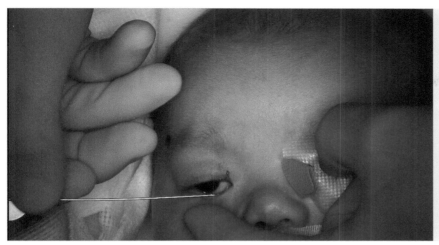

Fig. 26.4 A Ritleng probe for nasolacrimal intubation is being introduced through the lower punctum and is being advanced toward the nasolacrimal sac.

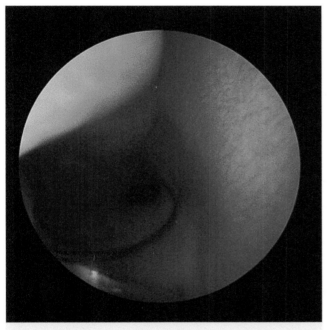

Fig. 26.5 Endoscopic view of the suture of the silicone tube after it has been advanced through a Ritleng probe.

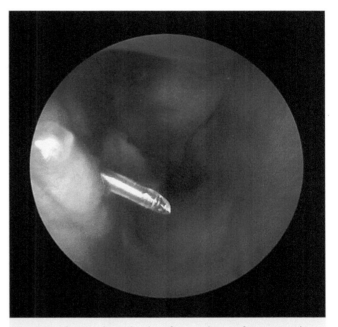

Fig. 26.6 Silicone tube under the inferior turbinate after excess tubing has been trimmed.

It is not uncommon for a dacryocystocele to recur after probing; ask the parents to continue performing Criggler massage and warn them that the child might require an additional probing. In cases of failed probing, the next step is to plan nasolacrimal intubation in the OR with marsupialization of the nasal aspect of the cyst (► Fig. 26.7).

26.9 What to Avoid

The most common mistake novice surgeons make is being too forceful when passing the lacrimal probe, as this can lead to a false passage being created. The probe should essentially glide along the nasolacrimal system. Along those lines, it is just as important to have reached a "hard stop" prior to rotating the probe inferiorly to direct it into the nasolacrimal duct.

26.10 Complications/Bailout/ Salvage

The main complication of P&I is recurrence, which can be as high as 50% if performed after 36 months of life.[3,4,5,8] If symptoms persist after traditional P&I, the use of nasolacrimal balloon dilation or intubation should be considered.[3,4,5,8,14] Patients who remain symptomatic despite nasolacrimal intubation should be evaluated for possible dacryocystorhinostomy, which can be done endoscopically in children.[15]

A false passage can be created if one is too forceful when passing a probe within the nasolacrimal system. If it is suspected that a false passage has been created then placement of a nasolacrimal stent should be considered.

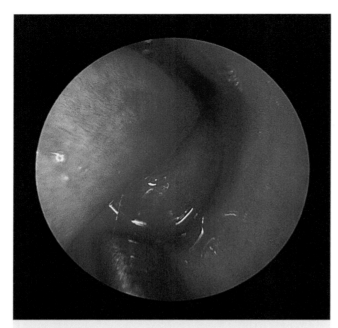

Fig. 26.7 Endoscopic view of the nasal aspect of a dacryocystocele that requires marsupialization.

Nasal bleeding can occur as a result of intranasal manipulation. If it occurs, spraying the nares with a nasal vasoconstrictor, such as oxymetazoline hydrochloride 0.05%, as well as placing neurosurgical patties soaked with the vasoconstrictor in the nose will usually suffice. If bleeding does not stop then nasal packing should be done. Patients who remain symptomatic should be evaluated by otolaryngology for possible cauterization of the bleeding source.

Postoperative infections and dacryocystitis are uncommon. However, should infection occur a culture should be obtained and the patient should be started on topical and systemic antibiotics that cover the usual pathogens for upper respiratory infections according to the guidelines of your hospital. Children under 1 month of life should be admitted for intravenous antibiotics.

A partially extruded nasolacrimal stent requires removal. Parents can tape the part of the stent that has extruded to the skin and bring the child to clinic.

26.11 Postoperative Care

Both P&I and nasolacrimal intubation require minimal postoperative care and most patients return to their usual daily routine almost immediately. A topical antibiotic/steroid combination can be used postoperatively for 5 to 7 days.

References

[1] Petris C, Liu D. Probing for congenital nasolacrimal duct obstruction. Cochrane Database Syst Rev. 2017; 7:CD011109

[2] Wong RK, VanderVeen DK. Presentation and management of congenital dacryocystocele. Pediatrics. 2008; 122(5):e1108–e1112

[3] Repka MX, Chandler DL, Beck RW, et al. Pediatric Eye Disease Investigator Group. Primary treatment of nasolacrimal duct obstruction with probing in children younger than 4 years. Ophthalmology. 2008; 115(3):577–584.e3

[4] Okumuş S, Öner V, Durucu C, et al. Nasolacrimal duct intubation in the treatment of congenital nasolacrimal duct obstruction in older children. Eye (Lond). 2016; 30(1):85–88

[5] Napier ML, Armstrong DJ, McLoone SF, McLoone EM. Congenital nasolacrimal duct obstruction: comparison of two different treatment algorithms. J Pediatr Ophthalmol Strabismus. 2016; 53(5):285–291

[6] Petersen RA, Robb RM. The natural course of congenital obstruction of the nasolacrimal duct. J Pediatr Ophthalmol Strabismus. 1978; 15(4):246–250

[7] Frick KD, Hariharan L, Repka MX, Chandler D, Melia BM, Beck RW, Pediatric Eye Disease Investigator Group (PEDIG). Cost-effectiveness of 2 approaches to managing nasolacrimal duct obstruction in infants: the importance of the spontaneous resolution rate. Arch Ophthalmol. 2011; 129(5):603–609

[8] Repka MX, Melia BM, Beck RW, et al. Pediatric Eye Disease Investigator Group. Primary treatment of nasolacrimal duct obstruction with nasolacrimal duct intubation in children younger than 4 years of age. J AAPOS. 2008; 12(5): 445–450

[9] Lee KA, Chandler DL, Repka MX, et al. PEDIG. A comparison of treatment approaches for bilateral congenital nasolacrimal duct obstruction. Am J Ophthalmol. 2013; 156(5):1045–1050

[10] Dotan G, Nelson LB. Congenital nasolacrimal duct obstruction: common management policies among pediatric ophthalmologists. J Pediatr Ophthalmol Strabismus. 2015; 52(1):14–19

[11] Khatib L, Nazemzadeh M, Revere K, Katowitz WR, Katowitz JA. Use of the Masterka for complex nasolacrimal duct obstruction in children. J AAPOS. 2017; 21(5):380–383

[12] Eustis HS, Nguyen AH. The treatment of congenital nasolacrimal duct obstruction in children: a retrospective review. [Epub ahead of print October 9 2017]. J Pediatr Ophthalmol Strabismus. 2017; •••. DOI: 10.3928/01913913–20170703–08

[13] Mocan MC, Gulmez Sevim D, Kocabeyoglu S, Irkec M. Prognostic value of metal-metal contact during nasolacrimal duct probing. Can J Ophthalmol. 2015; 50(4):314–317

[14] Casady DR, Meyer DR, Simon JW, Stasior GO, Zobal-Ratner JL. Stepwise treatment paradigm for congenital nasolacrimal duct obstruction. Ophthal Plast Reconstr Surg. 2006; 22(4):243–247

[15] Vanderveen DK, Jones DT, Tan H, Petersen RA. Endoscopic dacryocystorhinostomy in children. J AAPOS. 2001; 5(3):143–147

27 Punctoplasty

Larissa H. Habib

Summary

Punctoplasty is a surgical skill which is successful in the treatment of symptomatic epiphora in patients with punctal stenosis with a patent lacrimal system. This in-office procedure is used to widen the punctal opening allowing for more efficient tear drainage. There are minimal complications associated with the procedure. This chapter will discuss in detail the steps of the procedure as well as how to handle complications or restenosis.

Keywords: epiphora, punctal stenosis, punctoplasty

27.1 Goals

- To widen the punctal opening in patients with punctal stenosis.
- To maintain good punctal position against the tear lake.
- To preserve the function of the lacrimal pump.[1]

27.2 Advantages

The three-snip punctoplasty (TSP) is an essential surgical skill for the oculoplastic surgeon in treatment of the patient with symptomatic epiphora due to punctal stenosis with a patent nasolacrimal duct. The advantage of this procedure is that it is minimally invasive with few side effects and can be easily done in the office. TSP results in symptomatic relief in a majority of patients without placement of a foreign body.

27.3 Expectations

- Resolution of symptoms ranges in the literature from 57 to 92%. [2,3,4,5]
- With the subsequent placement of a stent, previously unsuccessful cases had resolution of symptoms in a study by Murdock et al. [2]

27.4 Key Principles

Punctal stenosis results in epiphora due to interruption of the tear drainage system by blocking the entry of tears into the nasolacrimal outflow system. The exact incidence is unknown and ranges in the literature from 8 to 54%.[6] The cause can be congenital or acquired. The most common acquired cause is involutional/idiopathic. Other secondary causes are chronic inflammation (blepharitis), dry eye, trauma, neoplasm, long-standing use of antiglaucoma or chemotherapeutic drops, and radiation.[2,7] In one study of presumed idiopathic punctal stenosis, 47.8% were found to have underlying etiologies for their stenosis through histopathologic examination and direct immunofluorescence.[8]

The clinical understanding of a "normal" punctum is poorly defined in the literature, and it likely is the reason for the wide range of symptomatic relief reported. Optical coherence tomography (OCT) and infrared (IR) imaging studies hope to better predict who will be successful. The diameter just within the punctum may be more predictive of success of the procedure rather than that of the punctal entrance. OCT is also able to measure the intrapunctal tear meniscus, which has been shown to be significantly higher in patients with epiphora when compared to controls, suggesting that there may be a distal obstruction not detected by irrigation alone.[3]

27.5 Indications

- Symptomatic epiphora due to punctal stenosis without distal obstruction and no active secondary process.

27.6 Contraindications

- Ongoing inflammatory process.
- Anatomic abnormalities.
- Suspected neoplasm in the area of punctum.
- Ocular cicatricial pemphigoid in a non-immunomodulated patient.
- Significant dry eye syndrome where punctual occlusion is desirable.

27.7 Preoperative Preparation

The size of the punctal opening should be assessed for stenosis. A thorough ocular exam should be performed to assess for a secondary process resulting in stenosis and which must be treated prior to surgical intervention. The Munk scoring system for epiphora was developed to objectively follow symptoms that range from 0 (no watering) to 5 (constant watering).[9] The nasolacrimal duct must be probed and irrigated to evaluate for distal obstruction.

27.8 Operative Technique

The procedure is most often performed in a minor procedure room setting with local anesthesia. The patient is placed in a supine position. Local anesthetic consisting of 1% lidocaine with 1:100,000 epinephrine is injected to the pericanalicular area. The punctal opening is enlarged circumferentially with a punctal dilator (▶ Fig. 27.1).

A triangular opening is created by three cuts using a Vannas scissor. The first cut is made beginning at the punctal opening extending vertically (▶ Fig. 27.2). A cut is then made along the horizontal canaliculus (▶ Fig. 27.3). The two cuts are then connected to create a triangular enlargement of the punctum (▶ Fig. 27.4). Hemostasis is achieved with direct pressure to the area.

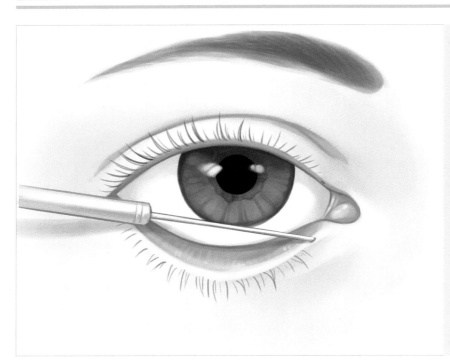

Fig. 27.1 Dilation of the punctum.

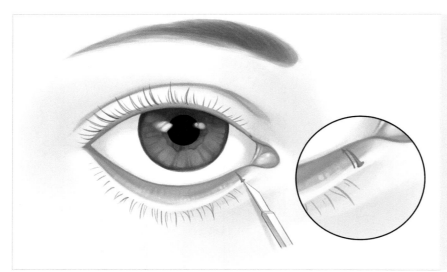

Fig. 27.2 Vertical incision beginning at the punctal margin.

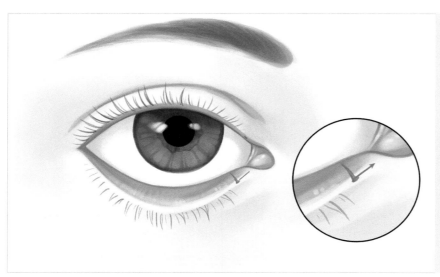

Fig. 27.3 Horizontal incision along the canaliculus.

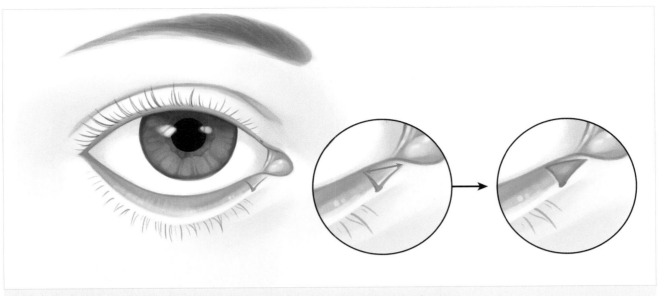

Fig. 27.4 Incision along the base of the tissue flap connecting the two incisions and excising the tissue.

27.9 Tips and Pearls

- In patients with restenosis after punctoplasty due to cicatrix, an in-office redilation of the punctum has been shown to achieve a 95.5% resolution of symptoms and 100% anatomic success.[10]
- A variety of techniques have been described in the literature to attempt to avoid scarring.
  - A rectangular opening can be created with two vertical incisions and a horizontal incision to connect them at the base rather than the traditional triangular excision described above.
  - A Kelly punch has also been used to create the opening.[11]
  - Placement of a monocanalicular stent, such as a mini-Monoka tube, with suture fixation, if needed, may result in a more perfectly round punctum after the procedure and prevent restenosis. The stent is removed 2 to 3 weeks after surgery.

27.10 What to Avoid

It is important to avoid excising too much tissue. This may result in damage to the lacrimal pump mechanism, leading to an increase in functional epiphora.

27.11 Complications/ Bailout/ Salvage

- Restenosis due to healing and scarring at the apposed edges occurs in about 5 to 14% of patients.[2,4] Options for prevention of restenosis include mitomycin C, bicanalicular stent, or mini-Monoka placement.[12,13,14]
  - In a comparison of TSP alone versus in combination with a bicanalicular stent, Calvatzis et al. found better functional

and anatomical results in the stent group; however, 25% required reintroduction of the stents.[12]
- Damage to the lacrimal pump can result in functional epiphora in as high as 10.3%.[4] To avoid this, a rectangular TSP can be considered. Chak et al found a higher success rate with this procedure when compared with the traditional triangular approach as described above, though it was not statistically significant.[15]

27.12 Postoperative Care

Direct pressure is done immediately after the procedure for hemostasis. An antibiotic/steroid combination drop should be used three times a day for 1 week to guard against infection and aggressive inflammation. The patient should be watched closely to assess for symptomatic improvement and the need for further intervention.

References

[1] Kashkouli MB, Beigi B, Astbury N. Acquired external punctal stenosis: surgical management and long-term follow-up. Orbit. 2005; 24(2):73–78

[2] Murdock J, Lee WW, Zatezalo CC, Ballin A. Three-snip punctoplasty outcome rates and follow-up treatments. Orbit. 2015; 34(3):160–163

[3] Timlin HM, Keane PA, Rose GE, Ezra DG. The application of infrared imaging and optical coherence tomography of the lacrimal punctum in patients undergoing punctoplasty for epiphora. Ophthalmology. 2017; 124(6):910–917

[4] Ali MJ, Ayyar A, Naik MN. Outcomes of rectangular 3-snip punctoplasty in acquired punctal stenosis: is there a need to be minimally invasive? Eye (Lond). 2015; 29(4):515–518

[5] Caesar RH, McNab AA. A brief history of punctoplasty: the 3-snip revisited. Eye (Lond). 2005; 19(1):16–18

[6] Soiberman U, Kakizaki H, Selva D, Leibovitch I. Punctal stenosis: definition, diagnosis, and treatment. Clin Ophthalmol. 2012; 6:1011–1018

[7] Kashkouli MB, Beigi B, Murthy R, Astbury N. Acquired external punctal stenosis: etiology and associated findings. Am J Ophthalmol. 2003; 136(6):1079–1084

[8] Reddy AK, Baker MS, Maltry AC, Syed NA, Allen RC. Immunopathology and histopathology of conjunctival biopsies in patients with presumed idiopathic punctal stenosis. Br J Ophthalmol. 2017; 101(2):213–217

[9] Munk PL, Lin DT, Morris DC. Epiphora: treatment by means of dacryocystoplasty with balloon dilation of the nasolacrimal drainage apparatus. Radiology. 1990; 177(3):687–690

[10] Fraser CE, Petrakos P, Lelli GJ, Jr. Adjunctive re-dilation for early cicatrization after punctoplasty. Orbit. 2012; 31(5):313–315

[11] Wong ES, Li EY, Yuen HK. Long-term outcomes of punch punctoplasty with Kelly punch and review of literature. Eye (Lond). 2017; 31(4):560–565

[12] Chalvatzis NT, Tzamalis AK, Mavrikakis I, Tsinopoulos I, Dimitrakos S. Self-retaining bicanaliculus stents as an adjunct to 3-snip punctoplasty in management of upper lacrimal duct stenosis: a comparison to standard 3-snip procedure. Ophthal Plast Reconstr Surg. 2013; 29(2):123–127

[13] Konuk O, Urgancioglu B, Unal M. Long-term success rate of perforated punctal plugs in the management of acquired punctal stenosis. Ophthal Plast Reconstr Surg. 2008; 24(5):399–402

[14] Hussain RN, Kanani H, McMullan T. Use of mini-monoka stents for punctal/canalicular stenosis. Br J Ophthalmol. 2012; 96(5):671–673

[15] Chak M, Irvine F. Rectangular 3-snip punctoplasty outcomes: preservation of the lacrimal pump in punctoplasty surgery. Ophthal Plast Reconstr Surg. 2009; 25(2):134–135

28 External Dacryocystorhinostomy (DCR)

Suzanne K. Freitag and Michael K. Yoon

Abstract

External dacryocystorhinostomy is a traditional lacrimal bypass surgery used to treat epiphora or dacryocystitis due to nasolacrimal obstruction at the level of the lacrimal sac or nasolacrimal duct. It requires a patent and functioning upper lacrimal system. The surgery has a steep learning curve, and many peri- and intraoperative considerations are important to help ensure a high rate of success.

Keywords: DCR, external dacryocystorhinostomy, dacryocystitis, epiphora, lacrimal, nasolacrimal obstruction

28.1 Goals

The purpose of dacryocystorhinostomy (DCR) is to alleviate epiphora or dacryocystitis and restore lacrimal outflow by anatomically bypassing a distal lacrimal obstruction via a fistula from the lacrimal sac to the middle meatus of the nose.

28.2 Advantages

External DCR was first described in 1904 by Toti and over the subsequent decades has become a mainstay of treatment for complete or significant partial nasolacrimal obstruction causing epiphora and/or infection of the lacrimal sac. Unlike endoscopic DCR, external DCR does not rely on expensive, highly technical instrumentation and electronic endoscopic video systems. External DCR can be performed with a basic instrument set, which is particularly useful in areas where there may be few resources.

28.3 Expectations

Although the procedure has a steep learning curve and requires a solid understanding of the anatomy of the nose, lacrimal outflow system, and medial canthus, once the basics are mastered, a high success rate is expected. It has become a routine procedure in the armamentarium of the ophthalmic plastic surgeon, and has the benefit of over 100 years of commonplace use, resulting in a vast body of knowledge and medical literature. The success rate of this surgery is reported to be over 90%, based on a variety of outcome measures including relief of epiphora, resolution of infection, and demonstration of lacrimal patency with dye disappearance testing or lacrimal irrigation. This is generally 10% higher than the reported rates for endoscopic DCR, although in highly experienced hands and with modern endonasal technology, the rates may be similar.

28.4 Key Principles

- Preoperative planning with lacrimal irrigation, and in select cases CT scan, is important to arrive at an appropriate diagnosis.
- Hemostasis is critical for intraoperative visualization, minimization of surgical duration, and anatomic success.
- A larger osteotomy (and corresponding mucosal fistula) may contribute to a higher success rate.

- Gentle handling of mucosal tissues is key to minimize undue iatrogenic inflammation of the flaps that may incite scarring and reduce fistula size.
- Placement of silicone lacrimal stents is important for anatomic success, and these stents are left in place between 3 and 8 weeks on average.

28.5 Indications

DCR is indicated for nasolacrimal obstruction resulting in epiphora or dacryocystitis. It is important to note that the majority of patients with complaints of epiphora do not have nasolacrimal obstruction, but rather one of the myriad causes of epiphora including secondary hypersecretion or, less commonly, proximal lacrimal outflow obstruction. In cases of epiphora without obvious infection, lacrimal irrigation in the office setting is essential to confirm and localize anatomic obstruction (► Fig. 28.1). When dacryocystitis is suspected, the diagnosis is

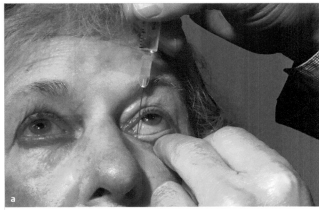

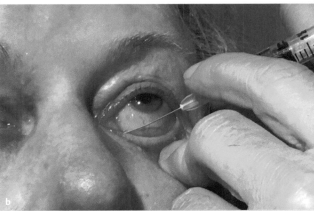

Fig. 28.1 Nasolacrimal irrigation is performed with a saline-filled 3 mL syringe and 26-gauge lacrimal cannula. **(a)** With the lower lid on stretch, the cannula is vertically inserted into the punctum. **(b)** The cannula is then oriented horizontally and advanced to the mid-canalicular area and the plunger is depressed. (From Bleier B, Freitag S, Sacks R. Endoscopic Surgery of the Orbit: Anatomy, Pathology, and Management. New York: Thieme Medical Publishers; 2018.)

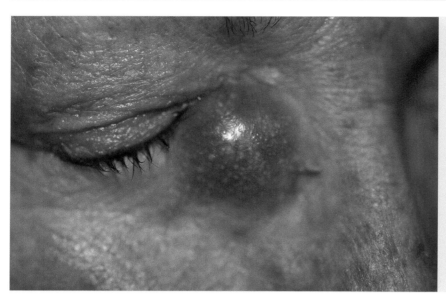

Fig. 28.2 External photograph demonstrating right dacryocystitis. The lacrimal sac is distended with overlying cutaneous erythema.

confirmed when there is pain, erythema, or palpable mass in the area of the lacrimal sac with purulent discharge expressed from the puncta with pressure on the lacrimal sac (▶ Fig. 28.2). It is best to allow a hyperacute infection to improve with systemic antibiotics prior to undertaking external DCR, as the inflamed, friable tissues may tear when they are handled, may not hold sutures well, or could scar together, resulting in a decreased chance of surgical success.

28.6 Contraindications

DCR success requires a functioning upper lacrimal system including puncta, canaliculi, and common canaliculus. Patients with upper system obstruction may be candidates for conjunctivodacryocystorhinostomy (CDCR) with Jones tube, as this creates a bypass of the entire lacrimal system from ocular surface to nose. A functioning lacrimal pump is also required to move tears into the lacrimal sac; hence, patients with epiphora secondary to facial paralysis should not expect to see improvement after DCR.

28.7 Preoperative Preparation

Careful planning with regard to many details is critical to ensure success in DCR surgery. Patients must be medically fit for a surgical procedure under anesthesia, typically general anesthesia. Maintaining hemostasis is important intra- and postoperatively; therefore, bleeding risks, including thrombocytopenia, clotting disorders, and use of anticoagulant or antiplatelet medications should be screened for prior to surgery. If DCR surgery is necessary, then steps should be taken to minimize these risks, including platelet transfusion, cessation of anticoagulant medications, and sometimes even consideration of type and crossing for possible transfusion. These should all be done with the permission and supervision of the primary medical doctor. Preoperative computed tomography (CT) scans are not universally necessary in cases of primary acquired nasolacrimal duct obstruction. However, in cases of known or suspected trauma, malignancy, chronic inflammation, visible/palpable mass, or in otherwise atypical presentations (e.g., unilateral tearing in a 20-year-old man), sinus or maxillofacial CT scan protocol is recommended (▶ Fig. 28.3).

28.8 Operative Technique

After the patient is placed under general anesthesia, the incision site is marked. A traditional incision is started 1 cm medial to the medial commissure of the eyelids and extends inferior and lateral about 1.5 cm. Some surgeons prefer placement of the incision in the tear trough.[1] The area underlying the incision is infiltrated with local anesthetic with epinephrine. A vasoconstrictive agent such as 4% cocaine solution or oxymetazoline is placed on neuropatties in the middle meatus of the nose. Consideration should be given to intraoperative intravenous antibiotic, especially in cases of current infection. The patient is prepped and draped in a sterile fashion and a scleral protective cover is placed over the eye. The incision should be made when bipolar cautery and suction with a small Fraser tip are available. After the skin is incised with a 15-blade, blunt scissors are used to spread to the periosteum of the anterior lacrimal crest. The periosteum is incised with a 15-blade and a Freer elevator is used to lift the periosteum attached to the lacrimal sac off the bone of the lacrimal sac fossa. With the sac reflected laterally, an instrument such as a small curved hemostat is used to gently fracture the lacrimal bone with care to preserve the nasal mucosa. A Kerrison rongeur is used to create an approximately 1 cm osteotomy involving the lacrimal sac fossa including the anterior and posterior lacrimal crests. A bicanalicular silicone lacrimal tube is placed into the upper and lower canaliculi and is used to tent the lacrimal sac away from the common canaliculus. An 11-blade or 15-degree cataract incision blade is used to incise the lacrimal sac and make H-shaped incisions to create anterior and posterior flaps. The neuropatties are removed from the nose, and a blade and Westcott scissors are used to make corresponding H-shaped nasal mucosal incisions to create anterior and posterior flaps. The metal probe ends of the

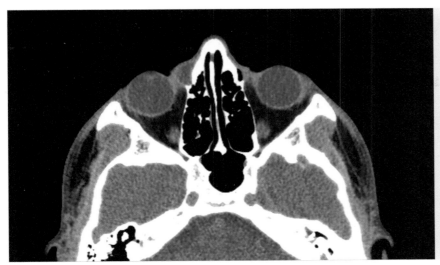

Fig. 28.3 Axial computed tomography of a 20-year-old male with clinical evidence of dacryocystitis, demonstrating distention of the right lacrimal sac.

silicone tubes are passed through the newly created openings and out the nose. The metal probes are removed and the tube is carefully tensioned and fixated. Absorbable suture such as 4–0 chromic gut on a small curved needle such as a P-2 or G-2 is used to anastomose the flaps. Often the posterior flaps are not sewn, but the anterior lacrimal sac flap should be sutured to the anterior nasal mucosal flap. The muscle and skin are closed in two layers using absorbable suture. Topical antibiotic is applied to the incision. ► Fig. 28.4 demonstrates the steps of the procedure.

28.9 Tips and Pearls

- Meticulous intraoperative hemostasis is important for both expedient and successful DCR surgery. Operative times directly parallel time spent controlling bleeding. Further, bleeding results in more difficult visualization of the narrow and deep operative field, and can result in less technical precision and a lower chance of surgical success. Appropriate measures should be taken preoperatively to safely discontinue anticoagulant medications and screen for a history of bleeding disorders or thrombocytopenia. Intra- and postoperative blood pressure control is important. Placement of nasal vasoconstrictive agents such as 4% cocaine solution or oxymetazoline on ½ x 3 inch neuropatties is important. Injection of local anesthetic containing epinephrine into the involved mucosal surfaces is also useful.
- General anesthesia is preferred for DCR surgery for a number of reasons. Sedated patients who are having pain will develop an associated rise in blood pressure, resulting in more bleeding. Also, there is the potential for blood loss into the nasopharynx and airway in DCR surgery and patients who are sedated but not intubated may be at risk for aspiration. However, if a patient has medical comorbidities that make general anesthesia highly risky, then external DCR may be performed with monitored anesthesia care plus local anesthesia.
- Osteotomy patency plays a critical role in DCR surgical success. A common teaching is that the osteotomy will shrink by about 50% after surgery; hence, a large osteotomy is required in order to retain patency long term.[2] Many recommend a 1 cm osteotomy, although there are regional trends for much larger openings. With this comes a higher risk of damage to adjacent structures and cerebrospinal fluid (CSF) leak.
- Consideration should be given to sending a small sample of lacrimal sac tissue, and possibly nasal mucosal tissue as well, for histopathologic evaluation. Studies have shown that between 3.3[3] and 8.2%[4] of specimens will have a specific diagnosis other than acute and chronic inflammation. In addition, if purulence is found upon opening of the lacrimal sac, a swab should be sent to microbiology for Gram stain, aerobic and anaerobic cultures, and sensitivities so that antimicrobial therapy can be tailored.
- Once the osteotomy has been started and the rongeur has removed sufficient bone to allow for visualization of the intact nasal mucosa, local anesthetic containing epinephrine may be injected into the nasal mucosa using a 30 gauge ½ inch needle to provide hemostasis for when the mucosa is incised to create flaps. Since epinephrine takes 10 minutes to provide vasoconstriction, injection as soon as the mucosa is visualized is recommended for maximal effectiveness.
- Careful creation of nasal mucosal flaps is often quite difficult in DCR surgery due to the friable nature of the tissue. Placement of an instrument such as a Freer elevator up the nostril and directly adjacent to the intact nasal mucosa at the osteotomy site will allow for a more controlled incision.

28.10 What to Avoid

One of the most common mistakes of the novice (and experienced!) DCR surgeon is damaging the nasal mucosa at the time of bone puncture during initiation of the osteotomy. This can make creation of nasal mucosal flaps nearly impossible, which some feel decreases the chances of surgical success. Further complicating this step, there is variability among patients with regard to the thickness of this bone, with younger patients and those with flat nasal bridges having thicker bone than others.

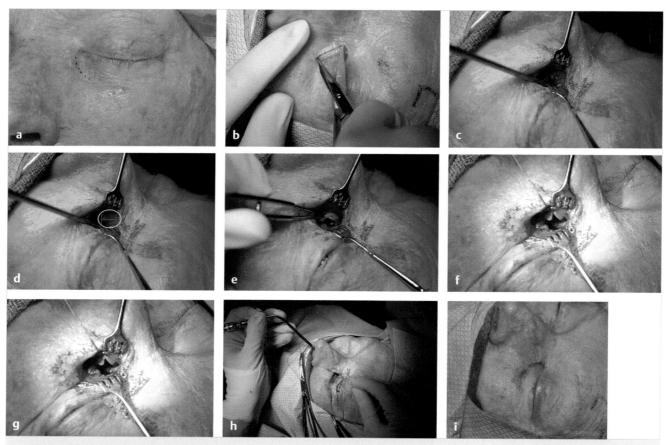

Fig. 28.4 **(a)** A tear trough incision is marked. It is placed in the medial aspect at the junction of the thin eyelid skin and the thicker cheek/nasal skin. **(b)** After the incision is made, blunt dissection is made through the orbicularis oculi muscle to the periosteum of the medial inferior orbital rim. **(c)** The osteotomy is complete. The anterior lacrimal crest has been removed. The intact nasal mucosa is intact and has been infiltrated with local anesthetic giving a blanched appearance. **(d)** The same figure with a yellow line outlining the bounds of the osteotomy. The planned "H" shaped incision is drawn in blue. **(e)** Following the incision through the nasal mucosa, it is reflected toward the incision. The anterior nasal mucosal flap is grasped with forceps. The posterior nasal mucosa flap is seen below this. The blue line deep to the nasal mucosa is the colored portion of the nasal packing. **(f)** After the nasal mucosa and the lacrimal sac have both been incised with flaps created. The posterior flaps have been sutured together and is seen deeper in the incision. **(g)** The same figure with markups. The # marks a 4–-0 chronic gut suture through the anterior nasal mucosa flap. The ^ marks a 4–-0 chromic gut suture through the anterior lacrimal sac flap. The * marks the suture apposing the posterior nasal mucosa and lacrimal sac flaps. **(h)** Prior to suturing the anterior flaps, the lacrimal stent is introduced through the upper punctum and canaliculus. It is then directed through the fistula. A suction tip is introduced through the nares and up to the fistula site. The stent is directed into the suction tip to aid in an atraumatic removal of the stent. **(i)** After closure of the anterior flaps, the skin is closed with an interrupted 6–0 fast-absorbing gut suture.

There are several options for making a controlled point of entry into the bone of the lacrimal sac fossa. Some surgeons use a powered drill to thin this bone, while most surgeons use an instrument such as a curved hemostat to carefully infracture the bone while exerting control to not allow the instrument to pass more than a millimeter or so into the nasal cavity.

28.11 Complications/Bailout/Salvage

Potential complications of DCR surgery include failure to solve the problem, resulting in recurrence of epiphora or dacryocystitis; intraorbital hemorrhage; epistaxis; wound dehiscence; medial canthal webbing/cutaneous scarring (► Fig. 28.5); intranasal synechiae; corneal abrasion; ocular irritation from stent tube; orbital emphysema; slit puncta; medial tube migration; tube extrusion; premature loss of tube; punctal inflammation or granuloma formation from tube; lacrimal sump syndrome.

If a patient is found to have a recurrence of epiphora in the early postoperative period, lacrimal irrigation may be performed with the tube in place to determine the patency of the system. If there is poor flow of irrigant, consideration may be given to topical steroid and/or antibiotic to shrink swelling within the system and to eradicate any bacterial overgrowth. If dacryocystitis occurs in the postoperative period, cultures may be considered and oral antibiotics prescribed. Consideration should be given to leaving stent tubes in place during such episodes, as the risk of surgical failure is high if the stents are removed when the system is inflamed.

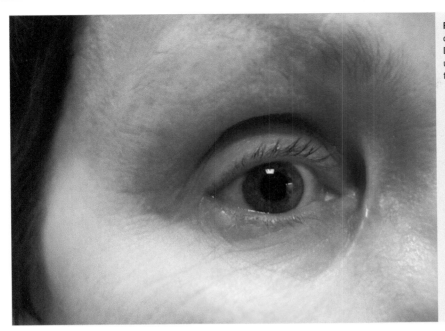

Fig. 28.5 External photograph demonstrating cutaneous web formation 1 year after external DCR. The web extends from the incision site upward through the medial canthus and exerts traction in the sub-brow area.

Postoperative epistaxis often occurs when there is inadvertent damage to uninvolved areas of the nose, such as the middle turbinate or the nasal septum. Meticulous dissection is key to prevent this. In addition, careful placement of the packing of middle meatus with adequate neuropatties can prevent inadvertent injury to these areas during nasal mucosal incision.

With regard to stent tube migration and extrusion, prevention is the best option. Careful fixation of the tube at the appropriate tension at the time of surgery is critical to maintenance of optimal tube position during the postoperative period. Options include suture fixation of the stent to the nasal side wall, tying multiple knots in the stent at a carefully determined location, or placing a sliding foam bolster (retinal scleral buckle sponge) at a location resulting in the desired tube tension and then tying a series of knots below the bolster. If a tube is migrating medially or causing punctal irritation or granuloma formation (▶ Fig. 28.6), recommendation is for early tube removal. If the tube loop is extruding (▶ Fig. 28.7), it may be reposited with forceps or, if this fails, may be grasped via the nose with endoscopic guidance.

Lacrimal sump syndrome occurs after surgery in which there is a large residual cavity that collects tears and mucoid debris. This can occur if there is a large amount of lacrimal sac left in place, or if the osteum is too superior or small. Additional surgery may be required to alleviate this problem.

28.12 Postoperative Care

- Patients should avoid drinking hot beverages and taking hot showers in the immediate postoperative period to avoid the risk of vasodilation and epistaxis.
- Patients should limit strenuous physical activity for 2 weeks after surgery to avoid hemorrhage.
- Ice packs may be gently placed over the cutaneous incision for the first 48 hours after surgery.
- Eyeglasses should be worn with care, if at all, in the days following surgery if the nosepiece of the glasses rests close to the cutaneous incision.
- Oral antibiotics for 5 to 7 days postoperatively should be considered, especially if purulent material is found in the lacrimal sac at the time of surgery.
- Topical ophthalmic ointment is helpful during the first week after surgery to lubricate the ocular surface, making the tube loop more comfortable; the moisture will help moisturize the cutaneous incision during healing.
- Patients should avoid nose blowing for several weeks after surgery due to the risk of hemorrhage, blowing air via the osteotomy into the orbit resulting in orbital emphysema (which can cause diplopia and pain), and stretching the stent tubing resulting in slit puncta and migration of the tube loop.
- Anticoagulant medications should be resumed as planned preoperatively in consultation with the prescribing physician.

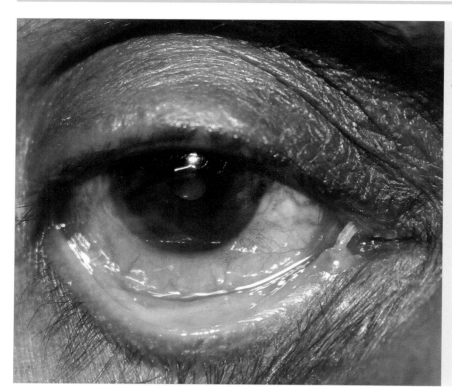

Fig. 28.6 External photograph with manual distraction of the right lower eyelid demonstrating granuloma formation around a silicone bicanalicular lacrimal tube. Photo courtesy of Dr. Mohammad Javed Ali.

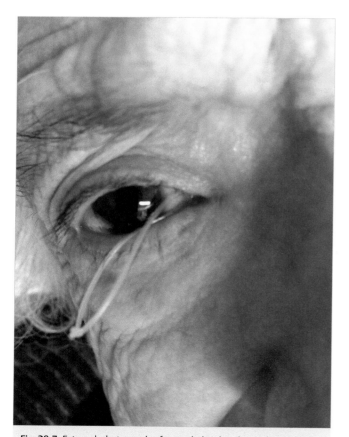

Fig. 28.7 External photograph of extruded right silicone bicanalicular lacrimal tube.

- Postoperative pain management should not include non-steroidal anti-inflammatory drugs, as this increases the risk of postoperative hemorrhage.
- Patients should follow up in several weeks and then again in approximately 2 months for stent tube removal. They should be reassured that the cutaneous incision will fade in most individuals to being nearly invisible within weeks to months.

References

[1] Davies BW, McCracken MS, Hawes MJ, Hink EM, Durairaj VD, Pelton RW. Tear trough incision for external dacryocystorhinostomy. Ophthal Plast Reconstr Surg. 2015; 31(4):278–281

[2] Ben Simon GJ, Brown C, McNab AA. Larger osteotomies result in larger ostia in external dacryocystorhinostomies. Arch Facial Plast Surg. 2012; 14(2): 127–131

[3] Bernardini FP, Moin M, Kersten RC, Reeves D, Kulwin DR. Routine histopathologic evaluation of the lacrimal sac during dacryocystorhinostomy: how useful is it? Ophthalmology. 2002; 109(7):1214–1217, discussion 1217–1218

[4] Anderson NG, Wojno TH, Grossniklaus HE. Clinicopathologic findings from lacrimal sac biopsy specimens obtained during dacryocystorhinostomy. Ophthal Plast Reconstr Surg. 2003; 19(3):173–176

29 Endoscopic Dacryocystorhinostomy

Daniel R. Lefebvre

Summary

Endoscopic dacryocystorhinostomy (DCR) is becoming ever more popular as patients seek minimally invasive options for surgical procedures. As instrumentation and surgical techniques have advanced, the success rates of endoscopic DCR performed by experienced surgeons is at least equivalent to that of traditional external DCR surgery. Many oculoplastic surgeons, in transitioning from external to endoscopic technique, may employ the use of a "light pipe" to transilluminate the lacrimal sac fossa endonasally. This can be helpful, but can also potentially misdirect the surgeon to make the osteotomy more inferiorly and posteriorly than is ideal if one does not fully understand the relevant anatomy. This chapter serves to outline some of these considerations, as well as to describe the author's surgical technique, to aid the surgeon engaging in endoscopic DCR surgery.

Keywords: endoscopic dacryocystorhinostomy, endoscopic DCR, dacryocystorhinostomy, DCR, nasolacrimal duct obstruction

29.1 Goals

Dacryocystorhinostomy (DCR) is the standard surgical correction for nasolacrimal duct obstruction in the setting of patent canaliculi to resolve problematic epiphora. The basic surgical concept dates back over one-hundred years,[1] and has been modified over time. The majority of DCR surgery over the past few decades has been performed externally (extDCR) via a skin incision placed near the tear trough/lower medial canthal region with generally great success. As patients and surgeons alike have aimed for more minimally invasive approaches, endoscopic DCR (enDCR) has become more popular. There was a period when enDCR was considered a second-rate "trade-off" procedure in which the patient was exchanging lack of a skin incision scar for a lower surgical success rate; however, with modern instrumentation and technique, this is no longer the case, as success rates for extDCR and mechanical enDCR are equivalent.[2] Today, both external and endoscopic DCR are excellent procedures and both are within the standard of care to be offered to patients based upon patient preference and surgeon comfort and personal outcome measures.

Note that the present report concerns mechanical enDCR only, not laser-assisted DCR.

29.2 Advantages

The most oft-cited advantage of enDCR over extDCR is lack of a "scar"; however, it must be acknowledged that the extDCR incision generally heals quite well with high patient satisfaction.[3] The author considers the main advantages of enDCR to be lack of external facial incision (and thus lack of external bruising, edema, or potential wound infection); lack of disruption of orbicularis oculi muscle and potential tear-pump dysfunction[4]; wide-view, magnified, high-definition visualization of the surgical site; potential to address other intranasal factors relevant to surgical success such as nasal septal deviation, concha bullosa of middle turbinate, etc.

29.3 Expectations

As in all surgical procedures, it is important to set patient expectations ahead of time. While modern enDCR performed by an experienced surgeon with the right equipment has very high success, this is not true if performed by a novice surgeon transitioning from extDCR. The success rates quoted in the literature do not apply to that individual; thus, an individual surgeon should have a sense for his or her personal success rate. The goal should be to reliably achieve success at least comparable to the reported literature, and to do so may require training courses, practice, mentorship, etc.

If one assumes a 90% success rate, it still means that one out of ten patients will "fail" the surgery, meaning they will continue to experience problematic tearing. This can be in the setting of a scarred DCR ostium, or in the setting of a patent DCR ostium (in which case the tearing is multifactorial, and particularly difficult to remedy). This should be discussed with patients preoperatively. The author will often use the example that the DCR surgery involves creating a hole in the blocked tear drain—the body views this hole as a wound and tries to "heal" it closed, and when it does close the surgery fails. This is one of the reasons stents and absorbable packing materials, etc. may be placed within the ostium—that is, to prevent the body from "healing" the ostium (fistula) closed.

Patients should also be warned about the possibility of early stent prolapse or loss, epistaxis, nasal congestion, sinusitis, cerebrospinal fluid leak, the possibility of air reflux from a lacrimal punctum when blowing the nose, and possible need for additional surgery, whenever preoperative counseling is performed.

29.4 Key Principles

The main principle of DCR, whether external or endoscopic, is to establish a patent and permanent internal fistula between the lacrimal sac and the nasal cavity for effective tear drainage.

29.5 Indications

enDCR is appropriate for any and all patients with nasolacrimal duct obstruction whether congenital, primary acquired, or secondary. The author no longer performs extDCR.

29.6 Contraindications

DCR, whether external or endoscopic, should be delayed when there is a recent history of cancer excision surgery in the medial canthal/lacrimal sac area in adherence to the oncologic principle of not violating bone and periosteum between a cavity involved with malignancy and cavity uninvolved, with the concern being that the DCR osteotomy could open a pathway for a cancer recurrence to enter the nasal cavity. The exact timeframe for which to wait between cancer treatment and lacrimal surgery ranges from 1 year to never, depending on the authority queried. The author addresses this situation on a case-by-case basis, and this analysis involves serial imaging (CT and MR), sometimes a surveillance biopsy, etc., with the earliest intervention occurring 1 year after cancer treatment.

In the setting of acute dacryocystitis, the author prefers to administer systemic antibiotics and treat the active fulminant infection and allow the inflammation to settle prior to undertaking surgery. Incision and drainage is performed if there is a pointing abscess or if the infection has failed empiric treatment.

29.7 Preoperative Preparation

A history of dacryocystitis connotes nasolacrimal duct obstruction, and thus the author does not routinely perform nasolacrimal irrigation on these patients.

The evaluation of the tearing patient otherwise includes the assessment of the tearing history (does it occur at all times? Intermittently? Every day? Is there discharge? Do the eyes itch or burn? Is there a history of trauma or prior surgery?) A history of radioactive iodine therapy, particularly high-dose radioactive iodine therapy as used for treatment of thyroid cancer, is highly associated with secondary nasolacrimal duct obstruction.[5] Eyelids are assessed for laxity, which if severe may be addressed at the time of DCR surgery. A history of chronic rhinosinusitis is ascertained; if present, a CT scan may be obtained, and if significant sinus disease is noted, enDCR may be performed in collaboration with an otolaryngologist for simultaneous functional endoscopic sinus surgery. Otherwise the author does not routinely obtain CT scan on all patients unless the patient has an unusual circumstance (young age; history of trauma or prior surgery; bloody tears; mass; etc.)

Nasal endoscopy is performed on all patients preoperatively. This is important for many reasons. First, the overall surgical anatomy may be assessed, in particular the status of the nasal septum (whether there is deviation blocking access to the nasal sidewall and maxillary line that would limit the ability to perform surgery and also raise the risk of postoperative scarring and surgical failure; whether there is a concha bullosa of the middle turbinate that blocks the maxillary line and would interfere with the DCR ostium). In addition, the general health of the nasal cavity can be assessed, looking for the status of the mucosa, evidence of polyps, mucopus, adhesions, ulceration, melanosis, bleeding, tumor, etc. It is important that any abnormality should be investigated by referral to an otolaryngologist. One can learn diagnostic nasal endoscopy technique by working with an otolaryngologist mentor and studying a rhinology atlas. Compact self-contained video-endoscopy units are available for the office setting that work quite well.

29.8 Operative Technique

- The patient is supine on the operating table and placed under general endotracheal anesthesia. A time-out is observed. The bilateral nasal cavities are packed with neurosurgical cottonoids soaked in oxymetazoline. The patient is draped in

the usual sterile fashion. If the patient has a prosthetic heart valve or joint, a systemic antibiotic is administered intravenously.
- A zero-degree rigid video endoscope system is used throughout the procedure, occasionally augmented with a 30-degree endoscope for better lateral visualization.
- The eyes are treated with a topical anesthetic such as proparacaine eye drops, and corneoscleral protecting shields are placed. The upper and lower puncta of the operative side are dilated.
- A light pipe (such as a 23-gauge vitrectomy endoilluminator) may be used to aid with endonasal confirmation of the lacrimal sac anatomy, although care must be taken with this step as will be described later. The light pipe is connected to a headlight light source and the light pipe can be advanced through the lower canaliculus to a hard stop with the pipe maintained in a horizontal position. The tip of the light pipe should be maintained against the hard stop and not allowed to rest within the soft tissues as thermal injury to the canaliculi could result. The light source should be kept on a relatively lower power setting such as 25% to further reduce the risk of thermal injury to lacrimal soft tissues.
- The nasal packing is removed and the endoscope is introduced into the nasal cavity. A bilateral intranasal examination may be performed. The transillumination may be visualized at this time, and reducing the endoscope illumination may be necessary temporarily to adequately see this. It is not uncommon to see all of the transillumination sharply posterior to the maxillary line, completely within the middle meatus under the middle turbinate (▶ Fig. 29.1). This is because the posterior lacrimal sac fossa (lacrimal bone) is quite thin and readily transmits the light, while the anterior lacrimal sac fossa (frontal process of the maxilla) is thicker and blocks light. Further, the light pipe will often have a posterior angulation due to the ergonomics of passing it over the ocular surface, brow, or cheekbone, which directs the

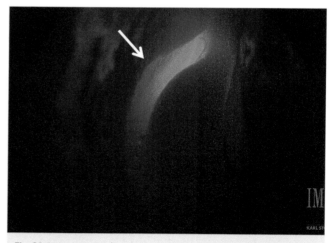

Fig. 29.1 An intranasal endoscopic view of right nasal sidewall. *Arrow* shows maxillary line. The endoscope light has been turned off to maximize visualization of lacrimal sac transillumination, which is seen occurring sharply posterior to the maxillary line. If the osteotomy was made only over the transillumination, this would be incorrectly limited to too inferior and posterior in location with increased likelihood of failure.

illumination posteriorly. Thus, it is important to note that the visualized light gives an accurate latitude or cranio-caudal position of the lacrimal sac, but the sagittal center of the lacrimal sac is not the visualized light but actually more closely the maxillary line (▶ Fig. 29.2).[6]

- The nasal septum, nasal sidewall at the maxillary line and root of the inferior turbinate, and middle turbinate are injected with 1% lidocaine with epinephrine 1:100,000 via a long 25-gauge needle. It is beneficial to wait 5 minutes to effect maximal hemostasis. Often the oxymetazoline cottonoids can be replaced at this time, and equipment, such as the drill, may be set up during this waiting period. The light pipe can be turned off during this time.
- Once the cottonoids are removed, surgery commences using a #15 blade to create bilobed interlacing posteriorly based rectangular flaps over the fundus of the lacrimal sac (extending from just anterior to the maxillary line posteriorly to the axilla of the middle turbinate) and then a vertical incision proceeding inferiorly along the maxillary line from the middle of the above flap down to just above the root of the inferior turbinate.[7] Alternatively, a singular posteriorly based flap can be created (▶ Fig. 29.3). A periosteal elevator is used to develop the flaps, and the superior flap is reflected posteriorly; the inferior flap is reflected anteriorly and inferiorly (if a single flap is employed, it is reflected posteriorly and may be "tucked" under the middle turbinate during surgery). This exposes a wide section of maxillary bone. The maxillary line is now well-visualized directly, and the light source may be turned on again, usually showing posterior to the maxillary line. The author begins drilling

away the thick bone of the anterior lacrimal sac maxillary bone with a diamond coated high-speed drill, working toward the lacrimal bone and light source posteriorly, thus staying out of the middle meatus directly. As the anterior lacrimal sac bone is thinned with the drill, light will begin to transmit through it. The light source may be turned off at this point.

- As the bone is further thinned it can be subsequently further removed with Kerrison rongeurs or Takahashi forceps.
- Once the ostium is adequately sized (approximately 1 cm diameter) the lacrimal sac is tented into the nasal cavity either with the light pipe or the stylet of the bicanalicular stenting system or a Bowman probe. A sickle knife is used to carefully open the lacrimal sac in a vertical sagittal incision, pulling in toward the nasal cavity to avoid directing cutting forces toward the orbit. Mucopus may be encountered at this stage and can be suctioned clear. If a dacryocystitis has been present, a culture may be obtained.
- Bellucci micro scissors or a comparable instrument may be used to perform horizontal cuts superiorly and inferiorly on either side of the vertical lacrimal sac incision to create anterior and posterior flaps of the lacrimal sac. A Kerrison rongeur can be used to remove a small segment of the lacrimal sac mucosa to be sent as a specimen to pathology.
- Bicanalicular silicone stenting is passed and retrieved endonasally and tied as a square knot approximately 1.5 cm from the DCR ostium.
- The surgical area is checked for hemostasis; generally hemostasis is not a problem as long as blood pressure is controlled and the patient is in a recumbent supine position.

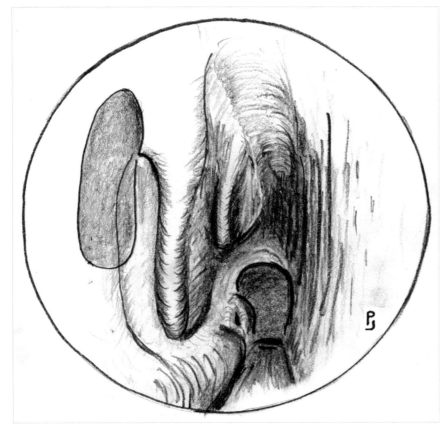

Fig. 29.2 Location of the lacrimal sac in relation to the maxillary line and middle turbinate. The shaded oval area represents the location of the lacrimal sac. Note that the maxillary line essentially bisects the lacrimal sac in the sagittal plane, and that the fundus of the lacrimal sac extends above the axilla of the middle turbinate. (From Wormald PJ. Endoscopic Sinus Surgery: Anatomy, Three-Dimensional Reconstruction, and Surgical Technique. 4th ed. New York: Thieme Medical Publishers; 2018.)

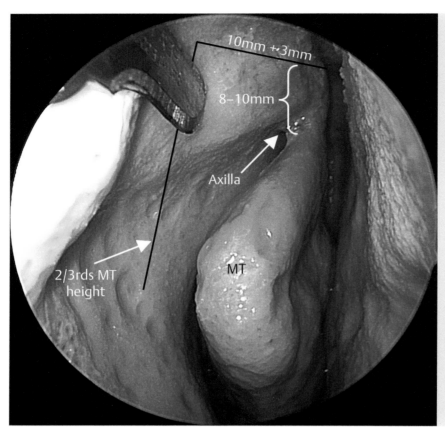

10mm +3mm

8–10mm

Axilla

2/3rds MT height

MT

Fig. 29.3 A posteriorly based mucosal flap is created with a scalpel, starting above the axilla of the middle turbinate, proceeding anteriorly for approximately 1 cm to travel anterior to the maxillary line, then proceeding inferiorly for approximately two-thirds the height of the middle turbinate. An inferior posterior relaxing incision may be made to aid with flap reflection. (From Wormald PJ. Endoscopic Sinus Surgery: Anatomy, Three-Dimensional Reconstruction, and Surgical Technique. 4th ed. New York: Thieme Medical Publishers; 2018.)

If cautery is necessary, suction monopolar cautery can be carefully administered, taking care to not cauterize directly over the area of the internal common punctum if this has been exposed (generally this would require a quite high/cranial exposure).

- The mucosal flaps are then redraped into their normal anatomical positions, which minimize any exposed bone and areas needed to heal by secondary intention. If double flaps are employed, the surgeon should take care that the flaps do not occlude the ostium. With the single posterior flap, a central portion of mucosa is excised with through-biting forceps to correspond to the underlying marsupialized lacrimal sac (▶ Fig. 29.4).
- The author prefers to place MeroGel nasal packing (Medtronic, Minneapolis, MN, USA) soaked in triamcinolone 40 mg, as small pieces placed within the DCR ostium, within the middle meatus, and between the middle meatus and nasal septum, as an added measure to combat adhesion formation.
- Shells are removed, the eyes are treated with an ophthalmic lubricant ointment, the patient is extubated from anesthesia, and taken to the recovery room.

Note that if a septoplasty is required it is performed as follows: Both sides of the nasal septum have been decongested with neurosurgical cottonoids soaked in oxymetazoline. A 0-degree endoscope is used to identify the site of septal deflection to allow for planning of placement of the cartilaginous incision. Next a Killian incision is made contralateral to the DCR side

with a #15 blade from posterior to anterior along the root of the septum, taking care not to score the underlying cartilage. A Cottle elevator is used to develop a submucoperichondrial plane ipsilateral to the Killian incision. The endoscope is placed under the mucosal flap and the flap is continued to be elevated posteriorly just beyond the osteocartilaginous junction of the septum. At this point the endoscope is again used to verify the site of septal deflection and an angled beaver blade is used to score the cartilage approximately 5 mm anterior to the site of deflection, ensuring that a caudal strut of at least 1 cm is kept intact to prevent a saddle nose deformity. A Cottle elevator is then used to create a full-thickness cartilaginous incision, taking care to prevent perforation of the contralateral mucosal flap. A straight-through cutting forceps is used to create a cartilaginous window to allow for the introduction of the endoscope into the contralateral submucoperichondrial flap. The contralateral flap is then raised posteriorly beyond the level of the deflection. A swivel-blade is then used to create a controlled superior incision in the cartilage to prevent torsion on the superior aspect of the septum at the site of its insertion at the skull base. The remainder of the inferior aspect of the region of deflection is then removed using a combination of straight-through cutting forceps, Takahashi forceps, and Jansen Middleton rongeurs. Once the deflection is fully removed, the mucoperichondrial flaps are redraped over the remaining cartilage and inspected to ensure that there are no regions of opposing perforations or areas of active bleeding. The mucosal flaps may be allowed to co-apt naturally or may be secured with a 4–0 plain gut suture on a Keith needle as a quilting stitch. If the

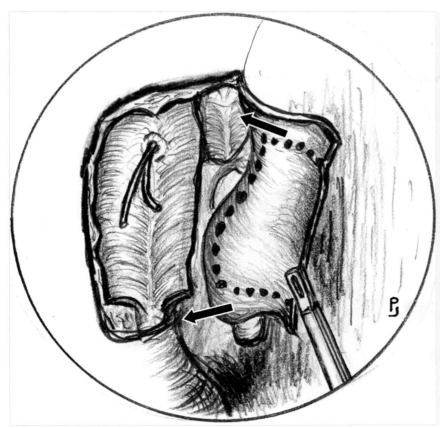

Fig. 29.4 The lacrimal sac has been opened and anterior and posterior flaps made. The posteriorly based nasal mucosal flap is being prepared to be redraped over the opened lacrimal sac by removing a section of mucosa (dotted line) with through-biting forceps. (From Wormald PJ. Endoscopic Sinus Surgery: Anatomy, Three-Dimensional Reconstruction, and Surgical Technique. 4th ed. New York: Thieme Medical Publishers; 2018.)

septum has a tendency to bow in one direction, silicone Doyle splints may be placed and secured anteriorly with a 4–0 polypropylene suture through the columella.

29.9 Tips and Pearls

- The operating surgeon by convention stands (or sits) on the patient's right side, regardless of operative side (right or left). The endotracheal tube, therefore, is best positioned to the left to maximize space around the nasal entrance.
- The use of a self-irrigating drill system can provide for cooler bone drilling temperature and a cleaner, better visualized surgical site intraoperatively.
- If a light pipe is used for transillumination of the lacrimal sac and visualization is difficult, moving the light pipe around within the lacrimal sac can help. It is important to maintain the light pipe against the hard stop of the lacrimal sac fossa to optimize visualization and to avoid soft tissue thermal injury. Use of the light pipe is not mandatory, and with experience the surgeon can reliably locate the lacrimal sac intranasally based on the landmarks of the axilla of the middle turbinate and the maxillary line.
- Dimming ambient/room lighting enhances video screen visualization.
- Hemostasis may be enhanced by a reverse Trendelenburg or lounge-chair positioning of the patient.
- For a right-sided procedure, turning the patient's head slightly to the patient's right improves surgeon ergonomics and access to the right nasal sidewall endoscopically.

- Take care when redraping the mucosal flaps to ensure that the silicone stent has been left long enough to not heal under the flap, and that the flaps do not entirely block the ostium. Some flap trimming may be needed.
- Occasionally, the patient has a thin quality mucosa or the superior flap is abraded and damaged by the drill during surgery. If the flap is in poor condition it should be excised as otherwise it may migrate and heal incorrectly, creating a problematic adhesion.

29.10 What to Avoid

- When using the light pipe, one must be careful not to be directed too posteriorly within the middle meatus at the cost of not removing bone of the anterior lacrimal sac fossa (which does not easily transilluminate). The light will preferentially shine through posterior lacrimal sac fossa because the lacrimal bone is thin and the light pipe will often have a posterior angulation as a result of clearing the globe/corneal scleral protecting shield.
- Avoid excessive manipulations within the nasal cavity that could abrade the nasal mucosa. Minor mucosal trauma can lead to intranasal adhesions. The use of proper intranasal instrumentation and round-tipped suction canulae, etc. is preferred.
- If fat is encountered during the procedure, the dissection has strayed outside the correct zone, and the fat is either facial or orbital fat, a pause should be taken and the surgeon should take note of landmarks and confirm spatial awareness within

the nasal cavity—dissection should be redirected appropriately.

- Bone removal should not proceed much above the level of the axilla of the middle turbinate, as the skull base can be nearby in some patients and a cerebrospinal fluid leak is a possibility. In addition, dissection should not proceed too posteriorly within the middle meatus unless one is prepared to perform a proper uncinectomy, as it is possible to create scarring that could lead to sinus outflow obstruction and sinusitis.
- Septoplasty is an advanced technique that should only be performed with proper training. Complications include septal hematoma, septal perforation, scarring, breathing difficulties, saddle-nose deformity, and cerebrospinal fluid leak. The perpendicular plate of the ethmoid should never be "twisted" or torqued for removal, as this can potentially lead to fracture of the cribriform plate leading to cerebrospinal fluid leak, pneumocephalus, and/or meningitis.

29.11 Complications / Bailout / Salvage

- Like any surgery, enDCR can fail. Most cases of failure are due to ostium stenosis or scarring. Nasal endoscopy can determine the status of the ostium. Revision surgery may be performed either as a 5-mm balloon dacryoplasty and placement of large diameter stenting, or formal excision of scar tissue and placement of stenting, both with the possible application of mitomycin-C to the ostium mucosa.
- Significant epistaxis may be encountered either intraoperatively, immediately postoperatively (in recovery), or delayed. Intraoperatively, one must ensure that blood pressure is controlled. Suction cautery can be used if a clear source of bleeding is identified. Loose bleeding mucosa may be excised. Reinsertion of neurosurgical cottonoids with oxymetazoline may be useful for vasoconstriction. In the recovery room or at home ice packs and pinching the nose and leaning forward for 5 minutes should stop most cases of epistaxis. If this is not sufficient, sometimes oxymetazoline may be sprayed into the nostril and then external pressure applied. Very brisk epistaxis in the recovery room generally deserves return to the operating theater for exploration and cautery. A patient who has delayed bleeding may need to be brought to the emergency ward for evaluation, where if conservative measures fail, options would include return to operating room or placement of an expandable nasal tampon such as Merocel (Medtronic, Minneapolis, MN, USA). Placement of an expandable nasal packing can be painful and often needs to be left in place for a number of days prior to removal, which obstructs the nasal airway and is again painful upon removal with a risk of repeat bleeding. While in place, the patient should be treated with prophylactic antibiotics to guard against toxic shock syndrome.

- Cerebrospinal fluid (CSF) leak is a potential complication of enDCR or septoplasty. It is generally heralded by clear rhinorrhea and/or headache. Evaluation by a rhinologist is key when this is suspected. The patient may be instructed to collect the clear nasal discharge in a specimen cup for laboratory evaluation for beta-2 transferrin to confirm that the fluid is indeed CSF. Some CSF leaks can heal spontaneously; however, many may require surgery for repair.

29.12 Postoperative Care

Postoperatively patients are advised not to bend or strain, or blow their nose for 1 week. Saline nasal irrigation may be advised, such as in the form of a sinus rinse kit. The author has stopped prescribing eye drops or ointments as this frequently seemed to be a cause of lacrimal stent prolapse during patient instillation, although these may be used if requested by the patient for comfort. The patient is seen at postoperative week 2 for endonasal suctioning and debridement of crust and any residual packing material. Generally, the silicone lacrimal stenting is left in position for 2 to 3 months, but may be removed earlier if granuloma formation is noted at the DCR ostium, in which case a topical ophthalmic steroid drop such as prednisolone acetate 1% is prescribed tapering over 2 to 3 weeks and then a reexamination is performed to ensure resolution. A repeat endoscopic examination, including endoscopic dye test in which fluorescein drops are applied to the ocular surface and observed intranasally passing through the DCR ostium, is performed 3 months following removal of bicanalicular silicone stenting to ensure anatomical and functional patency, and then again in 6 months or as needed.

References

[1] Toti A. Nuovo metodo conservatore di cura radicale delle suporazioni chroniche del sacco lacrimale. Clin Mod Firenze. 1904; 10:385–389

[2] Grob SR, Campbell A, Lefebvre DR, Yoon MK. External versus endoscopic endonasal dacryocystorhinostomy. Int Ophthalmol Clin. 2015; 55(4):51–62

[3] Davies BW, McCracken MS, Hawes MJ, Hink EM, Durairaj VD, Pelton RW. Tear trough incision for external dacryocystorhinostomy. Ophthal Plast Reconstr Surg. 2015; 31(4):278–281

[4] Detorakis ET, Drakonaki EE, Bizakis I, Papadaki E, Tsilimbaris MK, Pallikaris IG. MRI evaluation of lacrimal drainage after external and endonasal dacryocystorhinostomy. Ophthal Plast Reconstr Surg. 2009; 25(4):289–292

[5] Kloos RT, Duvuuri V, Jhiang SM, Cahill KV, Foster JA, Burns JA. Nasolacrimal drainage system obstruction from radioactive iodine therapy for thyroid carcinoma. J Clin Endocrinol Metab. 2002; 87(12):5817–5820

[6] Shams PN, Wormald PJ, Selva D. Anatomical landmarks of the lateral nasal wall: implications for endonasal lacrimal surgery. Curr Opin Ophthalmol. 2015; 26(5):408–415

[7] Mueller SK, Freitag SK, Lefebvre DR, Bleier BS. Endoscopic DCR using bipedicled interlacing mucosal flaps. Laryngoscope. 2018; 128(4):794–797

30 Conjunctivodacryocystorhinostomy

Adam Weber and Michael T. Yen

Summary

Conjunctivodacryocystorhinostomy (CDCR) and glass Jones tube placement can be an effective means of treating proximal lacrimal system dysfunction. Patients with this condition can complain of significant epiphora that is challenging to manage. In this chapter, we discuss the preoperative assessment, surgical strategy, and postoperative management for CDCR. We highlight the endoscopic surgical approach, and special considerations for physicians performing this procedure. Potential complications and how to address such situations are also discussed.

Keywords: conjunctivodacryocystorhinostomy, Jones tube, lacrimal, endoscopic, surgery

30.1 Goals

The primary goal of conjunctivodacryocystorhinostomy (CDCR) is to reestablish communication between the ocular surface and the nose to allow the passage of tears, thus resolving symptoms of epiphora. Secondary goals include good cosmesis, long-lasting functionality, minimal irritation, and easy maintenance. These goals are best achieved by placing a tempered glass Jones tube of the appropriate size in the proper location and orientation. This chapter discusses some strategies to help ensure good surgical results and patient satisfaction.

30.2 Advantages

CDCR offers a complete bypass of the native nasolacrimal system. This is the preferred operative approach in cases of proximal lacrimal system pathology with total or severe canalicular obstruction, prior failed canalicular repair, tear pump failure, and prior dacryocystorhinostomy (DCR) with anatomic but not functional success. These scenarios can be due to a variety of causes: congenital agenesis, postinfection scarring and fibrosis, trauma, neoplasms, inflammation, chemotherapy, radiation, and facial nerve palsy.[1] In such cases, salvaging the native proximal lacrimal system is not possible. Additionally, placement of a Jones tube serves to maintain the patency of the surgically created pathway. It should be noted that the option of canaliculorhinostomy (creating an anastomosis between the canaliculi and nasal mucosa) is available if there is at least 8 mm of normal canaliculus extending from the punctum.[2]

30.3 Expectations

As with any surgery, a major key to a successful outcome is a thorough discussion of the procedure and expected postoperative course with the patient. As will be discussed later, the patient will need to ascribe to a maintenance regimen to preserve the function of the surgery. Most importantly, the patient should be prepared to have a glass tube in their medial canthus,

and they should be aware that this tube is intended to remain there permanently. He or she should be aware of the potential for the tube to require adjustments, either in the office or potentially in the operating room. The patient should also expect some mild eye irritation following surgery, but this is usually transient as patients tend to adjust well to presence of the glass tube.

The patient should expect swelling, bruising, and some discomfort in the operative area. This is rarely severe, and can be well-managed with oral medication taken at home. If an external approach is employed, then the patient should be aware of the risk for a scar. Regardless of approach, the patient should be prepared for a nose bleed the day following surgery, but this is usually low volume and mild. However, in rare cases the patient may require nasal packing.

30.4 Key Principles

The key to a successful CDCR is providing adequate drainage for the tears to drain from the eye into the nose. In order to subvert abnormal and nonfunctional anatomy, the surgeon must have a complete understanding of that anatomy. Especially important is the three-dimensional relationship between orbital and nasal structures. An understanding of the location of the thin lacrimal bone is crucial for proper osteotomy placement. Otherwise, the surgeon may find himself or herself attempting to pass through the thick maxillary bone leading to great intraoperative difficulty and an improperly placed Jones tube. An appreciation of the middle turbinate and nasal septum is also important to prevent tube occlusion and patient discomfort. Once the surgeon has facility with the anatomical structures involved, the CDCR can be performed in an efficient, safe, and effective manner.

30.5 Indications

The CDCR with glass Jones tube placement is indicated in patients with proximal lacrimal system dysfunction. If the site of dysfunction is upstream of the nasolacrimal sac, it is the procedure of choice. There are many potential etiologies for proximal lacrimal obstruction. In pediatric patients, canalicular agenesis is a common cause. The canaliculi may also have acquired fibrosis from recurrent infection, autoimmune inflammation, or drug reaction such as Stevens-Johnson syndrome. Iatrogenic causes such as chemotherapy, especially noted with docetaxel, and radiation therapy are also known. Canalicular trauma can lead to scarring and stenosis if the laceration is not repaired promptly or properly. Additionally, trauma to eyelid and orbicularis muscle can lead to lacrimal pump failure despite proper canalicular repair. Facial paralysis can also produce an ineffective pump mechanism.

If the patient has had a prior DCR with anatomic but not functional success (a patent osteotomy into the nose with flow with forceful irrigation but persistent symptomatic epiphora), CDCR may be considered.

30.6 Contraindications

The first priority of any surgeon is to do no harm. If comorbidities place the patient at undue risk, surgery should be deferred until the patient is medically stable and better able to tolerate the procedure. As we tell all of our patients, "No one has ever died from tearing."

The patient should discontinue any anticoagulant or antiplatelet therapy for an adequate duration for full reversal of the medication's effects. Increased bleeding not only places the patient at risk for systemic complications from the surgery, but also makes performing a good and effective surgery more difficult due to poor visualization.

Even in patients with no increased bleeding risk, we advocate against bilateral surgery on the same day. Nasal packing may be required for postoperative bleeding, and bilateral nasal packing is uncomfortable and may place the patient in respiratory compromise. If only one side requires packing, postoperative edema and congestion in the contralateral nose may still make the patient uncomfortable and unable to breathe adequately.

Some physicians may prefer to defer surgery in pediatric patients, as maintenance of the Jones tube tends to be more difficult in children. Due to the active nature of pediatric patients, the tube may also be more likely to become displaced. Additionally, adjustments can rarely be performed in the office and would require general anesthesia.

Abnormal nasal anatomy may make placement of the Jones tube more difficult. Some patients with severe deviated septum or nasal fractures may require surgical repair of these issues. We recommend that any planned nasal procedures are performed prior to attempting CDCR.

30.7 Preoperative Preparation

As part of the preoperative exam, the surgeon should inspect the medial canthus and caruncle to assess for any potential problems in tube placement. Conjunctivochalasis or a large caruncle may need to be addressed at the time of surgery to prevent tube occlusion. It is also beneficial to perform a nasal exam in the clinic to evaluate for septum deviation and any other issues that may complicate tube placement.

Before the date of surgery, the surgeon should ensure that all equipment potentially needed for the case is available. Equipment needs depend on the surgical approach elected for the procedure. There are also several types and modifications of tubes available. Whichever tube type is preferred by the surgeon, multiple lengths and diameters should be available.

Adequate anesthesia is crucial to a successful surgery. Pain leads to increased blood pressure, which leads to increased bleeding, decreased visibility, increased manipulation, and increased pain. The most effective way to stop this cycle is to prevent it. CDCR can be performed under general anesthesia or monitored anesthesia care (MAC) with local blocks to the medial canthus, caruncle, medial peribulbar region, and lateral nasal wall. The surgeon, anesthesiologist, and patient should have a collaborative discussion to choose the best type of anesthesia for the case.

30.8 Operative Technique

A CDCR can be performed by an external or endonasal approach. We prefer to perform the surgery endonasally with an endoscope. We utilize a technique similar to those previously published.[1,3,4,5,6]

30.8.1 Patient Preparation

Once general anesthesia or conscious sedation anesthesia has been administered, topical anesthetic eye drops are applied to both eyes. On the operative side, a block of lidocaine with epinephrine is injected in the medial canthus, caruncle, medial peribulbar region, and lacrimal sac. A mixture of local anesthetic and oxymetazoline is aerosolized in the nose on the operative side. The patient is then prepped and draped in the usual sterile fashion. In general anesthesia cases, the nose is prepped and draped into the field allowing access to the nares. In MAC cases, the whole face is prepped and draped into the field to prevent claustrophobia.

30.8.2 Osteotomy Creation

An endoscope is inserted in the nose and nasal anatomy is assessed. Anesthetic is injected into the lateral nasal wall at the root of the middle turbinate. We also prefer to inject the anterior bulb of the middle turbinate as well at this time for increased efficiency if a middle turbinectomy is required later in the case. The caruncle is then decapitated using Westcott scissors. A 14-gauge angiocatheter is then inserted through the opening in the caruncle directed inferior, medial, and posterior to the lacrimal bone. Alternatively, the path can also be made with straight iris scissors. The scissors can be opened to dilate the passageway. The needle is advanced through the lacrimal bone and nasal mucosa into the nose under visualization with the endoscope. The needle is then retracted from the sheath, leaving the end of the sheath in the nose (▶ Fig. 30.1).

At this point, the surgeon can assess if the middle turbinate will interfere with placement of the glass Jones tube. Often, the middle turbinate is in close proximity to the planned location for the end of the Jones tube, and a partial middle turbinectomy is performed with Takahashi forceps.

30.8.3 Jones Tube Placement

A Bowman probe is inserted through the angiocatheter sheath and used to approximate the length of the glass Jones tube needed. The probe and sheath are removed, and a gold dilator is used to enlarge the opening. However, one does not want to dilate the passage too much, as a snug fit is important for preventing tube migration. A Bowman probe is placed through the aperture of the selected tube and inserted through the opening in the caruncle into the nose. The Jones tube is slid into position under direct visualization with the endoscope. The opening of the tube in the nose should be at least 2 mm from any adjacent structure, and it should sit flush with the surrounding tissue in the medial canthus. If the tube is too long or too short, it is exchanged for the appropriate size. Once the correct tube is in place, the Bowman probe is removed (▶ Fig. 30.2).

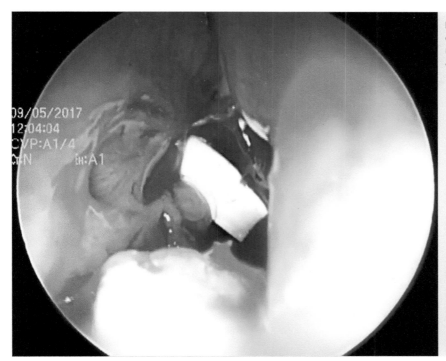

Fig. 30.1 Catheter sheath in place through osteotomy in lateral nasal wall. Partial anterior middle turbinectomy has been performed to allow for more space in nose.

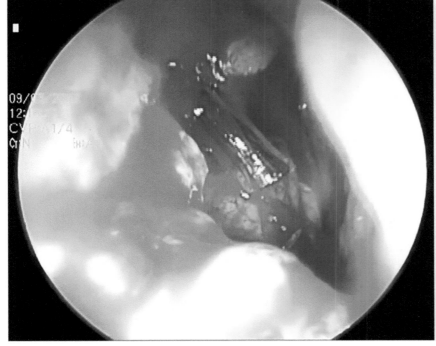

Fig. 30.2 Glass Jones tube in place with adequate space from nasal structures. A partial anterior middle turbinectomy has been performed.

Flow through the tube is assessed intraoperatively. Sterile water is dropped into the operative eye, and flow through the tube and into the nose is visualized with the endoscope. Sometimes flushing the tube or suctioning the nasal end of the tube may be needed to clear any clots. Once flow is confirmed with the tube in proper position, the tube can be affixed in the medial canthus with a 6–0 Vicryl suture passed through the medial palpebral conjunctiva and lassoed around the neck of the Jones tube.

30.9 Tips and Pearls

Every surgeon will and should adapt approaches of others into what he or she finds most comfortable. We can offer some advice from our experience that may be beneficial in future cases.

30.10 Nasal Preparation

Almost all reports in the literature utilize nasal packing with anesthetic and decongestant. While this is effective in producing anesthesia, hemostasis, and better operative space, it potentially distorts the nasal anatomy leading to an artificially widened nasal cavity. Decongestant alone shrinks the nasal mucosa, creating more space than normally present, and packing may further expand intranasal space. Therefore, the surgeon may choose a tube that is too long for the nose in its normal state.[5] Using an aerosolized spray delivers adequate medication to the nasal tissues without the potential physical displacement of nasal structures.

30.11 Endoscopic Approach

We strongly advocate the endoscopic approach to CDCR. This approach not only eliminates a skin incision and scar, but also allows for direct visualization of the nasal anatomy and surgical procedure. The surgeon can address nasal anatomical features that may jeopardize the success of the procedure when utilizing this approach. Visualization in the nose allows the surgeon to avoid placing the tube in or too close to the nasal septum and middle turbinate. The advantages of endoscopic endonasal CDCR have been documented in the literature, including high success rates, no skin scar, less blood loss, and shorter operating times.[3,4,5] Endoscopic visualization is especially helpful in revisions, where the nasal anatomy has already been distorted by prior surgery. We find a 30-degree scope most useful, as it allows the endoscope to stay inferior and does not interfere with the instruments manipulating the superior lateral nasal wall.

30.12 Osteotomy Formation

Using a 14-gauge angiocatheter needle greatly simplifies the procedure. This technique is well described in the literature.[6] This creates a tract wide enough for the Jones tube, but still snug enough to prevent migration. The plastic sheath is easy to identify in the nose and is flexible to prevent damaging other structures.

30.13 Partial Turbinectomy

Partial middle turbinectomy is an especially useful adjunct procedure during CDCR. The angle of insertion of the Jones tube often directs the distal opening of the tube into the anterior bulb of the middle turbinate. Rather than attempting to reposition or angle the Jones tube, it is easier and more successful to remove the offending portion of the turbinate, as has been validated in the literature.[1,6] As we routinely inject the middle turbinate with anesthetic and epinephrine at the beginning of each case, patient discomfort and bleeding are minimal. We advocate against cauterizing the resected margin of the middle turbinate. In our practice, we have found the increased tissue damage predisposes to scarring and fibrosis that jeopardize the procedure's success. Bleeding from the turbinectomy is usually minimal and resolves quickly without intervention.

30.14 Tube Selection

There is an abundance of different types and modifications of glass tubes available to the surgeon. There are glass tubes, silicone tubes, Medpor coated tubes, frosted tubes, angled tubes, flanged tubes, tubes with multiple flanges, and many other modifications. While literature states benefits from each different type of tube on the market, the most important factor in success is selecting the correctly sized tube. As discussed previously, a well-sized tube sits flush in the caruncle, with no tissue overriding and occluding the entrance, and the nasal end of the tube is at least 2 mm from any nasal mucosa. This space decreases the likelihood of scar tissue occluding the tube. In cases of abnormal nasal or midface anatomy, an angled Jones tube can be useful to get the desired clearance in the nose. The tube should sit snuggly in the passageway created through bone and soft tissue. This reduces tube movement and risk for tube migration.

30.15 Tube Fixation

There are also numerous methods to fixate the tube in the medial canthus. If the tube is held well by surrounding tissues, suture fixation may not be needed. However, if there is any concern that the tube may move, due to anatomical or patient concerns, a simple fixation is well worth the short amount of time required. We have had good success with 6–0 chromic gut anchoring the nasal tube to the medial palpebral conjunctiva. The suture dissolves around the same time that most scarring has completed forming and is not irritating to the patient.

30.16 What to Avoid

A solid understanding and application of the relevant anatomy is crucial to performing a safe surgery. Care should be taken to ensure that no damage to the eye occurs during the surgery. If the surgeon desires, a corneal-scleral protector can be placed on the operative eye.

If the external approach is chosen, the angular artery should be identified and avoided during incision and dissection. During osteotomy creation, the surgeon should take care not to

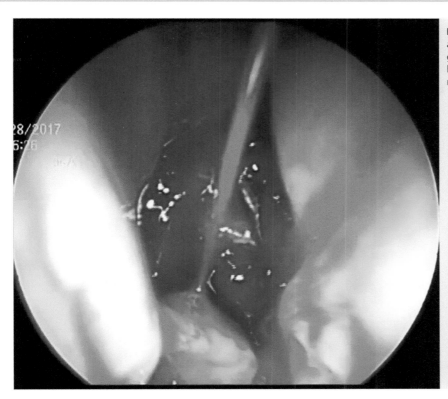

Fig. 30.3 Arterial bleeding following partial anterior middle turbinectomy. Nasal packing and gentle pressure is usually successful at stopping bleeding without cauterization, which can lead to more scarring.

twist rongeurs when engaged with bone. This can cause an uncontrolled break in the bone that may run up the ethmoid bone and involve the cribriform plate, and can cause a cerebrospinal fluid leak.

The surgeon should also be careful when sliding the Jones tube into position. The soft tissue surrounding the tract may make passage of the tube difficult. Exerting excess force can break the tube, and removing the broken pieces of glass from the canthus and nose can be very challenging. We use a cotton tip applicator to advance the tube, applying force over a wide area of the tube head. We prefer this to using forceps which focuses all force on a small area of the tube, increasing pressure and risk of fracture.

30.17 Complications/Bailout/ Salvage

30.17.1 Bleeding

The most common complication encountered during endoscopic CDCR is excessive bleeding. This compromises the surgeon's view, making performing the procedure more difficult. If performing the surgery under MAC, it makes the patient uncomfortable as the blood flows down the nasopharynx. The patient can cough or spit out the blood into the Yankauer suction. When performing the surgery under general anesthesia, the blood can accumulate on top of the airway. Preoperatively, the anesthesiologist should be made aware of the risk for bleeding and may choose to place an endotracheal tube instead of a laryngeal mask airway. It may also be prudent to aggressively suction prior to removing the airway to prevent aspiration.

High-volume bleeding usually stops quickly due to vasospasm. At times intranasal suction to clear blood can promote

more bleeding by agitating the tissues. Even in cases of arterial bleeding, nasal packing and pressure are very effective at achieving hemostasis (▶ Fig. 30.3). The most difficult thing for the surgeon may be waiting the 1 or 2 minutes for compression and local anesthetic to work and resisting the urge to resume tissue manipulation.

30.17.2 Tube Migration or Malposition

Perhaps the most common postoperative complication is tube migration or malposition.[5,7] This can be due to tube manipulation by the patient, poor fit of the tube, or scar tissue pushing the tube out of position. The tube can become displaced medially into the nose or laterally out of the medial canthus. If the tube is still present, it can often be adjusted back into proper position in the office. It is also helpful to have patients hold their finger over the end of the tube when they sneeze to prevent the tube from being pushed out by the increased intranasal pressure. If the tube is lost or continues to move out of proper position, tube replacement may be needed. This may be able to be performed in the office, but often the patient is more comfortable in the operating room with anesthesia. The tube should be checked for proper length and diameter, and any needed adjustments made.

30.17.3 Tube Obstruction

Tubes can also become blocked or obstructed. In the medial canthus, this may be due to excess tissue or pyogenic granuloma blocking the entrance to the tube. In the nose, the tube can be blocked by scar tissue (▶ Fig. 30.4), nasal tissue, or mucus. Mucus can also accumulate in the tube, blocking tear flow. Conjunctival inflammation can be treated with topical steroid, and conjunctivochalasis can be addressed with excision or

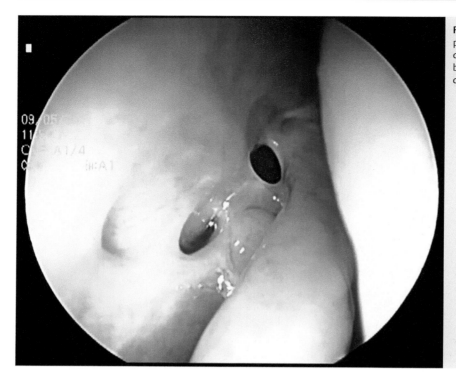

Fig. 30.4 Scarring of the lateral nasal wall in patient with failed prior conjunctivodacryocystorhinostomy. Fibrosis blocks outflow from the Jones tube and acts to displace the tube laterally out the medial canthus.

cautery. Irrigation with a cannula in the clinic can usually dislodge most mucus blockages. If the tube is blocked by nasal tissue, a tube exchange with or without additional nasal surgery may be indicated.

30.17.4 Infection

Infection is not a common postoperative complication, and usually responds well to antibiotic therapy.

30.17.5 Special Considerations

One special population of patients to be aware of is those with sleep apnea using continuous positive airway pressure (CPAP). These patients can complain of eye pain when sleeping from the air regurgitating up the Jones tube and onto the eye. This can lead to corneal epithelial damage. This can be addressed with lubrication ointment before sleeping, switching from a nasal mask to full-face mask CPAP, or switching to bi-level positive airway pressure.[8]

30.18 Postoperative Care

We place all patients undergoing CDCR on 1 week of oral antibiotics. We typically perform postoperative exams 1 week, 1 month, and 3 months following their surgery. At each exam, a nasal exam is performed to visualize the Jones tube, and patent flow through the Jones tube is confirmed. On postoperative days 7 to 10, we start patients on a nasal steroid spray two times a day for a month. We also advise our patients to use artificial tears at least once a day to preserve patent flow through the Jones tube. After the patient has completed a month of

nasal steroids, we recommend daily use of a nasal saline spray to prevent mucus build up around the tube.

We find it helpful to empower our patients with strategies to correct any mild issues they may have with their Jones tube. This includes increasing nasal saline spray and artificial tears use with upper respiratory tract infection symptoms or if they feel the tube is not draining as well. Patients can also occlude both nares and inhale to try to clear out the tube. Patients are also instructed to lightly cover the Jones tube when they sneeze to prevent expulsing the tube.

After the postoperative period, we continue to see our patients annually if there are no issues.

References

[1] Fang CH, Patel P, Huang G, Langer PD, Eloy JA. Selective partial middle turbinectomy to minimize postoperative obstruction following Lester Jones tube placement. Am J Otolaryngol. 2015; 36(3):330–333

[2] Lee JH, Young SM, Kim YD, Woo KI, Yum JH. Canaliculorhinostomy – indications and surgical results. Am J Ophthalmol. 2017; 181:134–139

[3] Kulwin DR, Tiradellis H, Levartovsky S, Kersten RC, Shumrick KA. The value of intranasal surgery in assuring the success of a conjunctivodacryocystorhinostomy. Ophthal Plast Reconstr Surg. 1990; 6(1):54–59

[4] Trotter WL, Meyer DR. Endoscopic conjunctivodacryocystorhinostomy with Jones tube placement. Ophthalmology. 2000; 107(6):1206–1209

[5] Chang M, Lee H, Park M, Baek S. Long-term outcomes of endoscopic endonasal conjunctivodacryocystorhinostomy with Jones tube placement: a thirteen-year experience. J Craniomaxillofac Surg. 2015; 43(1):7–10

[6] Devoto MH, Bernardini FP, de Conciliis C. Minimally invasive conjunctivodacryocystorhinostomy with Jones tube. Ophthal Plast Reconstr Surg. 2006; 22 (4):253–255

[7] Zilelioğlu G, Gündüz K. Conjunctivodacryocystorhinostomy with Jones tube. A 10-year study. Doc Ophthalmol. 1996–1997; 92(2):97–105

[8] Vicinanzo MG, Allamneni C, Compton CJ, Long JA, Nabavi CB. The prevalence of air regurgitation and its consequences after conjunctivodacryocystorhinostomy and dacryocystorhinostomy in continuous positive airway pressure patients. Ophthal Plast Reconstr Surg. 2015; 31(4):269–271

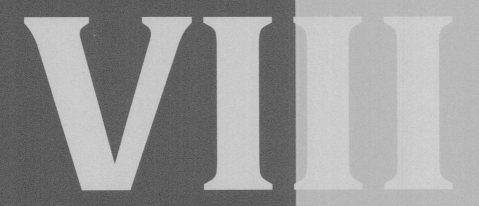

VIII

31 Orbital Floor Blowout Fracture Repair

Nicholas Mahoney

Summary

Orbital floor blowout fractures commonly occur as a result of blunt trauma to the orbit. Diplopia, enophthalmos, and infraorbital nerve hypoesthesia may result. Urgent surgical repair is indicated in the case of "white-eyed" blowout fractures with incarcerated muscle tissue within the fracture line. Early surgical repair (within 10 days) is recommended for large fractures, significant early enophthalmos, or intractable diplopia. Delayed surgical repair may also be performed for late enophthalmos, should this occur. The preferred surgical approach is transconjunctival with or without implant placement.

Keywords: orbital floor fracture, blowout fracture, enophthalmos

31.1 Goals

Orbital floor blowout fractures commonly occur as a result of blunt trauma to the orbit. The "blowout" occurs as the force of the trauma on the thick orbital rim transmits along the thin floor where buckling results in a fracture and posterior displacement of the globe results in pressurization of the orbital contents that displace this newly fractured floor segment outward. Diplopia can result from herniated entrapped muscle/soft tissues, muscle swelling, or cranial nerve injury. Early or late enophthalmos may also develop, particularly in larger fractures from an enlarged orbital volume but also from atrophy and displacement of orbital fat. Infraorbital nerve hypoesthesia may also occur. The goal of surgery is to free ensnared tissue and restore orbital volume. This results in correction of early enophthalmos, prevention of late enophthalmos, and correction of diplopia.

31.2 Advantages

Surgical repair in the case of the muscle entrapment within a non-displaced fracture can prevent permanent strabismus. Repair for large fractures or those with significant diplopia from displaced orbital tissue or ensnared orbital contents can result in a restoration of appearance and function. Early repair (i.e., within 10 days) has the advantage of an easier surgical field as fibrosis occurs within the orbit following trauma and progresses over the ensuing weeks and months. For patients who are not operative candidates due to other comorbidities or injuries, or do not seek medical care within this 10-day period, delayed repair may also be performed with good results. However, a longer operative time and possibility of less favorable outcomes may occur with delayed repair secondary to formation of scar tissue within the orbit.

31.3 Expectations

Surgical repair reposits prolapsed orbital tissues, restoring pre-injury orbital volume and resulting in correction of enophthalmos, prevention of late enophthalmos, and correction of diplopia. However, as diplopia often initially worsens after surgery due to surgical manipulation of tissues and a resulting increase in intraorbital edema, patients must be counseled that diplopia may take weeks to months to resolve. In addition, they must be counseled that if diplopia is due to muscle or nerve damage from the injury, it may not resolve, and strabismus surgery may be necessary in the future. Patients must be counseled as to the risks of surgery (see section "Complications"), and careful informed consent should be obtained.

31.4 Key Principles

- Orbital floor fracture repair should restore orbital volume by replacing orbital tissues to their anatomical position within the orbit and reconstructing the orbital bony anatomy.
- Any entrapped orbital tissues should be freed from the fracture site at the time of surgery, releasing any mechanical strabismus which should be verified at the end of surgery with forced duction testing.

31.5 Indications

Surgical repair of orbital blowout fractures is not always indicated, and smaller fractures without significant diplopia or enophthalmos may often be observed.

Urgent surgical repair is recommended for true muscle entrapment or "white-eyed blowout fractures."[1] These injuries are classically seen in children, where the flexible bone segment springs back into anatomic nondisplaced position, tamponades bleeding, ensnares the orbital contents, and can cause necrosis of extraocular muscles. As such, the presentation is that of a quiet-appearing eye with markedly restricted motility, guarding on motility exam and restricted forced ductions secondary to muscle incarceration. These patients may also display the oculocardiac reflex of bradycardia, nausea, vomiting, syncope, or heart block associated with ocular movements. Muscle ischemia can occur as early as 8 hours after injury and repair should be as early as possible.

Indications for early surgical repair (within 10 days) include large fractures (more than 50% of the orbital floor area), early enophthalmos or hypoglobus, and persistent diplopia without improvement over a short period of observation. However, individual patient characteristics and preferences must be considered in the decision whether to repair. For example, an elderly patient with multiple medical comorbidities, diplopia only in extreme upgaze and little concern with facial asymmetry from enophthalmos may not warrant surgical repair, but a young patient who is an athlete with a similar fracture and the same symptoms may desire or require repair.

31.6 Contraindications

With the exception of the true muscle entrapment in a nondisplaced blowout fracture, patients with relative medical contraindications to surgery may be observed given that they are counseled on the risks of persistent diplopia and enophthalmos. In patients with active or unstable ocular injuries such as a ruptured globe or retinal detachment, surgery should be deferred until the active ocular issues are treated and stabilized, and a retinal specialist clears the patient for surgery. Manipulation of the globe during fracture repair may worsen an existing retinal or globe injury. Monocular patients incapable of developing diplopia should also be aware of the indications for repair.

31.7 Preoperative Preparation

Preoperative oral antibiotics and steroids may be given depending on surgeon's preference with stronger indications for use in cases of preexisting sinus disease. Nose blowing should be avoided prior to surgery particularly if the medial wall is fractured. Perioperative intravenous antibiotics and steroids are preferred by the author. Informed consent is obtained, and the patient is given ample opportunity to ask questions about the surgery and expected postoperative course.

31.8 Operative Technique

Both eyes are prepped and draped in the typical manner for oculoplastic surgery. The surgery is begun with forced duction testing, which may be compared with the contralateral eye if indicated. A transconjunctival surgical approach is recommended, and this may be carried out in the preseptal or retroseptal planes (▶ Fig. 31.1). In the preseptal approach, an incision is made in the conjunctiva at the inferior border of the tarsus. Blunt dissection is carried down to the orbital rim in the preseptal plane. This has the benefit of preserving the septum which can keep the extraconal orbital fat out of the surgical field. It is slightly more cumbersome and given the periosteum is violated from the fracture in most cases, the orbital fat is often encountered nonetheless. In the retroseptal approach, the orbital rim is exposed and soft tissues displaced using a Desmarres retractor for the eyelid and malleable retractor for the orbital contents. An incision is made using Bovie cautery on a needle tip (Colorado Needle, Stryker, Portage, MI) in the conjunctiva, and dissection is carried down to the periosteum of the orbital rim posterior to the arcus marginalis in this fashion. In either approach, the periosteum is then incised with the Bovie cautery. A Freer elevator is used to dissect the periosteum off the orbital floor, taking care to preserve the integrity of the periosteum. The incision should extend from the lateral limbus to just medial to the punctum across the inferior orbital rim to fully access the fracture. This exposes the infraorbital nerve to the inferior oblique, both of which should be purposefully identified and protected. The infraorbital nerve is often unroofed as the lateral extent of the fracture typically ends at the infraorbital canal. The orbital contents often adhere to both the exposed infraorbital nerve and the sinus mucosa requiring careful blunt dissection. A blood vessel extending from the nerve to the inferior oblique is often encountered and can be ligated with cautery.[2] The inferior oblique can be disinserted with an elevator under the periosteum of its origin but should never be cut. If disinserted, it does not need to be reattached. The dissection is carried as far posteriorly, medially, and laterally as is necessary to identify all borders of the fracture. All prolapsed orbital

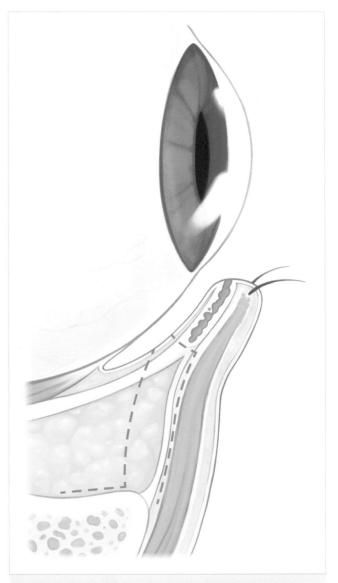

Fig. 31.1 Retroseptal and preseptal transconjunctival approaches to orbital floor fracture repair.

contents are gently lifted using the Freer elevator, taking care to avoid damage to the tissues. If further exposure is needed, the incision can be extended laterally into a lateral canthotomy and cantholysis or medially in a curvilinear manner into a retrocaruncular incision.

An implant is then placed. Several options are available, including porous polyethylene, titanium mesh, titanium mesh with porous polyethylene overlay, nylon sheets, silicone sheets, and absorbable materials (▶ Fig. 31.2). Titanium-containing materials are visible on postoperative imaging and hold a molded shape well. They can be custom bent by the surgeon freehand or with the assistance of a three-dimensional model. Pre-bent "anatomic" plates are available. Being rigid, if placed in the wrong location they can cause unintended damage to extraocular muscles or the optic nerve. Nonporous materials have the advantage of being flexible and as such can mold to the

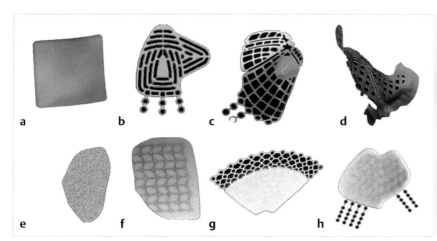

Fig. 31.2 Types of orbital implants. **(a)** Non-porous nylon Sheet, **(b)** flat, pre-cut titanium plate, **(c)** pre-bent, precut "anatomic" or "3d" titanium plate, **(d)** patient specific titanium implant, **(e)** porous polyethylene sheet, cut to size by surgeon, **(f)** porous polyethylene sheets embedded with titanium (PPTe), available with large or small pore sizes, **(g)** pre-cut fan shaped PPTe, **(h)** pre-cut, pre-shaped PPTe.

fracture site on their own. Being nonporous, they will not biointegrate and a capsule will form around them which can result in late infection or extrusion. Porous polyethylene sheets are rough enough to not require fixation and will biointegrate and, hence, once placed will not migrate. A theoretical downside to large pore porous materials and titanium has been orbital contents adherence, but this has not been demonstrated to be of clinical significance. Even so, dual layered implants exist that have smaller pore surfaces that face the orbital contents. Surgeon's preference largely dictates the materials selected and familiarity with multiple implant types is recommended.

The implant is selected and cut to size (if applicable), taking care to bend the posterior-most edge of the implant inferiorly to avoid impingement on the optic nerve. A small cutout at the anterior medial edge is also created to allow space for the inferior oblique muscle. It is then positioned such that it overlies the fracture defect, with its borders supported by stable bone, and the posterior edge resting on the posterior ledge of the fracture, taking care to ensure that no orbital contents are beneath the plate. If a titanium mesh implant is used, this is fixated to the orbital rim with 4- or 5-mm self-drilling titanium screws. If porous polyethylene is used, this does not necessarily require fixation if the implant is stable, but may be fixated in the same fashion if there is any doubt as to its stability. A nylon sheet can be fixated with a screw or by cutting a **U**-shaped tab at the anterior end and tucking this into the maxillary sinus. Forced duction testing is then repeated, and if any restriction is noted, the implant is checked thoroughly and any residual soft tissues trapped underneath are freed. If desired, a drain can be placed such as a ¼" Penrose drain to be removed the following day. It is not necessary to close a transconjunctival approach, although some surgeons do so with a single 6–0 plain gut suture. Some surgeons place a 6–0 nylon frost suture tarsorrhaphy to prevent chemosis, align the lid tissue, and protect the cornea from the drain. Patching has the benefit of helping with any bleeding to prevent retrobulbar hemorrhage but prevents checking vision postoperatively. Patients can either be discharged home or be admitted overnight for observation. A postoperative CT scan can be performed to assess implant placement, particularly if there is concerning motility postoperatively (e.g., a down gaze deficit from inferior rectus manipulation is normal but a severe upgaze deficit is of concern).

31.9 Tips and Pearls

- A transconjunctival approach to surgery is recommended.
- If fixating to the rim, try to place the screw inside the rim and avoid dissecting the arcus marginalis to prevent midface descent and adherence of tissues to the screw.
- Ensure that the posterior border of the implant rests on the posterior ledge of the fracture. You can find this ledge by removing the displaced orbital floor bone and then sweeping up along the maxillary sinus posterior wall with a Freer.
- Frequently assess the pupillary light response during surgery. Overzealous retraction will result in dilation from traction on the ciliary ganglion.
- Identify and protect the infraorbital nerve and inferior oblique muscle during dissection.
- The implant must be placed in the subperiosteal space. Limit periosteal dissection so that the implant will be less mobile.
- Angle the posterior border of the implant inferiorly, such that potential impingement on the optic nerve is avoided.
- Control any intraoperative bleeding during surgery. If there is concern for oozing at the end of the case, consider a drain.

31.10 What to Avoid

- Avoid prolonged traction on the optic nerve. Give frequent "rest" breaks to the eye.
- Avoid aggressive manipulation or transection of the infraorbital nerve during surgery.
- Avoid transection of the inferior oblique muscle—rather, if it must be moved, dissect its attachment in the subperiosteal plane.
- Avoid impingement on the optic nerve by the implant.
- Do not place the implant intraconally.

31.11 Complications

Complications of orbital floor fracture repair may include infection, implant migration, worsening diplopia, lower lid retraction or entropion, and vision loss or blindness.

Blindness is the most feared complication of orbital fracture repair. This occurs rarely, with a rate of 0.2 to 8.3%, but most studies report rates of less than 1%.[3] This may occur due to prolonged compression or stretch of the optic nerve during surgery or due to implant positioning or migration, orbital compartment syndrome due to retrobulbar hemorrhage or edema, or retinal arterial occlusion. Postoperative retrobulbar hemorrhage is rare, with a reported incidence of less than 0.5%.[4] This presents with sudden onset of pain, proptosis, elevated intraocular pressure, and decreased vision, typically within the first 24 to 48 hours following surgery. As a preventive measure, a drain may be placed for the first 24 hours following surgery, acting as a conduit to allow fluid or hemorrhage to leave the orbit. If orbital compartment syndrome with elevated intraocular pressure occurs, orbital exploration in the operating room should be performed as soon as possible, but immediate treatment with bedside lateral canthotomy and cantholysis is warranted. This should not be delayed while waiting for operating room availability.

Other complications include postoperative infection and implant migration or extrusion, both of which are rare. Porous polyethylene implants may have a lower rate of implant migration due to fibrovascular ingrowth.[5] Postoperative antibiotics are prescribed routinely to prevent infection. In the case of porous polyethylene implants, these may be soaked in antibiotic solution prior to implantation. In the case of postoperative infection, orbital hardware may need to be explanted.

Temporarily worsening diplopia is to be expected following orbital fracture repair due to postoperative edema, and typically resolves within weeks to several months. However, orbital tissue may be trapped beneath the implant causing mechanical restriction of motility. For this reason, careful forced duction testing following implant placement is crucial. The implant should be checked thoroughly to ensure that no tissues are incarcerated beneath the plate.

Eyelid malposition including ectropion, entropion, and lower eyelid retraction may occur due to scarring or disruption of the lower eyelid retractors. The risk of lower eyelid retraction and ectropion is greatest with a subciliary approach.[6] The risk of eyelid malposition is lower with a transconjunctival approach, but entropion may occur rarely.[7] The retroseptal conjunctival approach may have a slightly greater risk of eyelid malposition than the preseptal approach, but in the author's hands, the occurrence of postoperative eyelid malposition with the retroseptal approach and no wound closure is very low.

Despite an accurate anatomic repair, enophthalmos can still occur. This is partly because the orbital fat may atrophy after injury and partly because the trauma pressurized the intraconal orbital space, violating the fine septations separating the orbital fat compartments and displacing intraconal orbital fat extraconally. Even with perfect anatomic repair, particularly in delayed cases, additional enophthalmos correction may be needed.

31.12 Postoperative Care

Vision should be assessed immediately postoperatively once the patient has recovered from anesthesia.[8] If a patch is placed, the presence of a brisk response to light in the operative eye through the patch with the opposite eye completely occluded with a towel should be assessed. The author's preference is for the patient to be admitted for overnight observation, with frequent visual acuity reassessment. This allows for an intravenous steroid course and a reliable postoperative day 1 assessment when the surgical team removes the eye patch and the visual acuity and motility are reassessed. It is also our preference to obtain a postoperative CT scan, though this is certainly not standard in oculofacial surgery practices. This allows a reliable assessment of implant positioning and particularly when motility is abnormal and close follow-up is not always assured in traumatic patient populations, it can help ensure proper management. The patient then returns for a second postoperative visit 7 to 14 days after surgery.

If the patient is to be discharged home immediately following surgery, the eye patch should be removed prior to discharge and visual acuity assessed by the surgical team. The patient should be instructed in how to self-assess visual acuity by covering the fellow eye and should do so every few hours before bedtime. They should be instructed to call or return to the emergency department immediately should any worsening edema, pain, or change in vision develop.

References

[1] Jordan DR, Allen LH, White J, Harvey J, Pashby R, Esmaeli B. Intervention within days for some orbital floor fractures: the white-eyed blowout. Ophthal Plast Reconstr Surg. 1998; 14(6):379–390

[2] Patel AV, Rashid A, Jakobiec FA, Lefebvre DR, Yoon MK. Orbital branch of the infraorbital artery: further characterization of an important surgical landmark. Orbit. 2015; 34(4):212–215

[3] Joos ZP, Patel BCK. Reversible blindness following orbital fracture repair. Ophthal Plast Reconstr Surg. 2017; 33(3S) Suppl 1:S180–S183

[4] Cheon JS, Seo BN, Yang JY, Son KM. Retrobulbar hematoma in blow-out fracture after open reduction. Arch Plast Surg. 2013; 40(4):445–449

[5] Tabrizi R, Ozkan TB, Mohammadinejad C, Minaee N. Orbital floor reconstruction. J Craniofac Surg. 2010; 21(4):1142–1146

[6] Raschke G, Djedovic G, Peisker A, et al. The isolated orbital floor fracture from a transconjunctival or subciliary perspective—a standardized anthropometric evaluation. Med Oral Patol Oral Cir Bucal. 2016; 21(1):e111–e117

[7] Ridgway EB, Chen C, Lee BT. Acquired entropion associated with the transconjunctival incision for facial fracture management. J Craniofac Surg. 2009; 20(5):1412–1415

[8] Shew M, Carlisle MP, Lu GN, Humphrey C, Kriet JD. Surgical treatment of orbital blowout fractures: complications and postoperative care patterns. Craniomaxillofac Trauma Reconstr. 2016; 9(4):299–304

32 Medial Orbital Blowout Fracture Repair

Seanna Grob, Emily Charlson, and Jeremiah P. Tao

Summary

Medial orbital blowout fractures are a common sequela of blunt trauma and can be isolated or in combination with other fractures—namely, the orbital floor. Composed in part of the very thin lamina papyracea, the medial wall is most susceptible to fracture. Emergent repair is indicated for muscle entrapment which is rare along the medial wall. For all other cases, surgical invention or not is based on clinical exam findings once the acute soft-tissue swelling has subsided. Repair should be considered for persistent double vision/strabismus or to forestall disfiguring enophthalmos. Transcaruncular or transcutaneous approaches can be used to access the medial orbital wall. When an orbital floor fracture is also present, an additional swinging eyelid transconjunctival approach to the orbital floor can be performed. Combined medial wall and floor fractures can often be repaired with a single implant in a "wraparound" fashion. Complications of medial wall repair include lacrimal system damage, lower eyelid malposition, optic nerve compression, and globe restriction. With adequate planning and good surgical technique, outcomes after medial orbital wall blowout fracture repair are generally favorable with minimal visible scars.

Keywords: orbital fracture, orbital fracture repair, medial orbital wall fracture, combined medial and floor orbital fracture, blowout fracture, transcaruncular approach, swinging eyelid approach, wraparound technique

32.1 Goals

Medial orbital wall fractures are common after facial trauma. While not all medial wall orbit fractures require surgical intervention, ones that cause enophthalmos or eye movement abnormalities require repair. Surgery is generally performed within weeks of injury to successfully treat enophthalmos, globe malposition, strabismus, and large fractures. Rarely, if acute muscle entrapment is present, urgent surgical intervention in less than 24 hours is necessary.[1] Direct exposure of the entire fracture site, freeing of prolapsed orbital tissue from the fracture site, and reconstruction of the orbital wall with an orbital implant achieve the reconstructive goals of restoring extraocular muscle function, eye alignment, and globe projection.

32.2 Advantages

Repair of a medial orbital wall fracture is aimed at restoring the normal anatomy of the orbit, which in turn can normalize globe position and eye movement. Following fracture, repair is not always indicatedif the examination is normal, the fracture is small, or if there is no displacement of the fractured segment. If the examination is normal, the fracture is small, or there is minimal displacement of bone, fracture may not be indicated. Surgery can treat and prevent subsequent abnormalities. For example, should strabismus result from the trauma, strabismus surgery may improve diplopia, although single binocular vision in all fields of gaze is less likely than prevention with proper reduction of the fracture.

32.3 Expectations

Orbital appearance and globe function restored to the preinjury state can be expected in many cases with medial orbital wall fracture. Apart from soft-tissue edema, ecchymosis, and possibly some nasal congestion, many medial orbital wall fracture patients have minimal symptoms. Many medial wall fractures are incidentally discovered on facial imaging. Expansion of orbital volume causing enophthalmos (▸ Fig. 32.1) or restriction of orbital tissues with resulting strabismus are occasional sequelae of isolated medial wall fractures. When indicated, proper repair of medial wall fractures usually results in good outcomes with few complications and long-term stability. Importantly, many isolated medial wall fractures are associated with no morbidity and can be managed expectantly.

32.4 Key Principles

- Medial wall orbital fractures are common after trauma and often occur concomitant to ipsilateral orbital floor fractures.[2] Isolated medial wall fractures are often inconsequential clinically.
- Extraocular muscle entrapment is an indication for immediate repair.[1,3,2,3,4,5,6] Nausea, dizziness, or bradycardia with attempted eye ductions is suggestive of entrapment. Urgent repair is indicated to control the oculocardiac reflex as well as forestalling muscle necrosis. In other cases, fractures

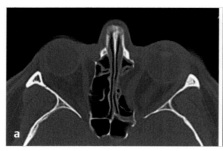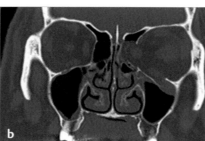

Fig. 32.1 Axial **(a)** and coronal **(b)** CT image showing a large medial orbital wall fracture with herniation of the medial rectus and orbital soft tissues into the fracture site.

may be observed for 1 to 2 weeks to allow soft tissue swelling to decrease. The primary indications for repair are nonresolving strabismus or enophthalmos, usually of 2 mm or greater.

- Medial fracture repair is most successful with direct exposure of the entire fracture perimeter, complete release of prolapsed orbital contents from the fracture site, and secure placement of a well-fitted orbital implant that re-creates the natural bony orbital wall contour and does not adhere or restrict the adjacent orbit.

32.5 Indications

Urgent repair (< 24 hours) is indicated for medial wall fractures with medial rectus entrapment. Entrapment often manifests as impaired horizontal eye movements, especially with abduction.[3,4,5] Other findings include bradycardia due to the oculocardiac reflex, nausea, or dizziness with attempted eye movements. Immediate repair is associated with an improved prognosis.[7]

In the absence of muscle incarceration, fractures can be observed for 1 to 2 weeks while spontaneous resolution of edema occurs, allowing for a more accurate assessment of extraocular movements and globe position.

Indications for repair of nonentrapped fractures include

- Enophthalmos > 2 mm or globe malposition, especially when inferior or posterior (however, formal exophthalmometry may be unreliable in the early injury phase due to edema).
- Persistent double vision, especially horizontal strabismus from medial rectus restriction in the setting of a medial wall fracture.[7]
- Large fracture (> 50% of the medial wall evidenced on neuroimaging) that is likely to result in globe malposition if left untreated.
- Concomitant orbital floor fracture needing repair.[2]

32.6 Contraindications

The major contraindication to medial wall fracture repair is concurrent severe ocular trauma such as corneoscleral laceration, rebleeding hyphema, compressive optic neuropathy from orbit compartment syndrome, or retinal detachment. As always, patients with an unstable general medical condition are not immediate candidates for surgery. Other concomitant injuries may be more urgent to address surgically prior to orbital fracture repair.

32.7 Preoperative Preparation

Informed patient consent should include possibilities of visual loss, infection, bleeding, implant extrusion, persistent diplopia, eyelid malposition, persistent or recurrent enophthalmos, and need for more surgery. CT imaging should be carefully reviewed. This provides information regarding the extent of the fracture site and concurrent orbital floor or other orbital or facial fractures that should be repaired simultaneously if possible (▶ Fig. 32.1). Importantly, muscle entrapment is a clinical diagnosis that can be missed on neuroimaging. If there is active sinusitis or other risk factors for infection, then antibiotics or nasal decongestants or both should be considered.

If clinical assessment indicates entrapment of a rectus muscle, surgery should be expedited to prevent ischemia to the muscle and permanent muscle damage. Otherwise surgical intervention may be deferred until soft-tissue edema has improved—approximately 1 to 3 weeks after injury.

32.8 Operative Technique

32.8.1 Approach to Medial Orbital Wall Fractures

Transcaruncular Approach to Medial Orbital Wall Fractures

Garcia et al first described the transcaruncular approach for medial orbitotomy.[8] The approach is popular for its good exposure and no cutaneous scarring.[9]

Anesthesia

Orbital fracture repair is usually performed under general anesthesia. The authors use 1% lidocaine with 1:100,000 epinephrine combined with 0.5% bupivacaine and sodium bicarbonate injected in the medial canthal area at the caruncle. Neurosurgical cottonoids soaked in Afrin can also be positioned into the nasal cavity to decongest the nasal mucosa.

Forced Duction Testing Under Anesthesia

A forced duction test may be helpful to evaluate for globe restriction due to entrapment or fibrosis. The authors believe edema in the acute setting may confound the forced duction findings and that visualization of the orbital fracture during repair is both sufficient and preferred.

Incision

A vertical snip incision is fashioned on the midcaruncle. Curved tenotomy scissors are used to bluntly dissect posteriorly to the area just posterior to the posterior lacrimal crest. Care is taken to avoid injury to the lacrimal sac. The periosteum is exposed in this area and incised with cutting electrocautery.

Exposure of the Medial Wall

A Freer or Cottle elevator is used to gently elevate the periosteum posteriorly into the orbit. Dissection is often started superiorly along the thicker and more stable frontal bone. The anterior and posterior ethmoid arteries are excellent landmarks for both inferior-superior (they lie generally at the level of the skull base) and anterior-posterior (anterior is ~ 24 mm and posterior is 36 mm from the orbital rim) position in the orbit. Exposure can proceed inferiorly to find the inferior edge of the fracture site. A malleable retractor can be used to protect the globe and elevate the orbital tissues for improved visualization. Orbital soft tissues are carefully elevated from the fracture site in a hand-over-hand technique. The orbital tissue that has herniated through the fracture site can be carefully elevated and retracted with a malleable retractor. The fracture site should be completely exposed, especially the posterior edge of the fracture to ensure that all herniated or entrapped tissue has been freed and reposited into the orbit.

Placement of the Medial Wall Implant

There are a wide variety of orbital implants that are available for orbital fracture repair. The authors prefer nonporous alloplastic thin implants such as nylon. This type of implant has been used to repair orbital blowout fractures since two case reports in 1961 by Browning and Walker.[10] They are available in thicknesses that range from 0.05 to 2.0 mm and the authors prefer the nylon foil implants of 0.35 mm or similar thickness. This thickness is flexible enough to conform to orbital walls, yet rigid enough to provide adequate support of the orbital contents. It is also useful in combined fractures of the inferior and medial orbital walls due to its flexibility (discussed later). Placement of a too large implant can cause displacement of the globe or can affect the function of the extraocular muscles. The size and flexibility of the nylon foil implant allows for reconstruction of the similar shape and structure of the original orbital walls. We also prefer the nonporous aspect of this implant and do not fixate the implant within the orbit. We believe fibrovascular ingrowth into the implant may also encourage cicatricial changes of the extraocular muscles and periorbita directly adjacent to the implant and subsequently induce diplopia. It is important to have the fracture fully visualized. The implant is cut to fit the medial wall of the orbit with enough overlap over the intact portions of the fracture edges. If further modification of the size is needed, the edges of the implant are trimmed until the ideal fit is achieved. The posterior aspect of the implant should rest on the orbital wall just posterior to the most posterior aspect of the fracture site. The anterior aspect of the implant rests comfortably inside the orbital rim. Implants well

seated across the perimeter of the fracture site with enough overlap onto the nondisplaced bone do not require fixation and a tamponade effect of orbital soft tissues further holds the implant as a scar capsule forms, which further stabilizes the implant. After the implant is placed, the surgeon should lift the orbital implant and view both sides of the implant to confirm no additional soft-tissue herniation prior to concluding the fracture repair. Forced duction testing at the end of repair should show free movement of the globe in all directions.

Closure

The conjunctiva is then closed with one to two interrupted 6–0 chromic or plain gut sutures. Ophthalmic antibiotic ointment is placed on the eye. No patch is placed to provide continued observation of the globe in the postoperative period. Orbital hemorrhage is the main concern in the more immediate postoperative period; so, careful vision monitoring is important.

Transcutaneous Approach to Medial Orbital Wall Fractures

The transcutaneous approach is similar to the transcaruncular except for the initial incision and wound closure.[11,12,13] It consists of an approximately 1.5- to 2.0-cm transcutaneous incision just anterior to the anterior ramus of the medial canthal tendon. The incision is only approximately 2 to 3 mm medial to the medial canthal angle, and is oriented vertically and centered over the medial canthal tendon (▶ Fig. 32.2). The cutaneous incision is made with the blade perpendicular to the nasal bone

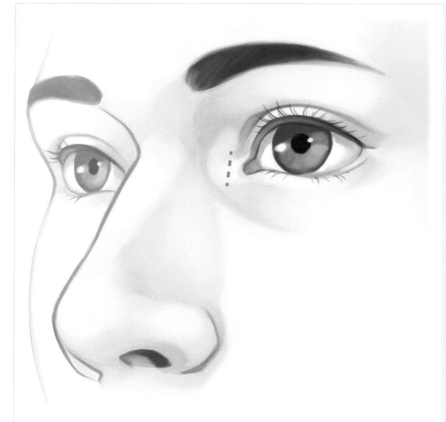

Fig. 32.2 Location of incision for a transcutaneous medial canthal tendon incision.

to avoid injury to the canthal tendon. Sharp dissection or electrocautery is carried down and through the periosteum just anterior to the anterior lacrimal crest. The anterior ramus of the medial canthal tendon and periosteum is then elevated with blunt subperiosteal dissection with a Freer or Cottle elevator and dissection is carried posteriorly to expose the medial wall. Care is taken to avoid damage to the lacrimal system as it is elevated and retracted laterally.

To prevent medial canthal dystopia, the medial canthal tendon along with periosteum is reapproximated with a 4–0 polyglactin suture which engages the medial periorbita, the medial canthal tendon, and skin edges. This helps tuck the medial canthus medially and posteriorly. The skin can then be closed with interrupted chromic, plain gut, or nylon sutures.

32.8.2 Combined Floor and Medial Wall Fractures

With combined fractures of the medial wall and the orbital floor, there may be loss of the inferonasal support to the orbit creating a challenging reconstruction of orbital volume. If the individual fracture sites are repaired separately, the repair may fail to approximate the inferonasal support of the orbital strut. Access to both the floor and medial wall is complicated by the origin of the inferior oblique muscle from the maxillary bone near the lacrimal fossa. Options for of the transition from the inferior to medial wall include a rigid implant fixed anteriorly or an even larger implant seated high on the medial wall and extending past the lateral floor defect such as nylon foil in a "wraparound" technique.[11]

Using a swinging eyelid approach, the orbital floor is exposed and the herniated orbital tissues are lifted out of the fracture site. Dissection is continued until the entire fracture perimeter is visualized. The medial wall is then exposed through a transcaruncular or transcutaneous approach. Dissection is continued to the periosteum, which is incised, and then elevated to expose the medial orbital wall. Orbital soft tissues are elevated from the medial orbital fracture site. Then an approximately 0.35- to 0.4-mm-thick nylon foil implant is cut in an ovoid shape to adequately span all of the fractures in a single unit. The average size of the implant is 4 cm × 2 cm. A 4–0 silk suture is then passed through the superior edge of the implant and tied. A hemostat is introduced through the medial orbitotomy approach inferiorly until the instrument tips are visualized from the transconjunctival lower eyelid approach. The suture attached to the implant is then grasped with the hemostat, and the implant is gently guided posterior to the inferior oblique origin to lay over both the medial and inferior orbital wall fractures. Once in place, the suture is removed from the implant. The implant is adjusted until all orbital tissues are free from the fracture sites and the implant is resting on stable bone (▶ Fig. 32.3). The incision sites are then closed.

If necessary, the inferior oblique can disinserted for improved view of both the inferior and medial orbital wall. A subperiosteal release of the inferior oblique origin is very safe, however, the authors prefer to avoid interrupting the muscle, if possible.

32.9 Tips and Pearls

The transcaruncular approach is popular due to its easy access and good exposure with no cutaneous scar.[9,14,15] The transcuta-

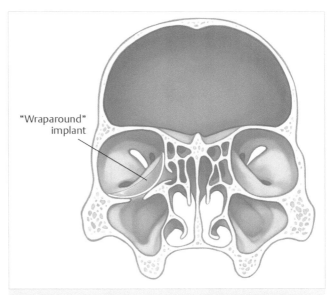

Fig. 32.3 Image of the placement of a nylon foil implant when using a "wraparound" technique for repair of combined floor and medial wall fractures.

neous approach offers access to the nasal bones if nasoethmoid fractures need to be repaired concurrently and may offer a wider medial orbitotomy view.[13] Finally, the "wraparound" method is especially useful in combined floor and medial wall fractures that are also lacking orbital strut support.

The key to any fracture repair is exposing the fracture site and all of the edges of the fracture perimeter, including the posterior ledge, as well as lifting and releasing all orbital soft tissue from the fracture site prior to implant placement. If this can be achieved with meticulous closure of the entry sites, then the patient will often have a good outcome.

32.10 What to Avoid

1. During medial orbital wall fracture repair, it is important to avoid damage to the lacrimal sac or lacrimal drainage system, as this can cause permanent tearing problems.
2. During the swinging eyelid approach for repair of a medial and floor fracture, it is important to minimize dissection of the lower eyelid tissues in order to prevent postoperative eyelid retraction or malposition.
3. While dissecting the posterior orbital tissues out of the fracture site, it is important to avoid compression of the orbital apex and optic nerve. This is also important during the shaping of the orbital implant, as not to create a too large implant that will impinge on the optic nerve and other orbit apical structures. Neuroimaging may be useful to plan surgery, but comfort with orbital anatomy and intraoperative identification landmarks such as the ethmoid arteries may be most important.
4. Insufficient release of orbital tissues from the fracture site may lead to persistent problems. All orbital soft tissues should be lifted out of the fracture site prior to orbital

implant placement. The surgeon should lift the orbital implant and view the both sides of the implant to confirm no additional soft-tissue herniation prior to concluding the fracture repair.

32.11 Complications

Visual loss following fracture repair is generally the result of retrobulbar hemorrhage in the acute presentation that causes an orbital compartment syndrome. In the case of an orbital compartment syndrome, the intraocular pressure is acutely elevated and can usually be relieved by a canthotomy and cantholysis procedure of the lower eyelid with or without the upper eyelid to control pressure. Some advocate high-dose steroids to help reduce additional free radical damage after acute injury akin to acute spinal cord injury; however, the evidence for use in optic nerve injury is not definitive. Cases of vision loss have also been reported from large implants that compress the optic nerve. Therefore, it is important not to place a patch or pressure patch after surgery, and patients should be monitored for orbital pressure and vision loss in the immediate postoperative period.

Diplopia may result from extraocular muscle ischemia or scarring due to the trauma or from persistent entrapment of the muscle. Neurogenic causes from trauma present with diplopia and full ductions on exam. In these cases, observation for a period of at least 6 months should be undertaken before any intervention, as neurogenic diplopia may resolve spontaneously without surgery. Persistent postoperative diplopia can be from incomplete reduction of orbital tissues. Adhesion to orbital implants can be considered in cases of late-onset diplopia and may require removal or revision of the implant.

Enophthalmos after orbital fracture can result in significant facial asymmetry. Failure to restore orbital volume after surgical correction, shifting of an orbital implant, or atrophy of orbital contents after trauma can lead to persistent enophthalmos. Failure to restore the normal orbital bony contours can also lead to persistent enophthalmos. Imaging may aid in the evaluation of persistent enophthalmos to guide possible revision of the fracture repair.

Infection after an orbital fracture is uncommon, and there is no consensus on the use of antibiotics after an orbital fracture. Infection or significant surrounding inflammation of an orbital implant generally requires removal of the implant.

Eyelid malposition including lower eyelid retraction, entropion, or ectropion may occur after severe trauma or poor orbitotomy technique. Care must be taken with orbital access and wound closure as to not cause adhesions or cicatricial changes to the eyelids and soft tissues.

32.12 Postoperative Care

Patients follow standard oculofacial postoperative instructions. Patients are monitored in the postoperative area for approximately 30 minutes to 1 hour to ensure no acute postoperative bleeding issues. They are discharged with ophthalmic antibiotic ointment to be used for 1 week and pain medications as needed. Cold packs should be applied to the area (20 minutes on then 20 minutes off), especially during the first 48 hours after surgery. Heavy lifting, straining, and strenuous activity are not permitted. Patients return for postoperative checks 1 week after surgery and then about 2 to 3 months, barring any complications or persistent problems. Patients should expect postoperative edema and ecchymosis for 1 to 2 weeks and may have postoperative diplopia that usually improves as orbital edema resolves. Patients should be given strict return precautions if there are any signs of infection or orbital hemorrhage.

References

[1] Jordan DR, Allen LH, White J, Harvey J, Pashby R, Esmaeli B. Intervention within days for some orbital floor fractures: the white-eyed blowout. Ophthal Plast Reconstr Surg. 1998; 14(6):379–390

[2] Dodick JM, Galin MA, Littleton JT, Sod LM. Concomitant medial wall fracture and blowout fracture of the orbit. Arch Ophthalmol. 1971; 85(3):273–276

[3] Rauch SD. Medial orbital blow-out fracture with entrapment. Arch Otolaryngol. 1985; 111(1):53–55

[4] Thering HR, Bogart JN. Blowout fracture of the medial orbital wall, with entrapment of the medial rectus muscle. Plast Reconstr Surg. 1979; 63(6):848–852

[5] Davidson TM, Olesen RM, Nahum AM. Medial orbital wall fracture with rectus entrapment. Arch Otolaryngol. 1975; 101(1):33–35

[6] Brannan PA, Kersten RC, Kulwin DR. Isolated medial orbital wall fractures with medial rectus muscle incarceration. Ophthal Plast Reconstr Surg. 2006; 22(3):178–183

[7] Jank S, Schuchter B, Emshoff R, et al. Clinical signs of orbital wall fractures as a function of anatomic location. Oral Surg Oral Med Oral Pathol Oral Radiol Endod. 2003; 96(2):149–153

[8] Garcia GH, Goldberg RA, Shorr N. The transcaruncular approach in repair of orbital fractures: a retrospective study. J Craniomaxillofac Trauma. 1998; 4(1):7–12

[9] Kim S, Helen Lew M, Chung SH, Kook K, Juan Y, Lee S. Repair of medial orbital wall fracture: transcaruncular approach. Orbit. 2005; 24(1):1–9

[10] Browning CW, Walker RV. Polyethylene in posttraumatic orbital floor reconstruction. Am J Ophthalmol. 1961; 52:672–677

[11] Nunery WR, Tao JP, Johl S. Nylon foil "wraparound" repair of combined orbital floor and medial wall fractures. Ophthal Plast Reconstr Surg. 2008; 24(4):271–275

[12] Nunery WR, Tao JP. Medial canthal open nasal fracture repair. Ophthal Plast Reconstr Surg. 2008; 24(4):276–279

[13] Timoney PJ, Sokol JA, Hauck MJ, Lee HB, Nunery WR. Transcutaneous medial canthal tendon incision to the medial orbit. Ophthal Plast Reconstr Surg. 2012; 28(2):140–144

[14] Lee CS, Yoon JS, Lee SY. Combined transconjunctival and transcaruncular approach for repair of large medial orbital wall fractures. Arch Ophthalmol. 2009; 127(3):291–296

[15] Shorr N, Baylis HI, Goldberg RA, Perry JD. Transcaruncular approach to the medial orbit and orbital apex. Ophthalmology. 2000; 107(8):1459–1463

33 Lateral Wall Orbital Decompression

Honglei Liu and Hunter Yuen

Abstract

Lateral wall orbital decompression is a form of bone removal orbital decompression. This can be done for functional and/or aesthetic rehabilitation for thyroid-associated orbitopathy (TAO). By removal of the lateral orbital wall, orbital volume is increased and proptosis can be corrected. This can be done alone, or in combination with medial wall and/or floor decompression and orbital fat removal. A customized approach should be done depending on the degree and severity of the TAO.

Keywords: lateral wall decompression, bone removal orbital decompression, thyroid-associated orbitopathy

33.1 Goals

- Functional and aesthetic rehabilitation for thyroid-associated orbitopathy (TAO) or Graves ophthalmopathy.[1,2,3,4,5,6,7,8,9,10] By surgical expansion of lateral orbital wall, the orbital cavity is expanded and hence, this will reduce orbital pressure, proptosis, and pressure on the optic nerve.[1,2,3,4,5,6,7,8,9]
- This chapter focuses on lateral orbital wall decompression which is the most common type of bone removal orbital decompression (BROD). Depending on the severity of the TAO, lateral wall orbital decompression may be used alone or in combination with multiple walls orbital decompression, and orbital fat can also be removed during the procedure for additional effect.

33.2 Advantages

- There are two main types of orbital decompression, BROD, and fat removal orbital decompression (FROD). Compared with FROD, BROD has broader indications and more effective results of proptosis reduction. In the BROD, theoretically, all four orbital walls could be removed for the decompression; however, lateral, medial, and floor decompression are routine choices for the clinical therapy. The orbital roof is usually spared.[1,11,12,13,14,15,16,17,18,19,20,21,22,23,24,25,26,27,28]
- Depending on the severity of the proptosis, lateral wall decompression could be customized by removing different areas and portion of the lateral wall.[11,12,13,14,15,16,17,18,19,20,21,22,23,24,25,26,27,28]
- The incidence of new-onset diplopia after pure lateral wall decompression is about 0 to 6%. The effect of ocular motility, as evaluated by the Hess screen, is minimal.[21,26,29,30,31,32]
- Balanced decompression refers to lateral wall decompression combined with medial wall decompression (i.e., lamina papyracea removal and ethmoidectomy). The orbital decompression effect is more than isolated lateral wall decompression. Compared with inferomedial orbital decompression or floor decompression, there are fewer complications such as hypoglobus, muscle imbalance, and hypesthesia.[33,34,35,36]

- Indications for lateral wall decompression include both type I TAO (fat predominant disease without muscle enlargement) and type II TAO (muscle predominant disease).[11,12,13,14,15,16,17,18,19,20,21,22,23,24,25,26,27,28]
- Compared to FROD, lateral wall decompression can achieve more proptosis reduction. Lateral wall decompression can also relieve compression in dysthyroid optic neuropathy (DON), improve exposure keratopathy, and reduce severe orbital congestion.[23,29,30,37,38,39,40,41,42,43,44,45,46]
- Favorable cosmetic outcomes can be achieved with an eyelid crease, swinging eyelid, or lateral canthal approach without a detectable cutaneous scar.[29,30,37,45]
- Lateral wall decompression may be combined with FROD to augment the degree of proptosis reduction.

33.3 Expectations

- Lateral wall decompression can improve the cosmetic appearance due to disfiguring proptosis for TAO patients who are in their inactive phase of the disease.
- For those TAO patients with active orbital inflammation and sight-threatening complications such as compressive optic neuropathy, corneal decompensation, or acute globe luxation, BROD such as lateral wall decompression can be helpful.
- Lateral wall decompression could achieve the proptosis reduction of 2.7 to 4 mm. When combined with fat removal, the proptosis reduction could reach 4.5 mm, especially for the patients with severe proptosis.[23,26,29,30,37,44,45,46]
- The percentage of new-onset diplopia is about 0 to 6%.[21,22,26,29,30,31,32]
- In active TAO without sight-threatening complications, the treatment aim is to control the orbital inflammation first, usually by means of steroid, immunosuppressive agents, or orbital irradiation. Orbital decompression should be deferred until inflammation settles.
- Patients may still need strabismus and eyelid surgeries for the complete ophthalmic rehabilitation after the lateral wall decompression.[47,48,49,50,51,52]

33.4 Key Principle

Preoperative high-resolution CT scans in both axial and coronal planes are mandatory for evaluating the amount of bone present in the great wing of the sphenoid, the amount of intraconal fat, the size of the extraocular muscles (EOM), and the size of sphenoid trigone.

- In our experience, the "skiving" of lateral wall is suitable for those cases with the proptosis less than 23 mm. For more severe cases with proptosis more than 23 mm, creating a lateral wall bony window is a more preferred approach, and sometimes with the combination of FROD. In patients with small trigone, lateral bone decompression alone will have limited effect on proptosis.
- When using the high-speed diamond tip burr for skiving the lateral wall, it is important to establish a safe depth, then

extend to the inferior and superior part of sphenoid when the inner table of the great wing of the sphenoid bone has been reached, the color has changed to a more pale appearance and the burr should not go deeper preventing tearing the dura causing the cerebrospinal fluid (CSF) leakage.

33.5 Indications

- Disfiguring proptosis, chronic pain, congestion, and corneal exposure in stable inactive TAO.
- Active and inactive TAO with compressive optic neuropathy or DON.

33.6 Contraindications

- Although not a true contraindication, active TAO is not treated with surgical decompression. Rather, anti-inflammatory treatment such as systemic corticosteroid, orbital irradiation, or immunosuppressive treatment should be administered to control the activity of the disease.
- Patients with severe cardiac disease, uncontrolled blood glucose, uncontrolled blood pressure, severe infection, bleeding tendency, and coexisting myasthenia gravis should be medically maximized prior to surgery.

33.7 Preoperative Preparation

33.7.1 Systemic Evaluation

- In patients with stable thyroid eye disease, the clinical ophthalmic examination should be stable for several months prior to surgery. In addition, result of thyroid hormone serologic tests should also be stable for at least 3 months prior to surgery, though this is not always possible for patients with sight-threatening condition such as severe corneal ulceration or DON.

33.7.2 Ophthalmic Evaluation

- Basic record of the original status of the visual function, including visual acuity, pupillary examination, degree of RAPD, visual field testing, color vision evaluation, IOP, and orbital pressure, should be recorded for the pre- and postoperative comparison.
- The TAO activity level (via the Clinical Activity Score or VISA score) and severity of TAO (e.g., NOSPEC) should be recorded. Other important information includes Hertel exophthalmometry reading, ocular motility and degree of strabismus, eyelid position, eyelid and orbital fat edema, color vision, and optic nerve function.
- It is mandatory to differentiate between type I and type II TAO by evaluating the orbital fat and extraocular muscle volume by CT scan or MRI scan.
- Pre- and postoperative photography is necessary. Adequate documentation of intraoperative details should be recorded such as the areas of bone removal, dural exposure, and the volume of orbital fat removal; also the real-time decompression effect could be recorded by intraoperative photographs.

33.7.3 Relevant Medical History

- Previous eyelid or orbital surgeries.
- Antithyroid medications or thyroxine replacement therapy.
- Anticoagulation or antiplatelet treatment.
- The presence of coexisting medical illness such as myasthenia gravis and other autoimmune diseases.

33.8 Operative Technique

- Surgery is generally performed under general anesthesia. Unilateral or bilateral surgery may be performed at the same setting/operative session depending on patient and surgeon preference. The incision may be placed in one of several locations: upper eyelid crease, coronal incision, swinging eyelid, or lateral canthal incision.[29,30,37,45] A wider surgical exposure can be achieved by coronal approach, but the process is time-consuming and with a large incision. The other incisions all allow for excellent exposure of the surgical site and aesthetic results.
- There are two general categories of lateral orbital decompression: one is to shave or skive the bone and the other is to create a lateral orbital window.
- Lateral wall "skiving" (shaving or burring) may be achieved by any of the previously described incisions. A subperiosteal dissection of orbital rim is created and a malleable retractor is used to expose the deep lateral wall. A lacrimal keyhole is performed by removing the superolateral orbital rim around the lacrimal gland region. This will facilitate the removal of deeper bone and improve upper lid swelling due to enlarged lacrimal gland. The superior orbital fissure is visualized and the area of greater wing of sphenoid is identified for decompression. Using the high-speed diamond burr, the decompression is started by drilling the inferior part of the greater sphenoid wing nearby the conjunction of the superior orbital fissure. After the diploic space is reached and a safe depth is established, the drilling is then extended to superiorly and inferiorly. Drilling should be continued until the bone turns pale, and then further drilling should be done with diamond burr with care, avoiding damage to dura which may lead to dural tear and CSF leakage. Once the bony decompression is complete, the periorbita is incised and excised by a sharp blade which will allow the orbital fat to prolapse into the newly drilled space on the great wing of sphenoid. If the bony decompression does not adequately reduce the proptosis, both extraconal and intraconal orbital fat can be excised at this time (▶ Fig. 33.1).
- The creation of the lateral orbital window of lateral wall allows for even further orbital expansion and decompression. In fact, there are five techniques to achieve the orbital window:
1. Standard marginotomy: A standard lateral orbitotomy incision is made followed by lateral orbital rim exposure by elevating the periorbita and temporalis muscle. A high-speed reciprocating saw is used to incise the orbital rim, the marginotomy should be performed at between the plane slightly above the frontozygomatic suture line and a plane parallel to the floor of the orbit, and the orbital rim is removed temporarily. Then, the thin anterior portion of the lateral wall is removed by a rongeur. The marrow of the

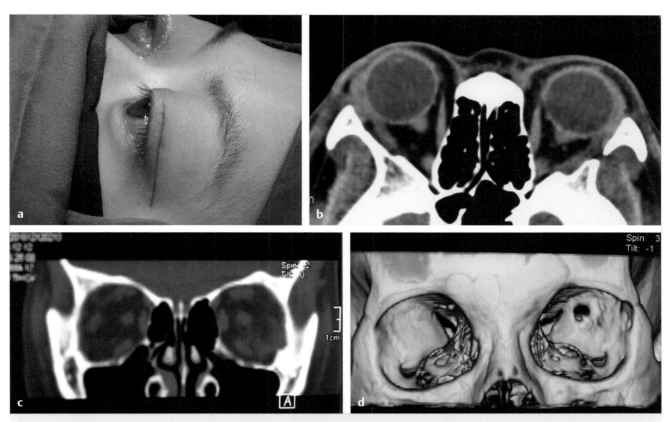

Fig. 33.1 (a) Upper eyelid crease approach; **(b,c)** lateral wall "skiving"; **(d)** area of the lateral wall skiving and keyhole shown by 3D reconstruction.

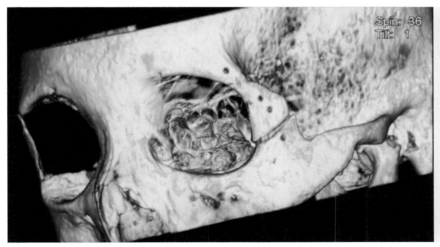

Fig. 33.2 Lateral wall decompression: window creation with orbital rim put back with the absorbable miniplate fixation.

diploic space of sphenoid bone is removed by high-speed drill. After adequate removal of the necessary parts of the lateral orbital wall, the orbital rim is replaced with the absorbable miniplate fixation (▶ Fig. 33.2).

2. Maximal marginotomy decompression: For the most severe case of proptosis or the DON case, a maximal lateral wall decompression is necessary. In these cases, it is necessary to remove the deeper lateral wall. All the bony structure of the lateral wall is removed until the dura is exposed about 2 cm. This complete bony removal allows the orbital apex structures to decompress laterally (▶ Fig. 33.3).

3. Intact orbital rim: Another method designed by Rose et al is to create a window with the intact orbital rim.[19] Following exposure of the lateral orbital wall by elevation of the periorbita and temporalis muscles, a window is created. A sagittal saw is used to make a rectangular opening in the wall. The window is then extended by a rongeur in the superior and inferior directions. Then, the periorbita is fenestrated by a sharp blade to allow the orbital fat to prolapse into the newly extended bony window (▶ Fig. 33.4).

4. Coronal transtemporalis approach: This is initiated by removing the lateral wall while leaving the orbital rim

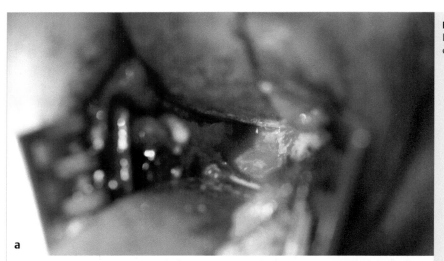

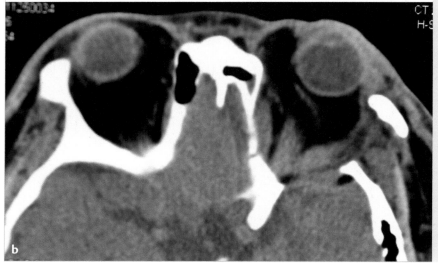

Fig. 33.3 (a) Dura exposure in the maximal lateral wall decompression intraoperatively; **(b)** dura exposure area shown in the axial CT image.

intact. The same bony space is accessed through the temporalis fossa, without a marginotomy. The lateral orbital rim is exposed and the dissection continues into the temporalis fossa, disinserting the muscle. A small amount of the lateral rim may be burred down in order to increase access posteriorly. A groove is created in the greater wing of the sphenoid exposing the diploic space posteriorly until the dura of the middle cranial fossa is observed. The diploic space is then removed from the lateral side. Finally, the thin bone overriding the orbit is removed from the posterior margin anteriorly to the lateral orbital rim.

5. Lateral wall decompression with lateral orbital rim removal (complete removal of the lateral orbit rim). This is similar to method 1 except that the lateral orbital rim is not replaced after its removal. Some surgeons feel that with the removal of the lateral rim, more proptosis reduction can be achieved.

33.9 Tips and Pearls

- To achieve optimal outcome, a suitable surgical approach should be selected for each patient according to the severity of the proptosis. For the mild and moderate proptosis, the skiving of lateral orbital wall is enough for proposes proptosis reduction; for moderate cases, an extended window can be created for greater prolapse of tissue into the temporalis fossa. For severe proptosis or DON, maximal decompression may be needed with aggressive removal of bone of the posterior lateral wall, exposure of dura, and possible removal of the lateral rim. Two-wall or three-wall decompression with fat removal may be required in some cases.

- There is a direct relationship between the volume of decompression and the degree of proptosis reduction. Deep lateral wall decompression ab interno without marginotomy may achieve 2.7 to 4.0 mm of proptosis reduction; via a temporalis ab externo technique with removal of the anterior bone overriding the temporalis muscle, similar results are achieved with proptosis reduction around 4.0 to 4.5 mm; by removing the orbital rim, an additional 1.5-mm decompression may be achieved.

- Lateral wall decompression combined with orbital fat removal enhances the proptosis reduction effect.

- Maximal decompression is not always necessary. Mild or moderate proptosis reduction may be sufficient for functional and cosmetic improvement for some patients.

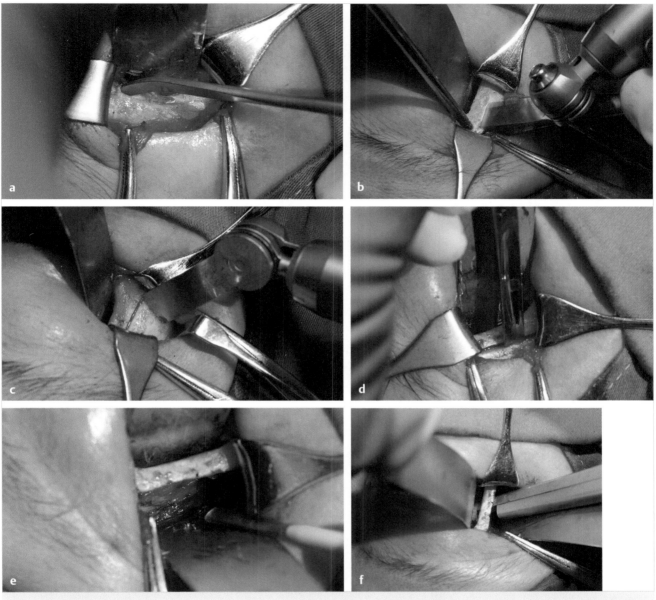

Fig. 33.4 (a) Orbital rim expose and periosteum dissection, (b–e) orbital window creation with orbital rim intact, (f) expanded the window with rongeur.

- Immediate ice packing and a short course of oral steroid after the surgery may help reduce postoperative edema.
- Inform patients that they may still need strabismus surgery and eyelid retraction correction later.

33.10 What to Avoid

- Damage to the optic nerve and the extraocular muscles can be avoided with excellent intraoperative visualization.
- Avoid the prolonged retraction and pressure on the globe.
- The pupil size should be monitored intraoperatively. Although pupil dilation does not occur even with direct damage to the optic nerve, sudden pupil dilation suggests pressure on the ciliary ganglion or traversing nerves.
- Because the drilling of the lateral wall is performed in a narrow space, persistent globe subluxation should be avoided (▶ Fig. 33.5).
- Caution not to drill too deep, risking laceration of the dura causing CSF leakage.
- Avoid thermal damage to surrounding structures by frequent irrigation during drilling and proper retraction of soft tissue away from powered instruments.

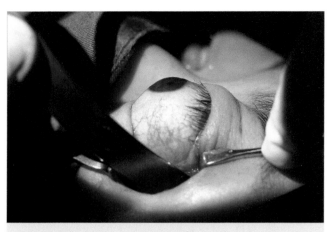

Fig. 33.5 Drilling in the narrow space of lateral decompression, the persistent globe subluxation should be avoided.

33.11 Complications/Bailout/Salvage

33.11.1 Possible Intraoperative Complications

- Intraoperative complications include CSF leakage in approximately 3 to 7%.[36,53,54,55,56,57,58,59,60,61,62,63] The CSF leaks can be managed intraoperatively with tissue glue, bone wax, orbital fat coverage, or dural patching. Postoperatively, conservative treatments such as best rest, head elevation, and avoidance of Valsalva maneuvers may lead to spontaneous resolution. Neurosurgical consultation should accompany any CSF leak.

33.11.2 Postoperative Complications

- Temple hypesthesia. This may be due to the ligation of zygomaticofacial or zygomaticotemporal neurovascular bundles that traverse the lateral orbital wall. This is a self-limited complication, although it may take months to recover.[19,22,44,63]
- Supraorbital nerve damage is possible with coronal or pretrichial dissections.[31,54,59]
- Alacrima could occur, in particular with the superolateral orbital *ab interno* dissection, if there is damage to the lacrimal nerve.
- Temporalis muscle wasting. This is an uncommon complication following dissection in the temporalis muscle fossa.
- Oscillopsia during mastication could occur due to the dissection of lateral wall overriding the temporalis.[54,64]
- Infections of surgical wounds. Although these infections are rare, the authors recommend systemic prophylactic antibiotics.[24,64]
- New-onset diplopia. With lateral wall decompression alone, the rate of new-onset diplopia is 0 to 6%, although combination with medial wall decompression increases the

rate to 30%. Secondary squint surgery may be necessary for the treatment of diplopia.[21,22,26,29,30,31,32]

33.12 Postoperative Care

- Dexamethasone and antibiotic eyedrops for 4 weeks.
- Oral prednisolone 30 mg daily for 3 to 5 days to reduce swelling.
- A 1-week course of oral antibiotic prophylaxis.

References

[1] Alper MG. Pioneers in the history of orbital decompression for Graves' ophthalmopathy. R.U. Kroenlein (1847–1910), O. Hirsch (1877–1965) and H.C. Naffziger (1884–1961). Doc Ophthalmol. 1995; 89(1–2):163–171

[2] Ogura JH, Walsh TE. The transantral orbital decompression operation for progressive exophthalmos. Laryngoscope. 1962; 72:1078–1097

[3] Walsh TE, Ogura JH. Transantral orbital decompression for malignant exophthalmos. Trans Am Laryngol Rhinol Otol Soc. 1957; 59:56–81

[4] Kennedy DW, Goodstein ML, Miller NR, Zinreich SJ. Endoscopic transnasal orbital decompression. Arch Otolaryngol Head Neck Surg. 1990; 116(3):275–282

[5] Baylis HI, Call NB, Shibata CS. The transantral orbital decompression (Ogura technique) as performed by the ophthalmologist: a series of 24 patients. Ophthalmology. 1980; 87(10):1005–1012

[6] Anderson RL, Linberg JV. Transorbital approach to decompression in Graves' disease. Arch Ophthalmol. 1981; 99(1):120–124

[7] Shorr N, Baylis HI, Goldberg RA, Perry JD. Transcaruncular approach to the medial orbit and orbital apex. Ophthalmology. 2000; 107(8):1459–1463

[8] MacCarty CS, Kenefick TP, McConahey WM, Kearns TP. Ophthalmopathy of Graves' disease treated by removal of roof, lateral walls, and lateral sphenoid ridge: review of 46 cases. Mayo Clin Proc. 1970; 45(7):488–493

[9] Olivari N. Transpalpebral decompression of endocrine ophthalmopathy (Graves' disease) by removal of intraorbital fat: experience with 147 operations over 5 years. Plast Reconstr Surg. 1991; 87(4):627–641, discussion 642–643

[10] Trokel S, Kazim M, Moore S. Orbital fat removal. Decompression for Graves orbitopathy. Ophthalmology. 1993; 100(5):674–682

[11] Dollinger J. Die druckentlastung der augenhöhle durch entfernung der äußeren orbitawand bei hochgradigem exophthalmos (morbus basedowii) und konsekutiver hauterkrankung. Dtsch Med Wochenschr. 1911; 37:1888–1890

[12] Lindholm J, Laurberg P. Hyperthyroidism, exophthalmos, and goiter: historical notes on the orbitopathy. Thyroid. 2010; 20(3):291–300

[13] Naffziger HC. Progressive exophthalmos following thyroidectomy, its pathology and treatment. Ann Surg. 1931; 94(4):582–586

[14] Naffziger HC. Progressive exophthalmos associated with disorders of the thyroid gland. Ann Surg. 1938; 108(4):529–544

[15] Goldberg RA, Kim AJ, Kerivan KM. The lacrimal keyhole, orbital door jamb, and basin of the inferior orbital fissure. Three areas of deep bone in the lateral orbit. Arch Ophthalmol. 1998; 116(12):1618–1624

[16] Rootman J. Orbital Surgery: A Conceptual Approach. 2nd ed. Philadelphia, PA: Wolters Kluwer Health/Lippincott Williams & Wilkins; 2014

[17] Hurwitz JJ, Birt D. An individualized approach to orbital decompression in Graves' orbitopathy. Arch Ophthalmol. 1985; 103(5):660–665

[18] Kennerdell JS, Maroon JC. An orbital decompression for severe dysthyroid exophthalmos. Ophthalmology. 1982; 89(5):467–472

[19] Mehta P, Durrani OM. Outcome of deep lateral wall rim-sparing orbital decompression in thyroid-associated orbitopathy: a new technique and results of a case series. Orbit. 2011; 30(6):265–268

[20] Wirtschafter JD, Chu AE. Lateral orbitotomy without removal of the lateral orbital rim. Arch Ophthalmol. 1988; 106(10):1463–1468

[21] Chang EL, Piva AP. Temporal fossa orbital decompression for treatment of disfiguring thyroid-related orbitopathy. Ophthalmology. 2008; 115(9):1613–1619

[22] Paridaens DA, Verhoeff K, Bouwens D, van Den Bosch WA. Transconjunctival orbital decompression in Graves' ophthalmopathy: lateral wall approach ab interno. Br J Ophthalmol. 2000; 84(7):775–781

[23] Ben Simon GJ, Schwarcz RM, Mansury AM, Wang L, McCann JD, Goldberg RA. Minimally invasive orbital decompression: local anesthesia and hand-carved bone. Arch Ophthalmol. 2005; 123(12):1671–1675

[24] Chu Ea, Miller NR, Grant MP, et al. Surgical treatment of dysthyroid orbitopathy. Otolaryngology–head and neck surgery: official journal of American Academy of Otolaryngology-. Head Neck Surg. 2009; 141(1):39–45

[25] Millar MJ, Maloof AJ. The application of stereotactic navigation surgery to orbital decompression for thyroid-associated orbitopathy. Eye (Lond). 2009; 23(7):1565–1571

[26] Nguyen J, Fay A, Yadav P, MacIntosh PW, Metson R. Stereotactic microdebrider in deep lateral orbital decompression for patients with thyroid eye disease. Ophthal Plast Reconstr Surg. 2014; 30(3):262–266

[27] Kroll AJ, Casten VG. Dysthyroid exophthalmos. Palliation by lateral orbital decompression. Arch Ophthalmol. 1966; 76(2):205–210

[28] Kalmann R, Mourits MP, van der Pol JP, Koornneef L. Coronal approach for rehabilitative orbital decompression in Graves' ophthalmopathy. Br J Ophthalmol. 1997; 81(1):41–45

[29] Ben Simon GJ, Syed HM, Lee S, et al. Strabismus after deep lateral wall orbital decompression in thyroid-related orbitopathy patients using automated Hess screen. Ophthalmology. 2006; 113(6):1050–1055

[30] Ben Simon GJ, Wang L, McCann JD, Goldberg RA. Primary-gaze diplopia in patients with thyroid-related orbitopathy undergoing deep lateral orbital decompression with intraconal fat debulking: a retrospective analysis of treatment outcome. Thyroid. 2004; 14(5):379–383

[31] Korinth MC, Ince A, Banghard W, Gilsbach JM. Follow-up of extended pterional orbital decompression in severe Graves' ophthalmopathy. Acta Neurochir (Wien). 2002; 144(2):113–120, discussion 120

[32] Liao S-L, Shih M-J, Chang T-C, Lin LL-K. Transforniceal lateral deep bone decompression–a modified technique to prevent postoperative diplopia in patients with disfiguring exophthalmos due to dysthyroid orbitopathy. J Formos Med Assoc. 2006; 105(8):611–616

[33] Leone CR, Jr, Piest KL, Newman RJ. Medial and lateral wall decompression for thyroid ophthalmopathy. Am J Ophthalmol. 1989; 108(2):160–166

[34] Unal M, Ileri F, Konuk O, Hasanreisoğlu B. Balanced orbital decompression in Graves' orbitopathy: upper eyelid crease incision for extended lateral wall decompression. Orbit. 2000; 19(2):109–117

[35] Alsuhaibani AH, Carter KD, Policeni B, Nerad JA. Orbital volume and eye position changes after balanced orbital decompression. Ophthal Plast Reconstr Surg. 2011; 27(3):158–163

[36] Sellari-Franceschini S, Berrettini S, Santoro A, et al. Orbital decompression in graves' ophthalmopathy by medial and lateral wall removal. Otolaryngology–head and neck surgery: official journal of American Academy of Otolaryngology-. Head Neck Surg. 2005; 133(2):185–189

[37] Goldberg RA, Perry JD, Hortaleza V, Tong JT. Strabismus after balanced medial plus lateral wall versus lateral wall only orbital decompression for dysthyroid orbitopathy. Ophthal Plast Reconstr Surg. 2000; 16(4):271–277

[38] Leone CR, Jr, Bajandas FJ. Inferior orbital decompression for thyroid ophthalmopathy. Arch Ophthalmol. 1980; 98(5):890–892

[39] Choe CH, Cho RI, Elner VM. Comparison of lateral and medial orbital decompression for the treatment of compressive optic neuropathy in thyroid eye disease. Ophthal Plast Reconstr Surg. 2011; 27(1):4–11

[40] Bingham CM, Harris MA, Vidor IA, et al. Transcranial orbital decompression for progressive compressive optic neuropathy after 3-wall decompression in severe graves' orbitopathy. Ophthal Plast Reconstr Surg. 2014; 30(3):215–218

[41] Wakelkamp IM, Baldeschi L, Saeed P, Mourits MP, Prummel MF, Wiersinga WM. Surgical or medical decompression as a first-line treatment of optic neuropathy in Graves' ophthalmopathy? A randomized controlled trial. Clin Endocrinol (Oxf). 2005; 63(3):323–328

[42] Day RM, Carroll FD. Corticosteroids in the treatment of optic nerve involvement associated with thyroid dysfunction. Arch Ophthalmol. 1968; 79(3):279–282

[43] Werner SC. Prednisone in emergency treatment of malignant exophthalmos. Lancet. 1966; 1(7445):10004–10007

[44] Liao SL, Chang TC, Lin LL-K. Transcaruncular orbital decompression: an alternate procedure for Graves ophthalmopathy with compressive optic neuropathy. Am J Ophthalmol. 2006; 141(5):810–818

[45] Rocchi R, Lenzi R, Marinò M, et al. Rehabilitative orbital decompression for Graves' orbitopathy: risk factors influencing the new onset of diplopia in primary gaze, outcome, and patients' satisfaction. Thyroid. 2012; 22(11):1170–1175

[46] Schaaf H, Santo G, Gräf M, Howaldt HP. En bloc resection of the lateral orbital rim to reduce exophthalmos in patients with Graves' disease. J Craniomaxillofac Surg. 2010; 38(3):204–210

[47] Shorr N, Seiff SR. The four stages of surgical rehabilitation of the patient with dysthyroid ophthalmopathy. Ophthalmology. 1986; 93(4):476–483

[48] Rootman DB, Golan S, Pavlovich P, Rootman J. Postoperative changes in strabismus, ductions, exophthalmometry, and eyelid retraction after orbital decompression for thyroid orbitopathy. Ophthal Plast Reconstr Surg. 2016

[49] Ben Simon GJ, Mansury AM, Schwarcz RM, Lee S, McCann JD, Goldberg RA. Simultaneous orbital decompression and correction of upper eyelid retraction versus staged procedures in thyroid-related orbitopathy. Ophthalmology. 2005; 112(5):923–932

[50] Fichter N, Krentz H, Guthoff RF. Functional and esthetic outcome after bony lateral wall decompression with orbital rim removal and additional fat resection in graves' orbitopathy with regard to the configuration of the lateral canthal region. Orbit. 2013; 32(4):239–246

[51] Lagrèze WA, Gerling J, Staubach F. Changes of the lid fissure after surgery on horizontal extraocular muscles. Am J Ophthalmol. 2005; 140(6):1145–1146

[52] Santos de Souza Lima LC, Velarde LG, Vianna RN, Herzog Neto G. The effect of horizontal strabismus surgery on the vertical palpebral fissure width. J AAPOS. 2011; 15(5):473–475

[53] Baril C, Pouliot D, Molgat Y. Optic neuropathy in thyroid eye disease: results of the balanced decompression technique. Can J Ophthalmol. 2014; 49(2):162–166

[54] Goldberg RA, Weinberg DA, Shorr N, Wirta D. Maximal, three-wall, orbital decompression through a coronal approach. Ophthalmic Surg Lasers. 1997; 28(10):832–843

[55] Graham SM, Brown CL, Carter KD, Song A, Nerad JA. Medial and lateral orbital wall surgery for balanced decompression in thyroid eye disease. Laryngoscope. 2003; 113(7):1206–1209

[56] Nadeau S, Pouliot D, Molgat Y. Orbital decompression in Graves' orbitopathy: a combined endoscopic and external lateral approach. J Otolaryngol. 2005; 34(2):109–115

[57] Sellari-Franceschini S, Lenzi R, Santoro A, et al. Lateral wall orbital decompression in Graves' orbitopathy. Int J Oral Maxillofac Surg. 2010; 39(1):16–20

[58] Unal M, Leri F, Konuk O, Hasanreisoğlu B. Balanced orbital decompression combined with fat removal in Graves ophthalmopathy: do we really need to remove the third wall? Ophthal Plast Reconstr Surg. 2003; 19(2):112–118

[59] Linnet J, Hegedüs L, Bjerre P. Results of a neurosurgical two-wall orbital decompression in the treatment of severe thyroid associated ophthalmopathy. Acta Ophthalmol Scand. 2001; 79(1):49–52

[60] Schick U, Hassler W. Decompression of endocrine orbitopathy via an extended extradural pterional approach. Acta Neurochir (Wien). 2005; 147(2):143–149, discussion 149

[61] Matton G. Resection "en bloc" of the lateral wall and floor for decompression of the orbit in dysthyroid exophthalmos. Eur J Plast Surg. 1991; 14(3):114–119

[62] Cruz AAV, Leme VR. Orbital decompression: a comparison between trans-fornix/transcaruncular inferomedial and coronal inferomedial plus lateral approaches. Ophthal Plast Reconstr Surg. 2003; 19(6):440–445, discussion 445

[63] Silver RD, Harrison AR, Goding GS. Combined endoscopic medial and external lateral orbital decompression for progressive thyroid eye disease. Otolaryngol Head Neck Surg. 2006; 134(2):260–266

[64] Fichter N, Guthoff RF. Results after en bloc lateral wall decompression surgery with orbital fat resection in 111 patients with graves' orbitopathy. Int J Endocrinol. 2015; 2015:860849

34 Orbital Decompression: Floor and Medial Wall Via an External Approach

José Luis Tovilla-Canales and Osiris Olvera-Morales

Abstract

Surgical orbital decompression is indicated for patients with compressive optic neuropathy, exposure keratopathy, globe luxation, uncontrolled elevation of intraocular pressure, or disfiguring proptosis secondary to thyroid eye disease. Multiple different techniques have been described to achieve effective orbital decompression. However, there is still controversy regarding the best surgical option likely to the variability in patient condition, patient anatomy, surgeon training, and available instrumentation.

The transconjunctival (for the floor) and transcaruncular approaches (for the medial wall) to the orbit are minimally invasive, provide excellent exposure, and leave minimally visible incisions.

Keywords: orbital decompression, compressive optic neuropathy, thyroid eye disease, transconjunctival approach, transcaruncular approach.

34.1 Key Principles

The transconjunctival decompression provides a wide exposure of the orbital floor, most of which is removed to allow expansion of the orbital fat into the maxillary sinus. During the floor removal, care needs to be taken with the inferior-orbital neurovascular bundle (V2) to avoid deep bleeding and paresthesia/hypoesthesia of the cheek.

Preservation of the orbital strut while removing bone decreases the incidence of new-onset diplopia secondary to a hypoglobus.

The transcaruncular approach provides excellent exposure of the medial wall in a minimally invasive manner. Through this route, the orbital apex can be widely decompressed to improve visual acuity in patients with compressive optic neuropathy.[1,2]

Excellent visualization of the orbit is imperative for effective decompression and avoidance of complications. Conjunctival incisions should be made large enough for proper retraction of the orbital structures. Maintaining orbital fat behind dissection planes (e.g., periorbital or orbital septum) and retractor instruments assists in this visualization.

34.2 Goals

The main aim of orbital decompression is to expand the orbital cavity to allow the orbital contents (eye, muscles, fat, nerves, and vessels) to herniate into the paranasal sinuses. This serves to reduce proptosis, alleviate exposure keratopathy, relieve compressive optic neuropathy, and provide better cosmesis to the patients.

Through the transcaruncular and transconjunctival approaches, these structures can be displaced into the ethmoidal and maxillary sinuses, respectively.

34.3 Advantages

- Via the conjunctiva, a skin incision is avoided. With careful dissection, the inferior orbital septum can be preserved, greatly reducing the risk of developing secondary lower eyelid retraction.
- Patients with compressive optic neuropathy need to have the orbital apex decompressed, which is well achieved through a transcaruncular dissection to remove the medial wall in the posterior-most aspect.
- The risk of postoperative new-onset diplopia is supposed to be less with decompression of the medial wall through the caruncle than with the endoscopic endonasal decompression.[1,2,3,4,5]
- The transcaruncular approach offers a reduced cost in equipment compared with the endoscopic endonasal decompression.[1,2]
- Advantages over other techniques include no external visible scar, less damage to adjacent tissue, and wide exposure to the entire medial and inferior orbital walls.

34.4 Expectations

Following surgery, proptosis may be reduced from 3 to 7 mm. By reducing proptosis, patients should experience improvement in symptoms associated with corneal exposure, such as foreign body sensation, tearing, and blurred vision. Also, a considerable reduction in vascular congestion of the periocular tissues is usually perceived (▶ Fig. 34.1).[1,2,3,4,5,6]

34.5 Indications

Orbital decompression is indicated in patients with
- Moderate to severe exophthalmos.
- Corneal exposure.
- Uncontrollable intraocular hypertension.

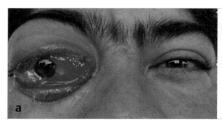
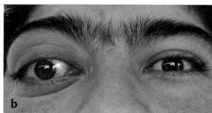

Fig. 34.1 (a) Preoperative and **(b)** postoperative clinical photograph of a patient with severe orbitopathy who was treated with a combined orbital decompression (through a transconjunctival and transcaruncular floor and medial wall approach).

- Globe luxation.
- Compressive optic neuropathy.
- Unacceptable cosmetic appearance.

Patients with mild exophthalmos (2–3 mm) are good candidates for a floor decompression alone. But when patients have severe visual loss due to optic nerve compression, a wide decompression of the posterior ethmoidal cells is mandatory, and in our experience, this can be best achieved through a transcaruncular approach.

34.6 Contraindications

Patients with active sinus infection need to be treated with antibiotics and/or antifungal medications before the orbital walls are disrupted. Also, if there is no severe visual loss that requires an urgent decompression, it is always preferred to perform surgery when the thyroid eye disease is in the inactive phase. Orbital decompression is also contraindicated in patients with an open globe or with a retinal detachment.

34.7 Preoperative Preparation

- As with all orbital surgery, patients need to have a complete systemic and ophthalmic examination.
- Unless decompression is urgent for vision salvage, the thyroid disease should be controlled and stable for 6 months prior to the surgery.
- Patients should stop smoking at least 4 to 6 months prior to the surgery.
- All patients need to have a CT scan with fine axial and coronal sections of the orbits to confirm that the sinuses are clear and to locate the position and height of the lamina cribrosa.
- In our personal experience, 50 to 80 mg of oral prednisolone, 2 to 3 days before the procedure, helps reduce postsurgical inflammatory edema.
- It is mandatory that patients stop aspirin or anticoagulant medication days before the procedure, as with any other

major surgery. This suspension of medication should be approved and ordered by the patient's primary care physician, cardiologist, or prescribing physician.
- It is important to preserve the lamina cribrosa to avoid cerebrospinal fluid leak.
- Prophylactic antibiotic is not standardized, and we do not routinely prescribe antibiotics prior to an orbital decompression surgery.

34.8 Operative Technique

Patients undergoing a transconjunctival and transcaruncular decompression are operated under general anesthesia.

34.8.1 For the Transconjunctival Approach Decompression

After infiltration of the lower eyelid in the subconjunctival space at the inferior fornix using 1% lidocaine with epinephrine 1:100,000, a 6–0 silk suture is passed in the lower eyelid margin just in front of the grey line, to allow the lower eyelid to be everted over a Desmarres retractor. Using a scalpel or a monopolar cautery, an incision is made inferiorly to the tarsal plate (▶ Fig. 34.2). Dissection is carried out through the lower eyelid retractors to the orbital rim in the preseptal plane to avoid fat herniation which may make visualization difficult (▶ Fig. 34.3). This is aided by the use of a malleable retractor to displace the globe and orbital tissues. Once the orbital rim is exposed, the periosteum is incised with electrocautery across the entire inferior rim (▶ Fig. 34.4). The periosteum is elevated with a periosteal elevator to gain access to the subperiosteal space of the orbital floor (▶ Fig. 34.5). After good exposure of the floor, using a periosteal elevator or a hemostatic clamp, a small opening in the bone is created medial to the infraorbital neurovascular bundle. With rongeurs, the bony decompression is enlarged in all directions (▶ Fig. 34.6). Care should be taken not to damage the infraorbital neurovascular bundle. It is preferred to leave

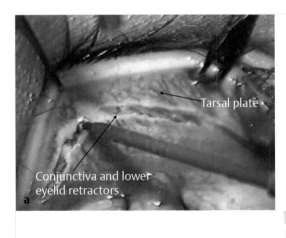

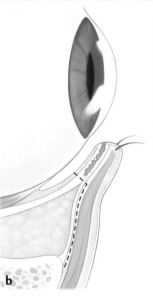

Fig. 34.2 (a,b) Transconjunctival approach for the orbital floor. The lower eyelid is everted over a Desmarres retractor and an incision is made below the tarsal plate, to separate conjunctiva and eyelid retractors.

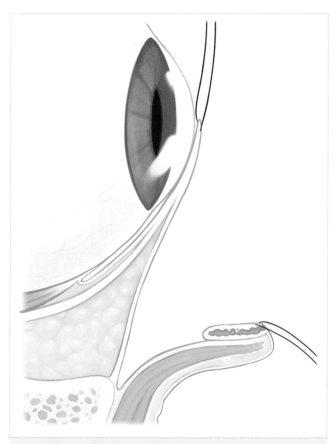

Fig. 34.3 Once the conjunctiva and retractors are separated, dissection is carried out downward to the orbital rim. Care needs to be taken to avoid disrupting the orbital septum as the orbital fat can herniate making the dissection more difficult.

the "orbital strut" (the junction of the maxillary and the ethmoidal sinuses) intact to reduce inferomedial displacement of the globe, hypoglobus, and postoperative diplopia. The periorbita needs to be incised to allow the orbital contents to herniate through the bone defect. The conjunctiva is typically closed with one buried 7–0 polyglactin suture in the central location.

34.9 For the Transcaruncular Approach Decompression

Lidocaine with epinephrine is injected subconjunctivally in the lower eyelid, caruncle, and medial canthus. A vertical incision is made behind the caruncle from the upper to the lower fornix in the subconjunctival space (▶ Fig. 34.7). Blunt dissection is then carried out to expose the periosteum at the posterior lacrimal crest (▶ Fig. 34.8). The periosteum is incised and reflected laterally (▶ Fig. 34.9). This dissection is continued superior, inferior, and posterior. Once the lamina papyracea is widely exposed, it is fractured and the bone is removed (▶ Fig. 34.10). With good exposure, the entire medial wall can be decompressed from the posterior lacrimal crest to the orbital apex and from the frontoethmoidal suture to the medial aspect of the orbital floor. Similar to the floor decompression, it is important to leave the inferior orbital strut intact to avoid postoperative hypothalamus and diplopia. At this point, the periorbita is incised in a horizontal fashion from anterior to posterior, and with gentle pressure to the globe the orbital fat herniates into the ethmoidal sinus. Finally, with a 6–0 absorbable suture (polyglactin), two interrupted sutures are placed to close the conjunctiva superiorly and inferiorly (▶ Fig. 34.11).

Combining the transcaruncular and the transconjunctival approaches, a wide decompression of the orbital floor and medial wall can be achieved to allow expansion of the orbital fat into the maxillary and ethmoidal sinuses (▶ Fig. 34.12).[1,2,3,4,5,6,7,8,9]

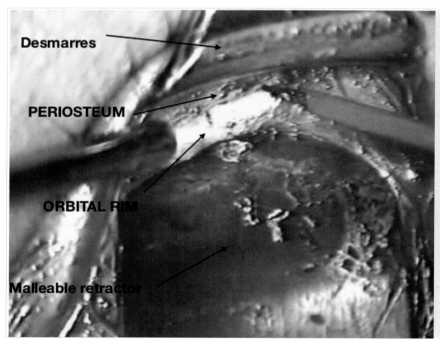

Fig. 34.4 The periosteum is incised with electrocautery across the entire inferior rim.

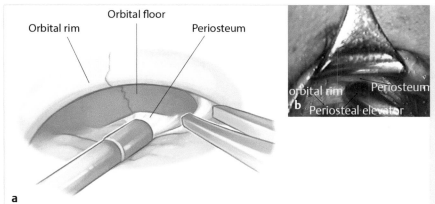

Fig. 34.5 (a,b) The periosteum is elevated with a periosteal elevator to gain access to the subperiosteal space of the orbital floor.

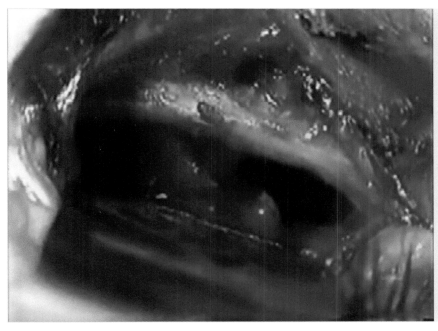

Fig. 34.6 Starting medially to the infraorbital channel, the floor is fractured and with rongeurs the bony decompression is enlarged in all directions. Care needs to be taken with the infraorbital neurovascular bundle.

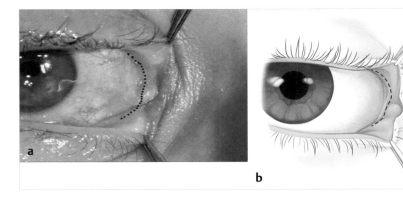

Fig. 34.7 (a,b) After lidocaine is injected, a vertical incision is made behind the caruncle from the upper to the lower fornix in the subconjunctival space.

34.10 Tips and Pearls

- When performing the floor decompression, use a periosteal elevator to remove the roof of the infraorbital channel. This has helped us reduce damage to the infraorbital neurovascular bundle.
- Using a small Kerrison rongeurs (1 or 2 mm) helps debulk the bony floor.
- For the transcaruncular technique, it is important to design a wide incision from the upper to the lower conjunctival cul-de-sac in order to have enough access to the medial wall.
- To avoid damage to the medial rectus, we use a curved Stevens tenotomy scissors with the tip pointing medially and bluntly dissecting toward the ethmoid sinus, posterior to the lacrimal sac.
- Thin malleable and Desmarres retractors are helpful to retract the orbital tissues and to maintain good visualization of the operating area.
- It is important to preoperatively evaluate the height and position of the lamina cribrosa in a CT to prevent from cerebrospinal fluid leakage.
- Closing the conjunctiva diminishes the risk of symblepharon formation and shortening of the fornices.

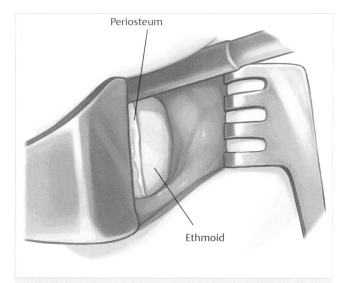

Fig. 34.9 The periosteum is incised to allow wide exposure of the lamina papyracea, and reflected medially.

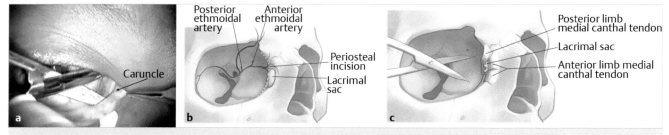

Fig. 34.8 (a–c) Blunt dissection is then carried out below the caruncle to expose the periosteum at the posterior lacrimal crest.

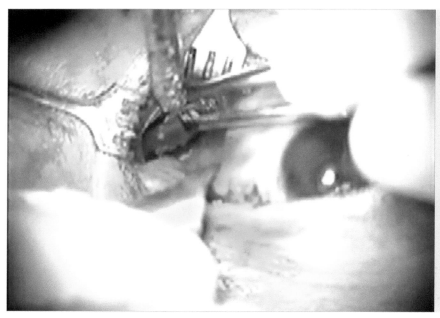

Fig. 34.10 Once the lamina papyracea is widely exposed, using a Kerrison rongeur and a freer thin ethmoidal bone is fractured and removed with forceps to create a wide opening through the entire medial wall.

34.11 What to Avoid

- Avoid resection of the orbital strut at the maxillary–ethmoid junction. By leaving this bony strut, the risk for inferomedial displacement of the muscle cone and postoperative diplopia is reduced.
- Avoid injuries to the infraorbital nerve/artery. Hypoesthesia and hemorrhage can occur.

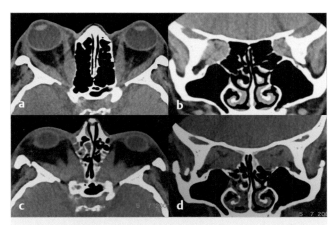

Fig. 34.11 **(a,b)** preoperative and **(c,d)** postoperative CT scan after transcaruncular orbital decompresssion of the medial wall in both orbits.

- For the transcarucular approach, start your periosteal dissection behind the lacrimal crest to avoid damage to the lacrimal sac.
- Avoid manipulation of and damage to the anterior and posterior ethmoidal arteries.

34.12 Difficulties Encountered

34.12.1 Transconjunctival Floor Decompression Considerations

In severely proptotic eyes, everting the inferior eyelid to expose the orbital rim may be difficult. In these cases, an external canthotomy and cantholysis help achieve better exposure.

If the orbital septum is transected during the dissection, the orbital fat may be difficult for visualization in the operative field. If this happened, the herniated fat can be contained with a malleable retractor to improve visualization of the orbital floor.

34.12.2 Transcaruncular Medial Wall Decompression Considerations

When the incision in the caruncle and conjunctiva is not wide enough, the operative field is reduced, making the surgery more challenging. Removing the posterior aspect of the ethmoid is limited by the reduced space in the posterior orbit. Special care needs to be taken with the anterior and posterior ethmoidal arteries as well as with the optic nerve.[1,2] If one of

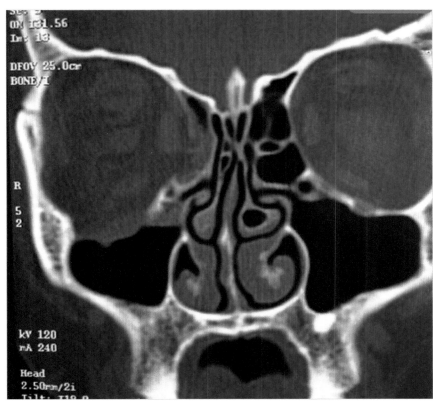

Fig. 34.12 Postoperative CT scan after a combined transcaruncular and transconjunctival floor and medial wall decompression of the right orbit.

the arteries is injured, it is important to cauterize it or ligate if necessary, as a severe hemorrhage can occur.

34.12.3 Complications/Bailout/Salvage

The most common complication reported after an orbital surgery is new-onset diplopia. Although spontaneous improvement could occur, strabismus surgery is generally necessary. Although rare, serious complication such as retrobulbar orbital wall decompression surgery is associated with retrobulbar hemorrhage and damage to the optic nerve at the orbital apex can occur, both causing loss of vision. Other reported major complications include infection, cerebrospinal fluid leakage, and subarachnoid hemorrhage.

Minor complications associated with transconjunctival and transcaruncular approaches include shortening of the conjunctival fornix, eyelid margin malposition (cicatricial entropion), suture granuloma, lower eyelid retraction, canthal dehiscence, canalicular laceration, conjunctival chemosis, and lacrimal sac laceration with associated dacryocystitis.

34.13 Postoperative Care

- After orbital decompression, some authors recommend to avoid patching the eyes to monitor visual acuity during the first postoperative hours.
- Oral steroids are prescribed in a tapered dose, starting with 50 to 80 mg of prednisone for 5 to 7 days. Tapering will depend on postoperative evolution.
- Use of prophylactic systemic antibiotics is controversial and may depend on each case and surgeon's choice.
- Ice compresses are useful to reduce postoperative edema.
- Patients need to be warned about the risk of postoperative diplopia and hypesthesia in V2 distribution.
- Avoid nose blowing, as orbital emphysema can be painful and rarely cause blindness.

34.14 Pitfalls

- Surgery on active thyroid eye disease. If orbital decompression is not urgent (e.g., severe visual loss due to optic nerve compression or risk of corneal perforation due to chronic exposure), delay surgery until the thyroid disease is controlled and stable.
- Ongoing smoking. Warn thyroid patients to avoid smoking. It is much better if this is achieved up to 6 months before the surgery.[10]
- Lack of imaging. CT scan is mandatory to evaluate the sinuses and lamina cribrosa.
- Sinus infection. In these patients with sinus infection, treat the infection before opening the periosteum.
- Removal of the inferior strut. This prevents an inferomedial displacement of the globe and postoperative diplopia.
- Incomplete posterior decompression. Patients with compressive optic neuropathy need to have the posterior aspect of the medial wall of the orbit decompressed. This can be achieved through the transcaruncular approach.
- Inadequate surgical exposure. For the transcaruncular decompression, it is important to design a wide incision from the superior to the inferior cul-de-sac.
- Damage to structures. Start your periosteal dissection behind the lacrimal sac and extend it to the orbital apex. Stay away from the anterior and posterior ethmoidal arteries.
- Keeping periosteum intact. After the bony decompression is done, open widely the periosteum to allow the orbital fat to expand into the paranasal sinuses.

References

[1] Shorr N, Baylis HI, Goldberg RA, Perry JD. Transcaruncular approach to the medial orbit and orbital apex. Ophthalmology. 2000; 107(8):1459–1463

[2] Liao SL, Chang TC, Lin LL. Transcaruncular orbital decompression: an alternate procedure for Graves ophthalmopathy with compressive optic neuropathy. Am J Ophthalmol. 2006; 141(5):810–818

[3] Mainville NP, Jordan DR. Effect of orbital decompression on diplopia in thyroid-related orbitopathy. Ophthal Plast Reconstr Surg. 2014; 30(2):137–140

[4] Fabian ID, Rosen N, Ben Simon GJ. Strabismus after inferior-medial wall orbital decompression in thyroid-related orbitopathy. Curr Eye Res. 2013; 38(1):204–209

[5] Boboridis KG, Bunce C. Surgical orbital decompression for thyroid eye disease. Cochrane Database Syst Rev. 2011(12):CD007630

[6] Cruz AA, Leme VR. Orbital decompression: a comparison between trans-fornix/transcaruncular inferomedial and coronal inferomedial plus lateral approaches. Ophthal Plast Reconstr Surg. 2003; 19(6):440–445, discussion 445

[7] Rootman DB. Orbital decompression for thyroid eye disease. Surv Ophthalmol. 2018; 63(1):86–104

[8] Reich SS, Null RC, Timoney PJ, Sokol JA. Trends in orbital decompression techniques of surveyed American Society of Ophthalmic Plastic and Reconstructive Surgery Members. Ophthal Plast Reconstr Surg. 2016; 32(6):434–437

[9] Siracuse-Lee DE, Kazim M. Orbital decompression: current concepts. Curr Opin Ophthalmol. 2002; 13(5):310–316

[10] Bartalena L, Piantanida E. Cigarette smoking: number one enemy for Graves ophthalmopathy. Pol Arch Med Wewn. 2016; 126(10):725–726

35 Fat Removal Orbital Decompression

Hunter Yuen and Shu Lang Liao

Abstract

Fat removal orbital decompression is a useful surgical option in the aesthetic rehabilitation of selected cases of thyroid eye disease (TED). The best candidates are those type I TED patients with mild to moderate proptosis in their inactive phase of disease. The low incidence of postoperative new-onset diplopia is the main advantage as compared with more traditional bone removal orbital decompression.

Keywords: fat removal orbital decompression, thyroid eye disease, proptosis, diplopia

35.1 Goals

- Aesthetic and/or functional rehabilitation for thyroid eye disease (TED) or Graves' ophthalmopathy are the main surgical goal. By removing orbital fat alone, the orbital volume is reduced, resulting in proptosis reduction.[1,2,3,4,5,6,7,8]
- In this chapter, the term fat removal orbital decompression (FROD) refers to orbital decompression by orbital fat removal only. However, during bone removal orbital decompression (BROD), orbital fat can also be removed to augment the orbital decompression effect.

35.2 Advantages

There are two main types of orbital decompression: BROD and FROD.[9,10,11] Due to modification of surgical techniques, the improved safety profiles of both procedures have successfully decreased postoperative complications in surgical decompression of the orbit.

However, postoperative diplopia is still an important potential complication. Between the two methods, FROD has a lower quoted incidence of new-onset postoperative diplopia, with studies quoting figures as low as 2.8%.[4] The exact reason of low incidence of postoperative diplopia is not entirely understood. Since the bony orbital walls are not removed in FROD, it is proposed that there is less alteration in the position of extraocular muscles. Yet selection bias may also contribute, as FROD is indicated in type I TED (fat predominant disease) where there is no muscle enlargement. These patients are intrinsically less prone to develop diplopia. In contrast, those with type II thyroid associated orbitopathy (TAO; muscle predominant disease) more commonly have baseline diplopia. In FROD, the degree of proptosis reduction may be more predictable by controlling the amount of fat removed.

In FROD, since the procedure is isolated to the orbit with orbital bones preserved, the possibility of serious life or vision-threatening complications such as cerebrospinal fluid (CSF) leakage, dura exposure, and secondary meningitis is reduced.[4,5,6,7,8] Other potential complications related to BROD such as sinusitis, infraorbital nerve and minor sensory nerve paresthesia or injury, and optic nerve trauma are minimized or even avoided.[9,10,11]

Besides being a high-benefit and low-risk procedure, FROD is also easy to perform in the hands of an experienced orbital surgeon.

35.3 Expectations

FROD can improve the cosmetic appearance due to disfiguring proptosis in type I TED patients (▶ Fig. 35.1) during the inactive phase of their disease.

In properly selected cases, the proptosis reduction usually ranges from 2 to 5 mm.[4,5,6,7,8] Therefore, FROD can be considered in patients with mild to moderate proptosis. However, in patients with severe proptosis, FROD alone may be inadequate.

The percentage of new-onset diplopia in pure FROD is about 2 to 3%.[4]

FROD is not the procedure of choice in active TAO patients when the disease is not yet stable. Operating while there is active orbital inflammation will increase bleeding, operative difficulty, and hence the risk of complications and morbidity. In active TAO, the treatment aim is to control the orbital inflammation first, usually by means of corticosteroids, immunosuppressive agents, or orbital irradiation.

Generally, FROD is not very helpful in TAO with compressive optic neuropathy. In such cases, BROD (commonly of the medial ± lateral wall) is usually required. In selected cases, FROD may be helpful in patients with TAO with optic neuropathy due to stretching of optic nerve.[9,10,11]

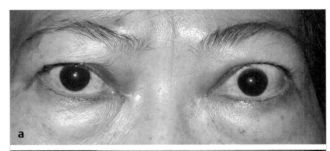
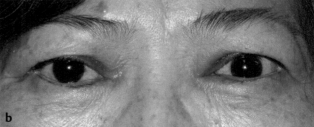

Fig. 35.1 External photographs. **(a)** Preoperative and **(b)** postoperative appearance of a type I TED patient treated with FROD.

Patients may still need strabismus and eyelid surgeries as part of the complete ophthalmic rehabilitation process.

35.4 Key Principles

In active TAO, inflammatory cells infiltrate the orbit with fibroblast activation and deposition of collagen and glycosaminoglycans (GAG) in the orbital and periorbital tissues. This is followed by scarring, fibrosis, and fat proliferation of the extraocular and levator muscles causing orbital volume enlargement. These changes in turn cause disfiguring proptosis from the limited confines of the bony orbital space. Some patients may develop more severe sight-threatening problems; for example, compressive optic neuropathy, exposure keratopathy, or diplopia.

Orbital decompression can be achieved either by expansion of the bony cavity (BROD) or removal of the orbital fat (FROD), or both.

In type I TAO, there is expansion of the orbital fat with minimal enlargement of extraocular muscles. By removing part of the orbital fat, there will be reduction in the retrobulbar orbital volume and hence proptosis.

In type II TAO, there is enlargement in extraocular muscles with less increase in orbital fat; hence, FROD is undesirable and BROD is the preferred option of orbital decompression in these cases.

35.5 Indications

FROD is indicated in type I TED patients (fat predominant type, ▶ Fig. 35.2a) with mild to moderate proptosis, in their inactive phase of disease, and require proptosis reduction for orbital rehabilitation.

Since FROD is an elective procedure, some patients may decline this surgery. This is in contrast to TED with compressive optic neuropathy where more aggressive treatment is required to salvage vision.

Other potential indications of FROD include globe retroplacement in patients with continued corneal exposure due to proptosis, anticipated keratoprosthesis, or to decrease lagophthalmos or pseudoproptosis in patients with high myopia or large eyeball.

35.6 Contraindications

- Active TED. In the active phase of disease, anti-inflammatory treatment such as systemic corticosteroid, orbital irradiation, or immunosuppressive treatment should be considered first to control the activity of the

disease. FROD should only be considered in the inactive phase of TAO.
  - Type II TED (muscle enlargement type, ▶ Fig. 35.2b), TED with compressive optic neuropathy, or malignant exophthalmos. In these situations, BROD is the preferred orbital decompression surgery technique.
  - For those patients with preexisting strabismus and diplopia, FROD may lose its advantage (i.e., inducing less postoperative diplopia); so, BROD may be considered.
  - In patients with severe proptosis greater than 5 mm, FROD may be inadequate. If complete proptosis correction is required, BROD should be considered.
- Preoperative preparation.
  - Systemic evaluation.
    – Thyroid status (hyper-, hypo-, or euthyroid), associated medical illness, e.g., myasthenia gravis, coexisting medical condition like diabetes, hypertension, or ischemic heart disease.
  - Ophthalmic evaluation.
    – Active or inactive TED (clinical activity score or VISA score), severity of TED (NO SPECS, Werner classification, or "NOSPECS" signifying No signs, Only signs, Soft tissue involvement, Proptosis, Extraocular muscle involvement, Corneal involvement, Sight loss), degree of proptosis by Hertel exophthalmometer, presence of strabismus (prism cover test), presence of upper eyelid retraction or lower eyelid scleral show (margin reflex distance, MRD_1/MRD_2), any prolapsed orbital fat, any signs of compressive optic neuropathy or globe compression.
    – It is mandatory to assess if the patient is having type I or type II TAO, either by CT scan or MRI scan.
  - Photography.
    – Pre- and postoperative photography is necessary.
  - Relevant medication history.
    – Any previous eyelid or orbital surgeries?
    – Is the patient on any antithyroid medications or thyroxine replacement therapy?
    – Is the patient on anticoagulation or antiplatelet treatment?

35.7 Operative Technique

Surgery is usually performed under general anesthesia with both eyes done at the same setting or operative session. A transforniceal conjunctival or transconjunctival incision beneath the lower margin of the tarsal plate is used. A wider surgical exposure can be achieved by swinging eyelid approach with lateral canthotomy and inferior cantholysis. However,

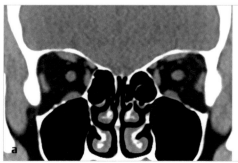
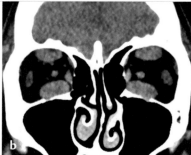

Fig. 35.2 Computed tomography, coronal plane: (a) type I vs. (b) type II TED.

lateral canthotomy and inferior cantholysis are not always necessary, especially for those patients with large palpebral fissure height.

The conjunctiva and the inferior retractors are incised. Traction sutures are then placed over the inferior cut end and the conjunctiva retraction complex is then pulled superiorly. Dissection is made at the orbital septum or the retroseptal plane (▶ Fig. 35.3a). The inferior oblique muscle is first identified between the medial and central fat pocket (▶ Fig. 35.3b). A silicone band segment can be passed underneath the inferior oblique muscle with the two ends sutured for its protection. Extraconal orbital fat is then prolapsed out and removed using the clamp, cut, cauterize technique: first clamping the fat to be excised with a small hemostat, then excision with scissors, and cauterization of the remaining clamped fat prior to releasing the clamp. The extraconal fat can be removed from the inferonasal or inferotemporal regions with more fat available at the latter (▶ Fig. 35.3c). This is then followed by removal of intraconal orbital fat which can be removed by blunt forceps (▶ Fig. 35.3d). Care must be taken not to damage the rectus muscles. The orbital fat is resected from the orbit using blunt surgical dissection to prevent damage to the surrounding tissues.[4,5,6,7,8]

Extraconal fat removal usually leads to a reduction in eyelid "bags" which are commonly seen in TED patients. On the other hand, one can preserve the extraconal fat with selective removal of intraconal fat if there are no prominent eyelid "bags" or preoperative tomography shows predominant intraconal fat expansion. All the fat removed is collected in a 5-cc syringe for measurement (▶ Fig. 35.4). In our experience, bleeding is usually mild and can be controlled by simple packing with ribbon gauze or bipolar cauterization.

The desired volume of orbital fat removal ranges from 3 to 7 mL, including 0.5 to 0.7 mL extraconal fat. For those patients with symmetrical proptosis on both sides, the same amount of orbital fat should be removed from both sides. However, intraoperative assessment of the globe position is essential.

For those with asymmetrical proptosis, more fat should be removed from the more proptotic eye to achieve better postoperative symmetry. A rough guide correlation for 1 mL of

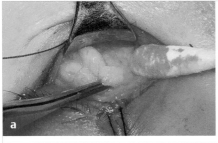
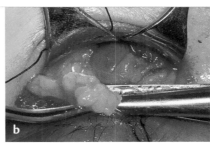
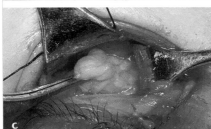
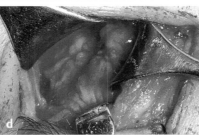

Fig. 35.3 (a) Intraoperative photograph, left orbit, surgeon's view. Dissection was made at the orbital septum or the retroseptum plane. The extraconal fat was exposed. **(b)** Intraoperative photograph, left orbit, surgeon's view. The inferior oblique muscle is identified between the medial and central fat pockets. Lateral extraconal fat is being removed. **(c)** Intraoperative photograph, left orbit, surgeon's view. After retraction of inferior oblique muscle, the extraconal fat and intraconal fat can be removed from the inferotemporal region. **(d)** Intraoperative photograph, left orbit, surgeon's view. After adequate removal of intraconal fat, only minimal intraconal fat left deep inside the orbit.

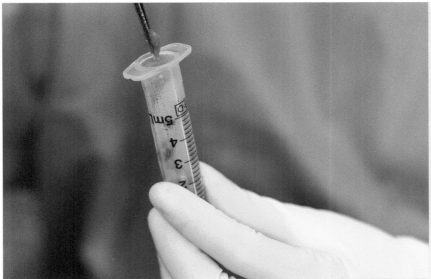

Fig. 35.4 All the removed fats are placed inside a syringe to measure the total volume of fat removed.

orbital fat removed, 0.8 mm of proptosis reduction is achieved.

Fat removal from the anterior one-third and middle one-third of the orbit is generally safe with a low-risk profile. Orbital fat removal from the posterior one-third of the orbit is associated with a higher complication including bleeding, mydriasis, and diplopia.

In some cases, the inflammatory TED has left the fat fibrotic and difficult to remove. In these cases, the amount of fat removed may be less than expected with insufficient proptosis reduction. BROD may be required for complete rehabilitation at the same setting or at a second stage depending on surgeon's and patients' choice.

35.8 Tips and Pearls

- Case selection is crucial for optimal result. Ideal patients are those with type I TED in the inactive phase of disease, with mild to moderate proptosis, who need improvement in their cosmetic appearance.
- A rough estimation is that for every 1 mL of orbital fat removed, there will be around 0.8 mm of proptosis reduction.
- Immediate ice packing and a short course of oral steroid after the surgery may help reduce postoperative swelling.
- Patients should be informed that eyelid surgeries (e.g., repair of eyelid retraction) may be needed for final rehabilitative effect.

35.9 What to Avoid

- Incorrect case selection (active TED, type II TED with muscle enlargement, TED with compressive optic neuropathy).
- Avoid damage to the extraocular muscles—this can be avoided with careful dissection and avoidance of sharp dissection.
- Overly aggressive fat removal at the posterior one-third of the orbit where there will be a higher chance of ciliary ganglion or cranial nerve injury.
- Though there is no direct correlation between the intraoperative pupil size and final visual outcome, pupil size can easily be assessed intraoperatively. One should exercise caution when pupil dilatation is seen.

35.10 Complications/Bailout/ Salvage

35.10.1 Possible Intraoperative Complications

- Generally, intraoperative complications are uncommon. Bleeding can be controlled by packing, pressure, and occasionally diathermy.
- In some cases, the orbital fat may be fibrotic. Excessive force and sharp dissection should not be used in these cases. Instead, additional bony decompression may be required, either at the same stage or as a second-stage procedure, to achieve adequate decompression effect.
- Other rare intraoperative complications include
  - Muscle damage—the torn muscle should be repaired.
  - Ciliary ganglion damage —from overly aggressive orbital fat removal in the posterior one-third of the orbit.
  - Optic nerve damage—very rare, strict intraoperative technique should be used.

35.10.2 Postoperative Complications

- Proptosis recurrence: This may be due to incorrect choice of patient, inadequate fat removal, reactivation of disease, postoperative fat regeneration, or age-related change in orbital fat volume.
- Retrobulbar hematoma: Lateral canthotomy and cantholysis may be required to relieve the pressure.
- Infection: Systemic antibiotics are recommended. The use of prophylactic antibiotics may help reduce the incidence of postoperative infection.
- New-onset diplopia: Secondary strabismus surgery may be needed.
- Pupil dilation: Usually it will spontaneously recover. Pilocarpine eyedrops may be useful in the short term to reduce light sensitivity.
- Optic neuropathy.

35.11 Postoperative Care

- Dexamethasone and antibiotic eyedrops on the operated eye for 1 to 4 weeks.
- Oral prednisone for 3 to 5 days to reduce swelling (optional).
- Oral antibiotic prophylaxis for 1 week (optional).

References

[1] Olivari N. Transpalpebral decompression of endocrine ophthalmopathy (Graves' disease) by removal of intraorbital fat: experience with 147 operations over 5 years. Plast Reconstr Surg. 1991; 87(4):627–641, discussion 642–643

[2] Adenis JP, Robert PY, Lasudry JG, Dalloul Z. Treatment of proptosis with fat removal orbital decompression in Graves' ophthalmopathy. Eur J Ophthalmol. 1998; 8(4):246–252

[3] Robert PY, Camezind P, Adenis JP. [Orbital fat decompression techniques]. J Fr Ophtalmol. 2004; 27(7):845–850

[4] Wu CH, Chang TC, Liao SL. Results and predictability of fat-removal orbital decompression for disfiguring graves exophthalmos in an Asian patient population. Am J Ophthalmol. 2008; 145(4):755–759

[5] Liao SL, Huang SW. Correlation of retrobulbar volume change with resected orbital fat volume and proptosis reduction after fatty decompression for Graves ophthalmopathy. Am J Ophthalmol. 2011; 151(3):465–9.e1

[6] Li EY, Kwok TY, Cheng AC, Wong AC, Yuen HK. Fat-removal orbital decompression for disfiguring proptosis associated with Graves' ophthalmopathy: safety, efficacy and predictability of outcomes. Int Ophthalmol. 2015; 35(3): 325–329

[7] Cheng AM, Wei YH, Tighe S, Sheha H, Liao SL. Long-term outcomes of orbital fat decompression in Graves' orbitopathy. Br J Ophthalmol. 2018; 102(1):69–73

[8] Al-Sharif E, Alsuhaibani AH. Fat-removal orbital decompression for thyroid associated orbitopathy: the right procedure for the right patient. Saudi J Ophthalmol. 2017; 31(3):156–161

[9] O'Malley MR, Meyer DR. Transconjunctival fat removal combined with conservative medial wall/floor orbital decompression for Graves orbitopathy. Ophthal Plast Reconstr Surg. 2009; 25(3):206–210

[10] Boboridis KG, Uddin J, Mikropoulos DG, et al. Critical appraisal on orbital decompression for thyroid eye disease: a systematic review and literature search. Adv Ther. 2015; 32(7):595–611

[11] Braun TL, Bhadkamkar MA, Jubbal KT, Weber AC, Marx DP. Orbital decompression for thyroid eye disease. Semin Plast Surg. 2017; 31(1):40–45

36 Endoscopic Orbital Decompression

Benjamin S. Bleier and Sarina K. Mueller

Abstract

Endoscopic medial orbital wall and floor decompression may be indicated for several reasons including thyroid eye disease, compressive or stretch optic neuropathy, and orbital tumors. Access to inferomedially based orbital tumors is also facilitated by the endoscopic approach. The greatest advantages of the endoscopic technique are the avoidance of scars, an improved visualization of certain landmarks, and the ability to address concomitant sinonasal pathology or perform optic canal decompression. In order to minimize postoperative diplopia, the inferomedial strut may be preserved.

Keywords: inferomedial strut, orbital tumor, medial/inferior decompression, thyroid eye disease, sinonasal pathology, optic nerve decompression, optic neuropathy, diplopia

36.1 Goals

When performing endoscopic orbital decompression for thyroid eye disease, indications may be compressive or stretch optic neuropathy requiring expansion of the orbital apex or recession of the globe. Thus, the goal is bony decompression (i.e., expansion of the bony orbit) to allow restoration of optic nerve function. In other cases, exposure keratopathy and cosmetic proptosis are the primary indications. In these cases, reduction of proptosis is the primary goal. Endoscopic decompression techniques may also be used to provide access to inferomedial tumors of the extra- and intraconal spaces.

36.2 Advantages

Advantages of endoscopic orbital decompression are the avoidance of external incisions, magnified visualization of certain landmarks, and the ability to address concomitant sinonasal pathology. To minimize postoperative diplopia, the inferomedial strut can be reliably preserved using angled drills and instrumentation. Lastly, in select cases, simultaneous optic nerve canal decompression in case of compressive optic neuropathy can be performed.[1]

36.3 Expectations

These depend on the individual patient's indication for the surgery. In patients with disfiguring proptosis or exposure keratopathy, the expectation is an improvement in exophthalmometry measurements. A mean ocular recession of 3.5 to 5.5 mm might be achieved with combined medial and inferior decompression. An additional 2 mm can be achieved through concurrent lateral decompression.[2,3,4,5,6,7] Additional recession can be achieved with fat removal. In a review of 45 decompressed orbits (medial + lateral or medial + lateral + floor), the mean reduction in proptosis was 3.89 mm.[8]

Regarding intraocular pressure, in patients with varying degrees of thyroid eye disease, decompression has been reported to decrease pressures from 19.3 ± 4.4 mm Hg to 17.0 ± 2.9 mm Hg at 1 week and to 15.9 ± 3.7 mm Hg at 6 months.[5,9]

Visual improvement for surgical orbital apex/optic nerve decompression can vary greatly depending on severity and duration of optic nerve compression. In series with a breadth of cases treated with surgery and with or without steroid therapy, improvement varied between 27 and 82%.[10,11,12]

Diplopia is a common, yet often unavoidable, outcome following endoscopic orbital decompression surgery. Rates of new-onset diplopia range from approximately 20 to 30%, although rarely resolution of diplopia may occur.[8] Additional strabismus surgery may be necessary for improvement of diplopia and patients should be routinely counseled on the potential need for corrective strabismus surgery.

36.4 Key Principles

- Provide wide endoscopic access to medial and inferior walls of the orbit through comprehensive adjacent sinus surgery.
- Protection of unopened sinuses against iatrogenic obstruction from orbital fat prolapse.
- Removal of the medial and inferior bony walls of the orbit ± inferomedial strut.
- Incision of the periorbita in order to allow feathering of extraconal fat, which facilitates orbital fat prolapse into the ethmoid and maxillary sinus cavities.
- Reduction of intraorbital pressure on the neurovascular structures caused by enlarged extraocular muscles, fat, orbital tumors, and other space-occupying lesions.

36.5 Indications

Orbital decompression is performed for several conditions and indications. The most common indication for orbital decompression is dysthyroid orbitopathy resulting from Graves' disease.

When enlarged extraocular muscles and fat increase in size due to the thyroid eye disease, compression of the optic nerve can result. Surgical decompression of the bony orbit relieves this compression and may allow for vision recovery. Other indications in patients with thyroid eye disease include the reduction of proptosis. Proptosis can lead to exposure keratopathy, corneal ulceration, and perforation which can ultimately result in vision loss. Additionally, the cosmetic disfigurement may cause psychosocial limitations in dysthyroid orbitopathy patients.

Other indications include providing endoscopic access to orbital tumors or lesions that cannot be safely accessed otherwise. These conditions may also cause compressive optic neuropathy, proptosis, and visual dysfunction.

36.6 Contraindications

Patients undergoing endoscopic orbital surgery must be candidates for general anesthesia.

36.7 Surgical Approach

36.7.1 Preoperative Preparation

A CT scan is generally obtained preoperatively to verify the bony anatomy of the orbit and the surrounding sinonasal structures. If Graves' orbitopathy is suspected, intravenous contrast should not be applied, as there are reported cases of orbitopathy exacerbation after the administration of iodine-containing intravenous contrast. MRI scans, particularly fat-suppression sequences, can be helpful in the identification and characterization of intraorbital pathology. Contrast enhancement may facilitate localization of the ophthalmic artery, which should be avoided during intraconal surgery due to its position adjacent the optic nerve.

36.7.2 Operative Technique

As with all sinonasal surgery, the surgery begins with decongestion and optimization of hemostasis. This can be achieved by elevating the head and topicalization using 1:1,000 fluorescein-labeled epinephrine-soaked neuropathies. Local anesthetic may also be injected into the axilla of the middle turbinate to further reduce bleeding from the anterior ethmoid arterial distribution.

The entire surgery may be performed with a 0-degree endoscope. However, angled scopes are useful in the setting of inferomedial strut preservation.[13,14] Septoplasty or middle turbinate resection may be performed as needed. However, middle turbinate resection should be performed only when necessary, since it carries the risk of olfactory disruption, frontal sinus obstruction, and postoperative epistaxis.

The first surgical step is the removal of the uncinate process at its insertion on the maxillary line. After the removal of the uncinate process, the maxillary sinus should be opened in all cases, even when no orbital floor decompression is needed, to avoid iatrogenic maxillary obstruction. The ethmoid bulla, basal lamella, and posterior ethmoid cells are removed entirely. It is important to extend the dissection to the entire skull base if maximal decompression is necessary. The sphenoid sinus does not have to be opened in all cases as the remaining superior turbinate will typically protect the sphenoid sinus from the obstruction by orbital fat. However, if a maximal orbital apex decompression is necessary, partial resection of the superior turbinate and wide opening of the sphenoid face are required. After complete opening of the sinuses, the mucosa may be stripped from the lamina papyracea to the lateral skull base in order to avoid postoperative mucocele formation. The removal of the lamina papyracea may be performed by first creating a micro infracture. Then upbiting Blakesley forceps and ball-tipped probe are used to carefully medially reflect and remove the bony fragments (► Fig. 36.1). Once completed, the periorbital fascial layer will be encountered (Fig. 36.2). At this point, the medial rectus muscle and several venous structures might be identified through the periorbita which should be spared during periorbital incision. Depending on the extent of decompression necessary, the degree of periorbital incision can be tailored. If a maximal decompression is desired, regardless of concerns for the induction of postoperative diplopia, the medial periorbita may be stripped completely (Fig. 36.3). To decrease diplopia rate, a strip of periorbita may be retained overlying the medial rectus muscle to function as a sling (Fig. 36.2).[15] Once the periorbita has been removed, the orbital fat may be feathered medially using blunt instrumentation (e.g., double ball probe or blunt sickle knife) as well as gentle pressure on the globe in order to disrupt the periorbital fascial bands and enhance the degree of decompression (Fig. 36.4).

The endoscopic decompression of the orbital floor requires a similar extent of adjacent sinus surgery. Though rarely

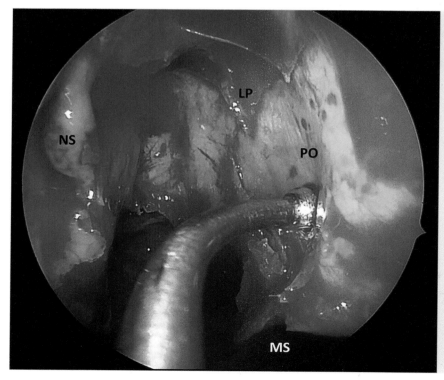

Fig. 36.1 Endoscopic view of the left medial orbit demonstrating use of a ball-tipped probe to resect the lamina bone. NS, nasal septum; LP, lamina papyracea; PO, periorbita; MS, maxillary sinus.

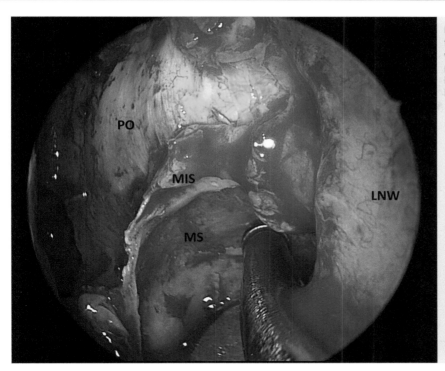

Fig. 36.2 Endoscopic view of the left orbit following removal of the medial and inferior bony walls with preservation of the inferomedial strut prior to periorbital incision. PO, periorbita; MIS, inferomedial strut; MS, maxillary sinus; LNW, lateral nasal wall.

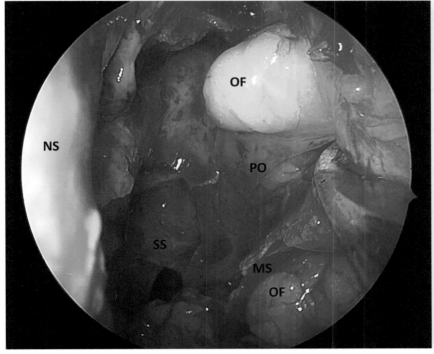

Fig. 36.3 Endoscopic view of the left orbit demonstrating controlled incision of the periorbita. NS, nasal septum; OF, orbital fat; PO, periorbita; SS, sphenoid sinus; MS, maxillary sinus.

performed, an isolated orbital floor decompression might be performed while preserving the basal lamella and posterior ethmoid air cells. Maximizing the vertical dimension of the maxillary antrostomy is important to ensure adequate access for orbital floor decompression. The superior maxillary sinus mucosa may be reflected laterally prior to bone removal to facilitate preservation and redraping after completion of the surgery. This procedure facilitates remucosalization, reduces

postoperative crusting, and expedites postoperative healing.[16] The removal of the orbital floor is performed with a curette and is limited to the area medial to the infraorbital canal. In patients without preoperative diplopia, the inferomedial bony strut may be preserved in order to limit globe prolapse and to reduce postoperative diplopia (Fig. 36.5).[8,13,17,18] This requires precise drilling of the orbital floor between the inferomedial strut and infraorbital canal, as down fracture using a curette risks

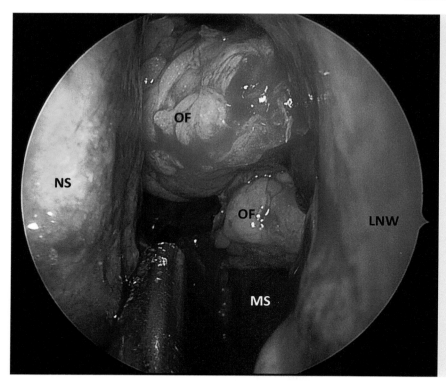

Fig. 36.4 Endoscopic view of left orbit demonstrating completed decompression with orbital fat prolapse and preservation of the inferomedial strut. SN, nasal septum; OF, orbital fat; MS, maxillary sinus; LNW, lateral nasal wall.

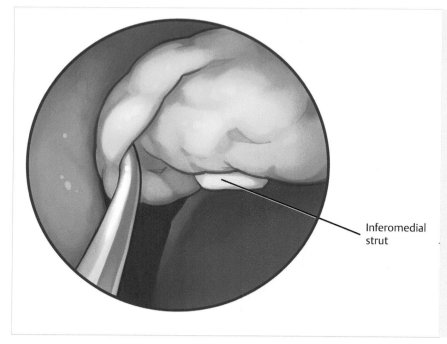

Fig. 36.5 Illustration of the left orbit demonstrating completed medial decompression with orbital fat prolapse and preservation of the inferomedial strut.

migration of the fracture line through the strut with consequential loss of structural support. Finally, as with the medial decompression, the exposed periorbita must be incised to release the orbital fat into the maxillary sinus while avoiding direct injury to the inferior rectus muscle. In order to increase the dissection corridor for further surgical steps e.g. for intraoperative tumor resection, the orbital process of the palatine bone (OPPB) may be resected (Fig. 36.6).[19]

36.8 Tips and Pearls

- Unlike in traditional endoscopic sinus surgery, the superior insertion of the uncinate process is left in place in order to protect the frontal recess from the secondary obstruction by orbital fat prolapse.
- The sphenoid suture line may be identified as the transition of the thinner lamina papyracea to the thicker sphenoid bone.

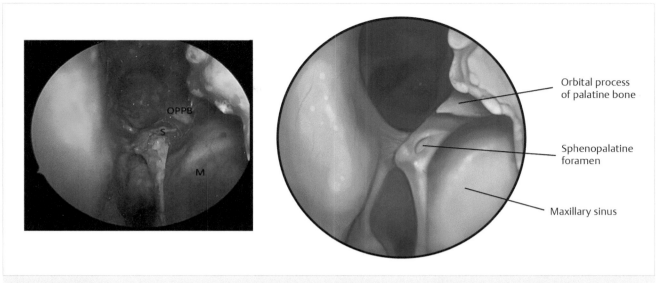

Fig. 36.6 Illustration of the left orbit demonstrating the surgical anatomy for OPPB (orbital process of palatine bone) resection.

- For inferomedial strut preservation during floor decompression, a 4-mm high-speed tapered 70-degree diamond bur (Medtronic, Jacksonville, Fl) is used to thin the bone from the lateral edge of the inferomedial strut to the medial border of the infraorbital canal under direct visualization using a 70-degree endoscope. A double ball probe may then be used to down fracture the bone away from the orbit. Further bony expansion or fine adjustments might be performed using a frontal sinus cobra through punch (Karl Storz, Tuttlingen, Germany).

36.9 What to Avoid

- Early uncontrolled penetration of the periorbita should be avoided, as herniated orbital fat may obscure visualization of the surgical field.
- Cauterization within the orbit should be avoided to prevent thermal damage to the sensitive orbital structures.
- Packing should be avoided postoperatively to minimize pressure on the orbit and allow accumulated blood to drain.
- Patients must refrain from nose blowing and should sneeze with an open mouth to minimize intrasinus pressure and reduce the risk of orbital emphysema.
- The eye should never be patched after orbital surgery so as to not obscure detection of postoperative vision loss or hemorrhage.

36.10 Postoperative Care

- Discharge medications may include an oral antistaphylococcal antibiotic and steroid taper if deemed necessary.
- Patients should have limited activity for 2 weeks and should not resume anticoagulant medications until several days after surgery.
- The first postoperative follow-up visit should be scheduled within 1 week after surgery. Twice-daily low-pressure nasal

saline irrigations should be initiated after the first follow-up visit.
- At 1 week, the inferior airway may be carefully debrided to assist with breathing and mucosal healing. Clot adjacent to the orbit or optic nerve should be left in place to be irrigated out by the patient over the subsequent 3 to 4 weeks.

36.11 Complications/Bailout/Salvage

General surgical complications may include infection, postoperative edema, and hemorrhage. To minimize the risk of orbital infection, intravenous antibiotics should be administered intraoperatively. Retrobulbar hemorrhage can quickly result in permanent visual loss if unrecognized or untreated. Use of intraorbital electrocautery within the orbit is not recommended. However, for well-visualized vessels in the orbital walls (e.g., infraorbital, anterior, or posterior ethmoid), bipolar cauterization can be vision preserving. Maintaining a conduit for blood egress (i.e., decompression) and saline lavage, however, are safer. Postoperatively, patients must refrain from exercise or strenuous activity for 2 weeks. Although agreement with a primary care physician or cardiologist is critical, initiation of anticoagulant medications should be delayed until several days after surgery. The eye should never be patched after orbital surgery, as it is critical that patients are able to monitor their vision postoperatively to be able to immediately report any changes.

When performing an endoscopic decompression, additional immediate complications may include high-flow arterial bleeding from sphenopalatine arterial branches or the internal carotid artery including the anterior and posterior ethmoidal branches. However, the latter is much less common.

A cerebrospinal fluid (CSF) leak may also occur during the ethmoid and sphenoid dissection or when resecting the lamina papyracea from the frontoethmoidal suture line. If this occurs, the site should be identified, cleared of mucosa, and repaired in an over and underlay fashion per standard CSF leak repairs.

Lastly, the periorbital incision might directly injure the extraocular muscles. This is best avoided using a sharp blade (e.g., disposable sickle knife) to minimize the amount of pressure needed to incise the periorbita and placing incision well above and below the expected course of the extraocular muscles. Once the periorbita has been incised, the feathering of orbital fat should be performed carefully and gently with a blunt probe to avoid damage to intraorbital structures.

A long-term complication includes postobstructive mucocele formation, reinforcing the importance of prophylactic sinusotomy, and meticulous mucosal stripping.

References

[1] Jacquesson T, Abouaf L, Berhouma M, Jouanneau E. How I do it: the endoscopic endonasal optic nerve and orbital apex decompression. Acta Neurochir (Wien). 2014; 156(10):1891–1896

[2] Hauser LJ, Ir D, Kingdom TT, Robertson CE, Frank DN, Ramakrishnan VR. Evaluation of bacterial transmission to the paranasal sinuses through sinus irrigation. Int Forum Allergy Rhinol. 2016; 6(8):800–806

[3] Ueland HO, Haugen OH, Rødahl E. Temporal hollowing and other adverse effects after lateral orbital wall decompression. Acta Ophthalmol. 2016; 94(8):793–797

[4] Kingdom TT, Davies BW, Durairaj VD. Orbital decompression for the management of thyroid eye disease: an analysis of outcomes and complications. Laryngoscope. 2015; 125(9):2034–2040

[5] Paridaens DA, Verhoeff K, Bouwens D, van Den Bosch WA. Transconjunctival orbital decompression in Graves' ophthalmopathy: lateral wall approach ab interno. Br J Ophthalmol. 2000; 84(7):775–781

[6] Siracuse-Lee DE, Kazim M. Orbital decompression: current concepts. Curr Opin Ophthalmol. 2002; 13(5):310–316

[7] Leong SC, Karkos PD, Macewen CJ, White PS. A systematic review of outcomes following surgical decompression for dysthyroid orbitopathy. Laryngoscope. 2009; 119(6):1106–1115

[8] Finn AP, Bleier B, Cestari DM, et al. A retrospective review of orbital decompression for thyroid orbitopathy with endoscopic preservation of the inferomedial orbital bone strut. Ophthal Plast Reconstr Surg. 2017; 33(5):334–339

[9] Takahashi Y, Nakamura Y, Ichinose A, Kakizaki H. Intraocular pressure change with eye positions before and after orbital decompression for thyroid eye disease. Ophthal Plast Reconstr Surg. 2014; 30(1):47–50

[10] Joseph MP, Lessell S, Rizzo J, Momose KJ. Extracranial optic nerve decompression for traumatic optic neuropathy. Arch Ophthalmol. 1990; 108(8):1091–1093

[11] Levin LA, Beck RW, Joseph MP, Seiff S, Kraker R. The treatment of traumatic optic neuropathy: the International Optic Nerve Trauma Study. Ophthalmology. 1999; 106(7):1268–1277

[12] Kountakis SE, Maillard AA, El-Harazi SM, Longhini L, Urso RG. Endoscopic optic nerve decompression for traumatic blindness. Otolaryngol Head Neck Surg. 2000; 123(1, Pt 1):34–37

[13] Bleier BS, Lefebvre DR, Freitag SK. Endoscopic orbital floor decompression with preservation of the inferomedial strut. Int Forum Allergy Rhinol. 2014; 4(1):82–84

[14] Yao WC, Sedaghat AR, Yadav P, Fay A, Metson R. Orbital decompression in the endoscopic age: the modified inferomedial orbital strut. Otolaryngol Head Neck Surg. 2016; 154(5):963–969

[15] Metson R, Samaha M. Reduction of diplopia following endoscopic orbital decompression: the orbital sling technique. Laryngoscope. 2002; 112(10):1753–1757

[16] Palmer N, Chiu A. Atlas of Endoscopic Sinus and Skull Base Surgery. 1st ed. Elsevier; 2013:255

[17] Goldberg RA, Shorr N, Cohen MS. The medical orbital strut in the prevention of postdecompression dystopia in dysthyroid ophthalmopathy. Ophthal Plast Reconstr Surg. 1992; 8(1):32–34

[18] Wright ED, Davidson J, Codere F, Desrosiers M. Endoscopic orbital decompression with preservation of an inferomedial bony strut: minimization of postoperative diplopia. J Otolaryngol. 1999; 28(5):252–256

[19] Mueller SK, Freitag SK, Bleier BS. Morphometric Analysis of the Orbital Process of the Palatine Bone and its Relationship to Endoscopic Orbital Apex Surgery. Ophthalmic Plast Reconstr Surg. 2018 May/Jun;34(3):254-257. doi: 10.1097/IOP.0000000000000940.)

37 Anterior Orbitotomy

Catherine Y. Liu and Vinay K. Aakalu

Summary

An anterior orbitotomy is a broad term to indicate entry into the orbit, generally to the orbit anterior to the equator of the globe. A multitude of techniques are available, and the ones discussed here are extensions of commonly used incisions fundamental to oculofacial plastic surgery. Access to the posterior orbit can be achieved with modification of the described techniques. In this chapter, we organize approaches based on location of the orbit: superior, inferior, lateral, and medial.

Keywords: anterior orbitotomy, lid crease incision, lid split, subbrow incision, Lynch incision, subciliary incision, transconjunctival incision, transcaruncular approach, subconjunctival space, swinging eyelid

37.1 Goals

The goals of the surgery are dependent on the problem being addressed, which is determined prior to surgery. In general, surgery performed should provide adequate access and visualization of the area, should minimize the risk of damage to the surrounding structures, and leave minimal visible scars. Preoperative planning should incorporate a detailed medical history, examination, and imaging to formulate a differential diagnosis. An anterior orbitotomy is performed to access areas anterior to the equator of the globe. Isolated, well-circumscribed lesions may warrant total excisional biopsy while infiltrative lesions may warrant incisional biopsy for tissue diagnosis. Anteriorly positioned abscesses can be evacuated via different anterior orbitotomy approaches.

37.2 Advantages

Many of the anterior orbitotomy approaches are extensions of common incisions used in oculoplastic surgery. Some of these approaches can also be used to access the posterior orbit. These incisions are commonly placed in areas that heal with imperceptible or minimal scarring.

37.3 Expectations

With correct selection of biopsy location, surgeons should expect excellent access to the relevant portion(s) of the orbit with minimal risk of damage to surrounding structures.

37.4 Key Principles

37.4.1 Location

Preoperative determination of the location of the lesion guides the anterior orbitotomy approach (▶ Fig. 37.1). Lesions located in the superior orbit can be accessed by an eyelid crease, subbrow, eyelid split, or fornix approach. The medial orbit can be accessed by a transcaruncular, transconjunctival, or Lynch incision. Lesions in the inferior orbit can be accessed by an external transcutaneous approach such as a subciliary, lower eyelid crease; direct orbital rim incision; or internal transconjunctival approach such as a conjunctival or fornix incision. The lateral orbit is typically accessed with a canthotomy and cantholysis (e.g., swinging eyelid incision). This may be necessary for lesions more posteriorly located in the orbit or for placement of large orbital implants.

Combined approaches (inferior fornix + swinging eyelid) are useful for large lesions that span two spaces (e.g., the inferior and lateral orbit). Accessing the subperiosteal location may be more easily achieved with certain approaches (e.g., subbrow or eyelid crease incision vs. superior fornix approach).

37.4.2 Well-Hidden Incisions

Although cosmesis is not the primary goal of orbitotomy procedures, utilization of approaches close to the lesion that hide incisions can lead to superior results without compromising access. Choices include the upper eyelid crease, palpebral conjunctiva, subciliary line, and subciliary brow.

37.4.3 Exposure

By utilizing an approach where the incision hides well allows the surgeon to comfortably create a wide incision for improved surgical exposure. When working deep in the orbit, maintaining a wide superficial incision improves visualization. Retraction of superficial structures with skin hooks, Desmarres retractors, and traction sutures and deeper structures with Sewall or malleable retractors helps exposure and dissection. Care should be taken to avoid prolonged or high pressure on the globe during retraction.

37.4.4 Hemostasis

A dry field makes exposing and removing an orbital lesion more manageable. Additionally, blood pressure, pain, and nausea should be well controlled during and after surgery. Herbal medications and supplements such as gingko biloba, vitamin E, and ginseng should be discontinued preoperatively. Intraoperative techniques to help control hemostasis include reverse Trendelenburg positioning, epinephrine injection (care should be taken to monitor for rebound bleeding after effects of epinephrine wear off), bipolar cauterization, and platelet-activating products such as absorbable gelatin (Gelfoam), oxidized regenerated cellulose (Surgicel), and thrombin (FloSeal). Paraffin wax can be useful for bony bleeding, although there are reports of retained wax causing granuloma formation or infection.[1] Cool compresses and gentle pressure are time tested and also well tolerated, if applied with caution (i.e., avoid prolonged ice packs

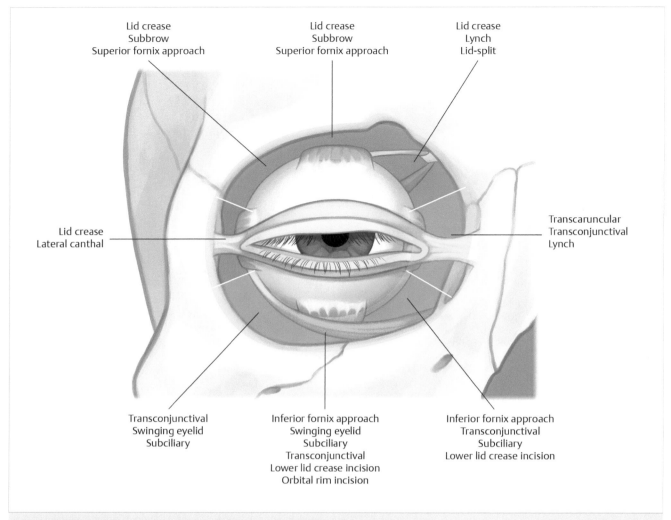

Fig. 37.1 Anterior orbitotomy approaches for various locations of lesions.

or excessive pressure). Intraoperative packing, such as neurosurgical patties, soaked with epinephrine-containing products can be used, but care should be taken to avoid excessive pressure, blood pressure changes with epinephrine, and retained packing material.

37.5 Indications

Anterior orbitotomy is indicated for access to lesions anterior to the equator of the globe. This may include the excision of orbital masses, incisional biopsies, drainage of abscesses, and removal of foreign bodies.

37.6 Contraindications

Contraindications to surgery are decided on a case-to-case basis. In general, access to deep orbital lesions may not be accessible with some approaches discussed here (see individual sections for more detail). An approach that does not provide

adequate exposure to visualize the surgical target or control bleeding is another relative contraindication.

37.7 Preoperative Preparation

The patient should be cleared medically prior to proceeding with surgery. Blood pressure should be controlled. Preoperative risk stratification and assessment for the possibility of discontinuing blood thinners perioperatively should be done in conjunction with the patient's primary care physician. Elective procedures should be avoided if blood thinners cannot be stopped. Herbal remedies (such as the ones discussed earlier) should also be discontinued.

The risks of the procedure should be thoroughly discussed and documented. In general, risks for anterior orbitotomies include infection, pain, postoperative edema and ecchymosis, ptosis, lagophthalmos, diplopia, and rarely postoperative orbital hemorrhage that can lead to permanent blindness. Rare complications include infection, orbital compartment syndrome, cerebrospinal fluid leak, or blindness.

37.8 Operative Technique

37.8.1 Superior Orbit

Upper Eyelid Crease Approach

This approach has the advantage of a cosmetically well-hidden incision (▶ Fig. 37.2a). It can be used to access the superior orbit either through the septum or the superior subperiosteal space.

Transseptal Approach

The patient is placed under local or general anesthesia. Corneal protectors are placed. The upper eyelid crease is demarcated with a marking pen. Local anesthesia (admixture of lidocaine and bupivacaine with 1:100,000 parts epinephrine) is infiltrated into the upper eyelid. An incision is made along the marked line sufficiently long for adequate exposure of the lesion. The orbicularis oculi muscle is then incised to expose the orbital septum. Meticulous hemostasis should be maintained. Once the septum is exposed, retractors (e.g., skin hooks) are centered over the lesion. Finger palpation of the lesion can help with localization. After horizontal incision through the septum, blunt dissection can locate, isolate, and remove the lesion. If the goal is an incisional biopsy, sufficient tissue for diagnosis should be removed. Clear communication with the pathologist including relevant history, clinical findings, and differential diagnosis is important for accurate diagnosis.

Subperiosteal Approach

The subperiosteal space can be accessed through this same incision. After the incision is made in the orbicularis muscle, a preseptal dissection plane is carried superiorly to the orbital rim, where sharp dissection can be carried to the periosteum. The periosteum overlying the frontal bone can then be incised and elevated to the arcus marginalis. Then, the superior subperiosteal space of the orbit is entered. Aggressive dissection at the arcus marginalis should be avoided, as periosteal violation can allow orbital fat to herniate into the field, limiting visualization. The eyelid crease incision can be extended medially, but should not cross any epicanthal folds or the medial canthal tendon, as contracture and formation of a medial canthal web may occur. In the superomedial orbit, there are numerous neurovascular structures (supraorbital bundle, supratrochlear bundle, trochlea, superior oblique) that should not be disrupted, if possible.

Subbrow Approach (Superior Subperiosteal Approach)

A subbrow approach can be used as a more direct approach to the superior subperiosteal plane or to access to the frontal bone for procedures such as mucocele removal, frontal sinus access, or limited frontal craniotomy (▶ Fig. 37.2b). This incision increases the chance of visible cutaneous scar, although placement of the incision adjacent to the cilia of the brow makes it generally well accepted.

The supraorbital notch is palpated at the medial superior rim and marked to avoid inadvertent injury to the supraorbital neurovascular bundle. Following infiltration with local anesthetic, this incision is made in the skin at the inferior brow cilia. Dissection is carried down to the periosteum about 5 mm superior to the orbital rim. An incision is then made through the periosteum using a blade or Freer elevator, and the periosteum is elevated off of the rim. The subperiosteal dissection continues inferiorly detaching the arcus marginalis and entering the superior subperiosteal space in the orbit. After completion of surgery, the periosteum may be closed with interrupted absorbable sutures, and the skin can be closed with interrupted absorbable sutures.

37.8.2 Inferior Orbit

Lower Eyelid Transcutaneous Approach

Inferior orbital lesions in the extraconal space can be approached via the subciliary skin or the inferior palpebral conjunctiva. These

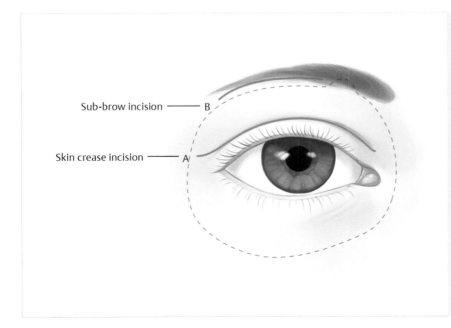

Fig. 37.2 Upper eyelid approaches. **(a)** Upper lid skin crease incision. **(b)** Subbrow incision.

Sub-brow incision ——— B

Skin crease incision ——— A

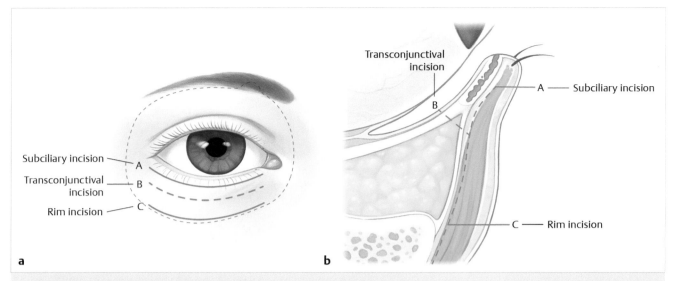

Fig. 37.3 (a,b) Lower eyelid approaches. (A) Lower lid transcutaneous incision. (B) Lower lid transconjunctival incision. *Dotted line* signifies incision made on the palpebral conjunctiva. (C) Rim incision.

offer excellent exposure to the orbit with low risk of postoperative eyelid malposition or visible scar. The lower eyelid crease incision or direct rim incision have been described; however, they routinely lead to disfiguring scars, and offer few advantages to the other access points (▶ Fig. 37.3).

The area can also be accessed by a conjunctival approach. An incision can be made a few millimeters inferior to the inferior tarsal border or it can be made in the fornix. These internal approaches generally give good cosmesis. Occasionally, releasing the capsulopalpebral fascia can lead to lower lid entropion or ectropion in those who already have eyelid laxity.

Subciliary Incision

The skin is marked horizontally 3 mm below the lower eyelid margin starting from the level of the punctum to the lateral canthus. A corneal protector is placed. Local anesthetic (equal parts lidocaine and bupivacaine with 1:100,000 parts epinephrine) is infiltrated. An incision is made in the skin. Sharp dissection is performed through the orbicularis oculi muscle and the orbital septum. Dissection is continued in the preseptal plane inferiorly to the orbital rim. Palpation of the lesion helps identify the rim. The orbital septum is incised overlying the area to be accessed. Blunt dissection is advocated for surgery within the orbit. Once meticulous hemostasis is obtained, the skin can be closed with a running 6–0 suture. No sutures are placed through the orbital septum. Antibiotic ointment is applied to the sutures.

Note that care should be taken when dissecting the septum as scarring can rarely lead to lower lid retraction or ectropion.[2]

Transconjunctival Approach

A corneal protector is placed, and local anesthetic is injected into the lower lid margin and the palpebral conjunctiva. A 4–0 silk traction suture is placed through tarsus at the margin. A Desmarres retractor is used to evert the lower eyelid to expose the conjunctiva. A horizontal incision is made in the conjunctiva and capsulopalpebral fascia across the width of the lower eyelid 2 to 3 mm inferior to the inferior tarsal border. Blunt dissection can be performed through capsulopalpebral fascia. A 4–0 silk traction suture is placed through the inferior cut edge of conjunctiva and retracted superiorly. Using blunt dissection technique, dissection in the preseptal plane can be carried inferiorly to the orbital rim. Note that the preseptal plane may be translucent with orbital fat pads sometimes visible through intact septum. Entry into the orbit and exposure of the relevant area are identical to the transcutaneous route. After hemostasis is obtained, the conjunctiva and capsulopalpebral fascia may be closed using three interrupted 6–0 fast absorbing gut sutures. Alternatively, it can be left open.[3]

Fornix Approach

The conjunctival fornix approach can be used to access the superior or inferior orbit (e.g., orbital floor, inferomedial, and inferolateral locations). Of note, a superolateral fornix incision should be avoided due to the presence of the lacrimal gland ductules. Transection can lead to dry eye or dacryocele formation.

Local anesthesia is infiltrated into the eyelid margin, and 4–0 silk traction suture placed to retract the eyelid away from the globe. Alternatively, Jaffe eyelid specula may be used. Local anesthetic is injected into the subconjunctival space. Traction sutures of 6–0 silk are placed at the corneal limbus to rotate the globe away from the area of interest. An incision is made in the conjunctiva at the fornix using Westcott scissors.

Tips

Occasionally, the lower eyelid fat pads are encountered immediately after incising the capsulopalpebral fascia. This occurs when the incision is made too inferiorly from the inferior tarsal border. Although the fat may require retraction for adequate exposure, surgery can be safely completed. Avoid injury to the inferior oblique muscle located between the medial and central fat pads.

Careful placement of the Desmarres retractor is essential to avoid unintended skin wound or cicatrix. If the skin and orbicularis oculi muscle are not completely retracted, they may fold under the instrument and be at risk of laceration. Distinction between the preseptal plane and an intramuscular plane can be made by assessing vascularity: the preseptal plane is relatively avascular while the orbicularis oculi muscle has a rich blood supply. Careful hemostasis at every step can help visualize the lamellae of the lower eyelid. Once the preseptal plane is reached, blunt dissection can further limit the risk of dissecting too anteriorly.

The transconjunctival approach is useful in that when larger exposure is needed, it can be continued medially to connect to a transcaruncular incision or laterally to connect to a lateral canthotomy/cantholysis incision.

37.8.3 Lateral Orbit
Canthus-Sparing Orbitotomy

This approach is excellent for anterior and small lesions of the lateral orbit. A horizontal incision is placed 1 to 2 mm lateral to the lateral canthus. Sharp dissection is continued through the orbicularis oculi muscle. Skin retractors can be positioned over the lesion, and then dissection can be used to access the area. After hemostasis, the incision is closed with buried interrupted 6–0 polyglactin sutures then 6–0 plain gut sutures for the skin.

Canthotomy Approach Orbitotomy

Alternatively, for greater exposure, a canthotomy and inferior cantholysis can be performed. First, a short horizontal line from the lateral canthus is marked. Following local anesthetic infiltration, the skin is incised. Dissection to the periosteum is made. The inferior crus of the lateral canthal tendon is severed until complete release of the lower eyelid is achieved. At this point, a subperiosteal or intraorbital approach can be used to access the relevant areas of the orbit. Please refer to Chapter 38 "Lateral Orbitotomy" for access to lesions in the deeper orbit.

Swinging Eyelid Approach

The lateral incision described earlier can be combined with a lower eyelid transconjunctival approach for wider exposure of the inferolateral orbit.

A lateral canthotomy and inferior cantholysis are completed as described earlier. Release of the tarsus and capsulopalpebral tissue inferiorly is done with closed curved Stevens tenotomy scissors inserted from the cantholysis incision just anterior to the capsulopalpebral fascia and pushed across the width of the eyelid. The blades are then opened to bluntly separate the tarsus. Next, an incision is made across the horizontal width of the conjunctiva and capsulopalpebral fascia 2 mm below the inferior tarsal border. The conjunctiva and capsulopalpebral fascia are retracted superiorly using 4–0 silk traction suture. A preseptal dissection is continued inferiorly to the orbital rim. If a subperiosteal dissection plane is desired, the periosteum is incised 1 to 2 mm from the orbital rim and then elevated.

Dissection is continued in the subperiosteal space over the arcus marginalis and into the orbit.

After completion of surgery, the periosteum is reapproximated with interrupted 6–0 absorbable suture. The capsulopalpebral fascia and conjunctiva may be closed with 6–0 absorbable sutures as well. The inferior crus of the lateral canthus is reattached to the orbital rim with 5–0 polyglactin or nonabsorbable suture, taking care to engage periosteal tissue. The lateral canthal angle should be reformed with interrupted 5–0 or 6–0 absorbable suture from the lower eyelid gray line to the upper eyelid gray line. The lateral canthus is closed with deep buried interrupted 6–0 polyglactin sutures and superficial 6–0 running suture.

Medial Orbit
Vertical Eyelid Split Incision

The vertical eyelid split approach can expose the superior and superomedial orbit, particularly the intraconal space. An advantage is deeper orbital access than a lid crease incision.

A vertical line is marked in the upper lid about one-third distance from the medial canthus (▶ Fig. 37.4). The lacrimal punctum and canaliculus can easily be avoided. A full-thickness incision is made along the mark extending superiorly above the tarsus (i.e., about 10 mm from the margin). A 4–0 silk traction suture is placed on both sides of the split eyelid at the margin to spread the incision. Additional exposure can be achieved with malleable or Sewall retractors or additional 4–0 silk traction sutures. Avoid damage to the superior oblique with this approach by using only blunt dissection. Following completion of the surgery, the eyelid is suture closed in standard fashion for eyelid margin incisions. We use 7–0 polyglactin suture through the margin tarsus in a vertical mattress fashion, a 6–0 polyglactin suture through partial-thickness tarsus, and 6–0 polyglactin suture for the skin.

Transcaruncular Incision

The transcaruncular approach has a well-hidden incision in the medial conjunctiva/caruncle[4] and affords access to the medial orbit (▶ Fig. 37.5). The incision can be extended superiorly or inferiorly and can even access the deep orbit.[2] This approach can be used for various conditions, including fracture repair, medial orbital decompressions, and fluid collection drainage.

Local anesthetic is injected to the medial conjunctiva and caruncle. A 4–0 silk traction suture may be placed in the conjunctiva and Tenon fascia to rotate the eye laterally. Westcott scissors are used to make an incision between the plica semilunaris and the caruncle. Stevens tenotomy scissors are used to bluntly dissect to the posterior lacrimal crest. An incision is made through the periosteum. A subperiosteal dissection plane can be developed by continuing posteriorly along the wall. The anterior and posterior ethmoid neurovascular bundles emerge through the medial orbital wall at the junction of the frontal and ethmoid bones. These serve as rough landmarks of the skull base. These vessels may bleed profusely or retract into their foramina; so, careful ligation should be performed using a vascular clip or thorough cauterization. The frontal bone superior to this location may be especially thin in elderly patients, increasing the risk of cerebrospinal fluid leak. After the surgery is complete, the conjunctiva can be closed with 6–0 polyglactin or plain gut sutures.

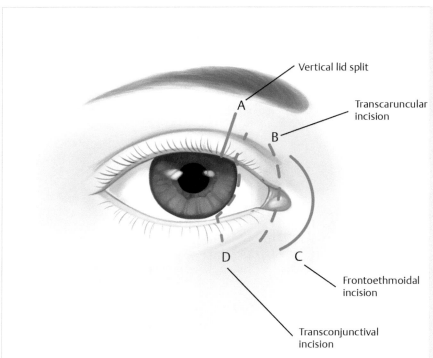

Fig. 37.4 Medial eyelid approaches. (A) Vertical lid split. (B) Transcaruncular incision. (C) Frontoethmoidal (Lynch) incision. (D) Transconjunctival medial orbitotomy incision.

Vertical lid split

Transcaruncular incision

A

B

D

C

Frontoethmoidal incision

Transconjunctival incision

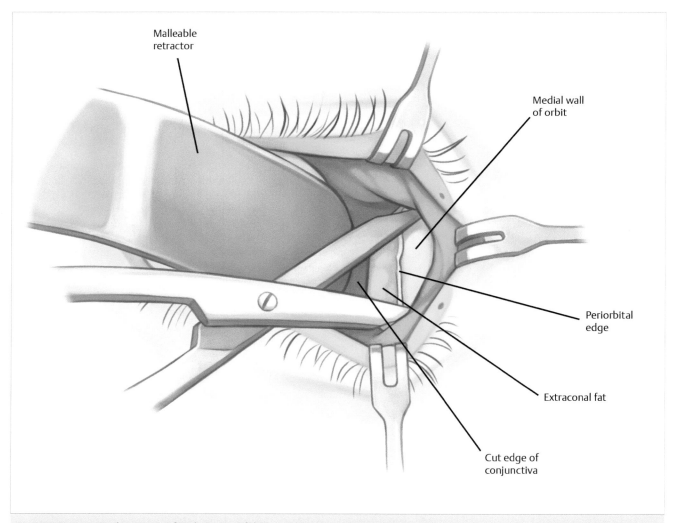

Malleable retractor

Medial wall of orbit

Periorbital edge

Extraconal fat

Cut edge of conjunctiva

Fig. 37.5 Transcaruncular incision. After distraction of the intraorbital content, an incision is made in the periorbita against the medial wall of the orbit just posterior to the posterior lacrimal crest. Dissection is then continued in the subperiosteal plane posteriorly.

Note that extraconal fat may enter the surgical field once an incision is made, obscuring visualization. A hand-over-hand dissection with malleable retractors and avoidance of excessive suction or manipulation can keep the surgical field clear. Careful placement of moistened neurosurgical cottonoids between orbital tissue and the retractors also helps maintain visualization.

Frontoethmoidal (Lynch) Incision

The Lynch incision gives the widest exposure of the medial extraconal space and subperiosteal space. However, it has been largely abandoned due to postoperative disfiguring scars causing and webbing in the medial canthal region. Large tumor resection in the midline or skull base may require such an incision.

A vertical curved line is marked midway between the medial canthal angle and the bridge of the nose. Local anesthetic is infiltrated. After the skin is incised, tissues are dissected apart in a lamellar fashion until the periosteum is reached. The periosteum is incised then elevated to access the desired portion of the orbit.

There are several structures that can limit exposure. If the superior oblique muscle is obstructing the field, it can be retracted away, or the trochlea lifted off the periosteum temporarily. Reapproximation can be considered, and the patient should be advised of the risk of diplopia postoperatively. If the lacrimal sac is obstructing the field, it can also be elevated within the lacrimal sac fossa and retracted laterally.

37.9 Limbal Conjunctival Orbitotomy

This approach can be used to access the anterior intra- and extraconal spaces, Tenon capsule space, and anterior optic nerve. It can be used to treat conditions such as prolapsed orbital fat, optic nerve sheath fenestration, and rectus muscle biopsy. This concept can be used to approach the superior, lateral, and inferior orbital spaces as well.

Local anesthetic is injected in the eyelid margin and subconjunctival space. A 4–0 silk traction suture is placed to retract the eyelid. Alternatively, a Jaffe eyelid speculum can be used. A limbal peritomy is made in the segment of orbit to be accessed. Generally, one-third of the corneal limbus is sufficient for most cases. Blunt-tipped scissors are used to elevate Tenon capsule from the sclera avoiding the rectus muscles. The intraconal space is then visible. For additional exposure, the rectus muscle can be detached. A 6–0 double-armed polyglactin suture is passed through the distal muscle, and then it is disinserted by cutting the tendon. A 4–0 silk traction suture can be placed on the stump, and the eye can be rotated to improve visualization. The muscle can be reattached back to the stump using the preplaced polyglactin suture when finished. It is rare for most patients to get diplopia postoperatively due to the horizontal fusional reserve. The conjunctiva can be closed with 6–0 or 8–0 polyglactin or gut sutures.

37.10 Tips and Pearls

37.10.1 Maintain Adequate Exposure

- Meticulous hemostasis is perhaps the most crucial principle of orbital surgery. Bleeding in the confined orbital space can quickly obstruct the field. Blunt dissection along tissue planes can minimize bleeding. Blood pressure should be monitored with hypertension quickly treated. Elevating the head of bed 5 degrees may help control bleeding.
- As dissection into the orbit continues deeper, the cutaneous exposure is also widened.[5] Use retractors (Sewall, Desmarres, malleable, skin hooks) or traction sutures.
- In the transconjunctival approach to the inferior orbit, blunt dissection is ideal for exposing the entire septum to the orbital rim.
- Avoiding monopolar cautery in the orbit is advisable.
- When dissecting in the subperiosteal plane, extra care should be taken at the rim, where the periosteum is tightly adherent to bone. Once the orbit is entered, the periosteum is less tightly adherent. The integrity of the periorbita should be maintained so that orbital fat will not herniate through and obstruct the view. Note that the periosteum in the elderly may be more attenuated; so, gentle tissue handling is advised.[6] During subperiosteal dissection, neurovascular bundles entering the orbit should be visualized, avoided, or ligated to prevent bleeding. These include the anterior and posterior ethmoid neurovascular bundles, the orbital branch of the infraorbital bundle, and the zygomaticofacial and zygomaticotemporal neurovascular bundles.
- Patients may have thin frontal bone of the orbital roof; so, application of pressure to the area should be minimized.

37.10.2 Orientation in the Anterior Orbit

- Finger palpation of the lesion is helpful for reorientation.
- Finding the orbital septum can also help orient how deep the dissection has been carried. The septum is relatively tough and offers resistance to pull with a toothed forcep.[7] It is sometimes confused with the loose connective tissue just anterior to the orbital septum. The septum is translucent and orbital fat can be seen deep to it. Identifying this layer will help guide dissection.

37.11 What to Avoid

- Do not patch the eye after orbital surgery as it prevents monitoring for signs of orbital hemorrhage, including vision loss, proptosis, and swelling.
- Avoid cauterization of lesions for biopsy, as thermal damage can confound pathologic evaluation.
- Avoid crushing and extensively manipulating surgical specimens. In some cases, such as in excision of a dermoid, a small amount of perilesional tissue can be left attached to the dermoid anteriorly for grasping with toothed forceps during dissection.

37.12 Complications/Bailout/Salvage

37.12.1 Orbital Hemorrhage

This is a true emergency that can lead to permanent blindness in a short period of time. To minimize risks preoperatively, medical conditions including hypertension should be controlled. Intraoperatively, materials such as surgical cellulose (Surgicel), gelatin foam-thrombin (Surgi-Flo), and bipolar cautery can be helpful to maintain meticulous hemostasis. If a clamp-cut-cauterize technique is done for hemostasis, attention should be made to make sure adjacent tissue including skin or other metal instruments are not in direct contact or else thermal burns in unwanted locations can occur. One technique is to place cotton-tipped applicators on either end of the clamp to elevate it above other tissues and create a margin of safety. Expansile hemostatic materials should not be left in the orbit as they can cause a compartment syndrome in rare cases. If possible, the patient should be woken up from deep anesthesia ("deep extubation") to avoid excessive Valsalva maneuvers. Drains in the orbit can reduce serosanguinous fluid accumulation. Postoperatively, the blood pressure, pain, and nausea should be controlled to prevent Valsalva maneuvers. Stool softeners should be considered, especially when used in conjunction with narcotics. The patient should self-assess to count fingers every hour while awake for 24 hours after surgery.[8] If an orbital hemorrhage is suspected, the incisions should be opened immediately, and the bleeding vessel identified.

37.12.2 Lagophthalmos

Sutures should never be placed through the orbital septum. Excessive manipulation of the orbital septum may lead to eyelid retraction due to inflammation.

37.12.3 Ptosis

The levator aponeurosis may be intentionally or unintentionally injured during surgery. Dissection in the superior orbit can rarely injure the superior division of the oculomotor nerve, resulting in a paralytic ptosis. Postoperative edema can stretch and disinsert the levator aponeurosis.

37.12.4 Protect the Cornea and Eye

Use corneal protectors and ophthalmic ointment to prevent corneal desiccation. If these are not used, intermittent balanced saline solution drops can be used.

37.12.5 Infections

Eyelid incisions rarely get infected due to a rich blood supply. In cases of a foreign body, however, prophylactic antibiotics should be administered. If an infection is suspected, surgical site exploration, wound culture, and lavage with copious antibiotic or saline irrigation should be performed. Blood cultures should be drawn and antibiotics started. If an abscess is present, drainage may be required.

37.12.6 Wound Dehiscence

If the dehiscence is superficial and small and without tension, observation, tape, or skin glue may be sufficient. Prophylactic topical antibiotic ointments can be considered. If a larger, deeper, or persistent wound dehiscence is present, infection, skin tension, or tumor recurrence may be causative; so, these should be evaluated. Once these are ruled out, the edges of the wound can be freshened and resutured or can be left to heal by secondary intention. Delayed reconstruction or tissue augmentation can be performed in the future.

37.13 Postoperative Care

- The patient should check vision of the operated eye every hour while awake for the first 24 hours. Should decreased vision, severe pain, proptosis, or a tense eyelid occur, the patient should go immediately to the emergency room.
- Avoid Valsalva maneuvers so that pain and nausea/vomiting should be controlled.
- Ice packs or cool compresses should be applied to the operative site for the first 24 hours.
- Antibiotic ophthalmic ointment should be applied to the incision two to three times a day for 7 to 10 days. Oral antibiotics can be considered for prolonged cases, known infections, contaminated wounds, or immunocompromised states.

References

[1] Katz SE, Rootman J. Adverse effects of bone wax in surgery of the orbit. Ophthal Plast Reconstr Surg. 1996; 12(2):121–126

[2] Rootman J, Stewart B, Goldberg RA. Orbital Surgery: A Conceptual Approach. Philadelphia, PA: Lippincott-Raven; 1995

[3] Lane KA, Bilyk JR, Taub D, Pribitkin EA. "Sutureless" repair of orbital floor and rim fractures. Ophthalmology. 2009; 116(1):135–138.e2

[4] Shorr N, Baylis HI, Goldberg RA, Perry JD. Transcaruncular approach to the medial orbit and orbital apex. Ophthalmology. 2000; 107(8):1459–1463

[5] Nerad JA. Techniques in Ophthalmic Plastic Surgery. Elsevier Inc; 2010

[6] Tse DT. Color Atlas of Oculoplastic Surgery. 2nd ed. Philadelphia, PA: Lippincott Williams & Wilkins; 2011

[7] Putterman AM, Urist MJ. Surgical anatomy of the orbital septum. Ann Ophthalmol. 1974; 6(3):290–294

[8] Putterman AM. Temporary blindness after cosmetic blepharoplasty. Am J Ophthalmol. 1975; 80(6):1081–1083

38 Lateral Orbitotomy

Edward J. Wladis

Abstract

While lateral orbitotomy requires more instrumentation than more anterior approaches and is more technically challenging, it affords excellent visualization of the deep lateral aspects of the orbit and facilitates excision of otherwise inaccessible lesions and is thus indicated in the management of deeper orbital masses. Comprehension of the technical aspects of the procedure and meticulous tissue handling allow for more precise interventions, and awareness of the potential complications of a lateral orbitotomy enables clinicians to avoid pitfalls. Additionally, close postoperative follow-up leads to early recognition and management of these problems. This chapter discusses the indications and contraindications of lateral orbitotomy, reviews the pre- and intraoperative steps necessary to achieve successful surgery, and considers possible complications and their appropriate treatments.

Keywords: lateral orbitotomy, orbitotomy, orbital tumor, piezo-electric, orbital hemorrhage

38.1 Goals

The goal of a lateral orbitotomy is to provide access to deep spaces of the orbit for surgical manipulation (i.e., biopsy, removal of lesion, etc.) with minimal external disruption. Despite the relatively invasive nature of this technique and extensive intervention inherent to this surgery, lateral orbitotomies can be accomplished without any lingering functional or cosmetic deficits.

38.2 Advantages

Certainly, anterior lesions of the orbit can be approached through transeyelid, transcaruncular, and transconjunctival approaches. Nonetheless, these techniques offer limited access to deeper orbital structures, and the manipulation that can be achieved through these tactics is limited by the size of the incisions.[1,2]

While a lateral orbitotomy represents a more challenging, instrument-intensive, and involved procedure, this technique provides outstanding visualization of the deeper orbit. Consequently, this technique provides unparalleled confidence and safety during delicate tissue dissection. Furthermore, when surgical approaches necessitate removal of intraconal lesions, deeper extraconal lesions, complete excision of the lacrimal gland, access to and manipulation of the posterior aspects of the optic nerve, and complete excision of the optic nerve, lateral orbitotomies can be safely employed with outstanding outcomes. Additionally, when lesions are too large to be safely removed through smaller-incision, anterior approaches, a lateral orbitotomy should be employed for complete removal.

38.3 Expectations

Through this technique, surgeons can achieve their primary goals (i.e., removal of a deep orbital tumor) that cannot be afforded with more anterior approaches, and without inducing functional deficits. Furthermore, patients can avoid the potential morbidities and prolonged recovery of more invasive procedures (i.e., transcranial approaches to the orbit).

38.4 Key Principles

- Lateral orbitotomies afford excellent access to the deep orbit, and afford surgeons the opportunity to safely address lesions with excellent visibility and safety.
- Meticulous tissue handling will enhance postoperative outcomes. Specifically, awareness of bony landmarks, meticulous bony resection, and anatomic bone replacement will provide outstanding postoperative realignment and will avoid postoperative pain. Furthermore, thorough handling of the orbital tissue facilitates enhanced safety.
- Careful awareness of potential complications will help surgeons avoid postoperative problems. In particular, ensuring meticulous intraoperative hemostasis diminishes the risk of potentially devastating postoperative hemorrhage formation.
- Fastidious bone replacement with excellent alignment is critical to improve postoperative outcomes.

38.5 Indications

Most orbital lesions can be safely approached through anterior approaches. However, intraconal lesions, deep extraconal masses, and lacrimal gland tumors that require either extensive debulking or complete resection are best served through a lateral orbitotomy.

38.6 Contraindications

Lesions of the orbital apex should not be approached through a lateral orbitotomy, as visualization of this region is limited through this technique. Instead, these lesions are best approached through a transcranial intervention.

Additionally, lesions along the medial aspect of the intraconal space are difficult to approach through a lateral orbitotomy, as such an approach would necessitate crossing the optic nerve. Such a mass would be better approached through a transethmoidal mechanism.

38.7 Preoperative Preparation

Patient counseling is absolutely necessary. Reviewing preoperative imaging with the patient often helps facilitate comprehension of the surgery and the decision to perform a more invasive approach. The risks, benefits, and alternatives to such an intricate operation must be discussed. Standard preoperative discussion should include an explanation of the possibilities of vision loss, double vision, damage to the orbital structures and eye, eyelid or temple numbness, orbital hemorrhage and the need for emergent evacuation, dry eye disease, and pupillary dilation. As part of the standard preoperative medical evaluation, management of anticoagulants should be specifically considered, and consultation with the patient's other physicians is required. Furthermore, patients should understand that time off from physical activity and work will be critical during the postoperative period.

The patient should be placed in a slight reverse Trendelenburg position. General endotracheal anesthesia is administered.

The lateral aspect of the left upper eyelid crease should be marked, and the marking should extend to the level of the lateral canthus. At this point, the crease, lateral orbital rim, and temporalis muscle are infiltrated with lidocaine with epinephrine. This aspect of the technique serves to provide postoperative analgesia, and, more critically at this juncture of the surgery, to decrease bleeding.

The patient is then prepped in a standard fashion with 5% povidone iodine for the periocular skin. Additionally, the conjunctiva and eyelashes are irrigated with this preparation, with the eyelashes scrubbed with iodine-soaked cotton-tipped applicators.

While the iodine dries, the surgeon should ensure that the patient's imaging is prominently displayed; of course, the location will depend on the particular offerings of each operating room.

Some surgeons advocate the use of an operating microscope for the intraorbital dissection. While I have not found this step to be necessary or advantageous, this juncture is an excellent time for preparation of the microscope, if you prefer its use.

Proper illumination is critical to enhance intraoperative visualization. Check to ensure sufficient position and intensity. Furthermore, the operating room headlights should be position with one directly superior to the site of the incision and the other at a 45-degree angle.

The patient should be draped. Given the need to dissect into the temporalis muscle, ensure wide draping.

Prior to making the initial incision, intravenous antibiotics should be administered, with the intent of targeting the saprophytic skin bacteria. Generally 1 to 2 g of cefazolin (for penicillin allergies 600 mg of clindamycin) may be used.

38.8 Operative Technique

1. Incise the eyelid crease with a 15 scalpel. Dissect deeply to the level of the periosteum, passing through the orbicularis muscle. The dissection should proceed laterally to delineate the temporalis muscle and fascia.
2. Expose the periosteum with a Cottle elevator, and incise it with cutting cautery. Using Desmarres retractors superiorly and inferiorly, demonstrate the bone. Dissect subperiosteally to expose the bone (▶ Fig. 38.1).
3. Dissect bluntly with a Cottle elevator to the lateral aspect of the lateral rim. At this point, incise the periosteum with

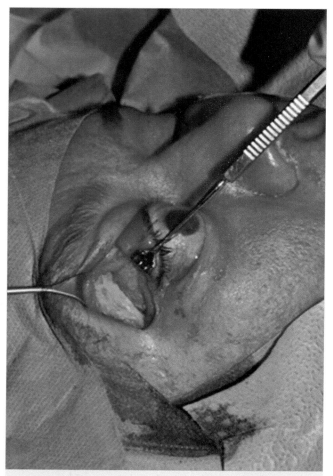

Fig. 38.1 The eyelid crease incision is advanced laterally to expose the lateral aspect of the orbit. The soft tissue is dissected to reveal bare bone.

cutting cautery and recess it from the rim. Extend the dissection into the temporalis fascia, exposing and elevating the muscle. This aspect of the procedure may induce bleeding from the cut edge of muscle; so, having suction readily available facilitates an improved view.

4. Similarly, dissect the periorbita away from the internal aspect of the lateral orbital rim with a Cottle elevator.
5. Identify and mark the frontozygomatic suture and the superior aspect of the union of the zygomatic arch and the lateral orbital rim. Of course, depending on the goal of the surgery, the extent of the bone removal may be customized.
6. Place a wide malleable retractor on the internal aspect of the lateral orbital rim to protect the orbital contents. Visually inspect the thickness of the bone prior to cutting it, so as to avoid extension of the osteotomy into the anterior cranial vault. With a bone saw, incise the pre-marked aspect of the bone in a full-thickness fashion (▶ Fig. 38.2). The saw becomes quite hot with extensive use, and the surgeon should either employ a self-irrigating saw or should irrigate

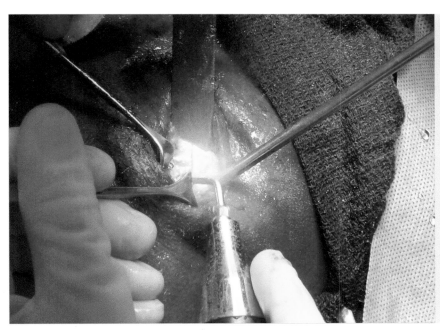

Fig. 38.2 A malleable retractor is placed along the internal aspect of the lateral orbit in order to protect the orbital contents. A saw is used to incise the desired length of bone.

the site of the osteotomy copiously. Additionally, the cut edges of bone rarely bleed, and these hemorrhages can obscure the surgeon's view. Have bone wax readily available, and apply it to the bleeding vessels within osteotomy site as needed.

7. Outfracture the incised bone with a straight rongeur. While the bone is quite thick, it should rock freely once the rongeur is clamped onto the bone. If the bone still seems rigid, check to ensure that the bony incisions have been created in a full-thickness fashion. Place the bone in sterile saline for later replacement.

8. Once the bone has been removed, the intact rim of periorbita should be visible (▶ Fig. 38.3). With a #15 scalpel or with Westcott scissors, incise the periorbita as an inverted T. Extend the incision along the entire length of the osteotomy. Reflect the flaps of the periorbita. If necessary, lyse any adhesions along the flaps with a Westcott scissors.

9. Dissect through the orbital fat with blunt instruments (i.e., cotton-tipped applicators, small malleable retractors, etc.) to approach the area of interest. The area of dissection will be determined by the location of the mass. If necessary, retract the lateral rectus muscle with a Desmarres retractor.

10. Once the lesion has been removed or biopsied, ensure meticulous hemostasis. The orbit must be completely dry.

11. Replace the bone. Pre-place drill holes, plates, and screws along the superior and inferior aspects of the outfractured bone. Ensure meticulous realignment of the bony architecture. Place screws through the intact bone superiorly and inferiorly. Tighten the screws, and re-inspect to confirm excellent position and a restoration of the normal alignment.

12. Close the periosteum and orbicularis layers with several interrupted 5–0 polyglactin sutures in a buried fashion. Close the skin incision with a running 6–0 fast-absorbing catgut suture.

13. Apply antibiotic ointment to the incision.[1,2,3,4]

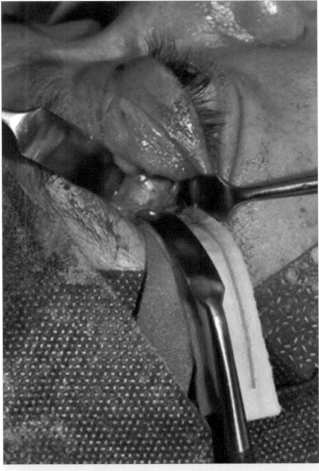

Fig. 38.3 Once the bone is removed, an intact rim of periorbita is visible.

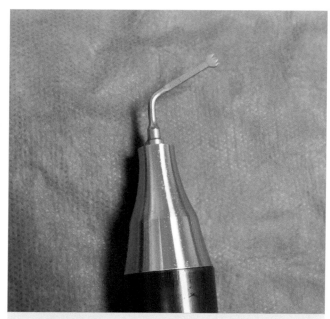

Fig. 38.4 Self-irrigating piezoelectric saws increase the margin of safety of this operation, as they incise mineralized tissue but spare the underlying soft tissue.

38.9 Tips and Pearls

- Meticulous hemostasis is critical. Beware of perforating blood vessels that may run through the orbital fat.
- Some surgeons advocate placement of a surgical drain that can be removed on postoperative day 2. This step is not frequently necessary.
- Many notable surgeons preplace drill holes along the intact bone and the outfractured bone, and then pass a Prolene suture to reattach the bone that is removed. The alignment and stability of the bone may be improved with a plating system.
- The periorbita does not need to be closed.
- Communicate with the anesthesia team. The recovery process needs to be very gentle to avoid postoperative hemorrhages, and patients may benefit from a deep extubation.
- Piezoelectric saws increase the margin of safety (▶ Fig. 38.4)[3]. These instruments oscillate at a frequency that is specific for mineralized tissue, and will thus cut freely through bone, but will leave the underlying soft tissue intact. Additionally, these saws are self-irrigating. As a result, some surgeons favor the use of piezoelectric saws for a surgeon's first few cases or in situations in which trainees (i.e., fellows, residents) will be performing the bone removal.
- During dissection, the orbital fat may obscure the surgeon's view. Careful application of cautery to the fat will successfully shrink the fat in a hemostatic fashion.
- Bleeding that arises from the cut edge of bone may be controlled with bone wax, although this intervention is rarely required.
- Hemostatic agents (i.e., thrombin-coated Gelfoam) should be available, and are quite useful in cases of extensive bleeding. However, prior to closure, the surgeon should be certain to remove these packs, as expansion and orbital compartment syndrome are possible complications.

- Bony alignment is critical to ensure proper reconstruction. Visual and digital inspection of the alignment along the superior and inferior edges ensures excellent apposition of the bony structures. Surgeons must be patient and should not be afraid to remove and reinsert sets of plates and screws until they are completely satisfied with the smooth, well-aligned lateral aspect of the orbit.

38.10 Complications

Patients should be examined immediately after surgery. Check the patient's vision, pupils, motility, and intraocular pressure. The patient should be checked again several hours later. A retrobulbar hemorrhage is a feared complication of this procedure. Should such an event occur, the bone flap can be safely removed and the hemorrhage must be evacuated immediately.

With extensive manipulation in the lateral orbit, the lateral rectus muscle function may be diminished. In fact, limited abduction of the globe is quite common after lateral orbitotomy. This issue resolves spontaneously, and, barring intraoperative damage to this muscle, observation for resolution of this problem is the standard of care; no surgical intervention is required immediately after surgery. If the patient suffers from postoperative diplopia, consider the use of prisms or occlusive patches.

Infections are quite rare after lateral orbitotomy. Routine use of postoperative antibiotics is not demonstrated to be necessary.

Trismus may theoretically arise with improper bony alignment. Particular attention should be paid to ensure excellent intraoperative position. At the first postoperative visit, patients should be interviewed regarding difficulty with chewing. Furthermore, the region of the bone that was removed intraoperatively should be examined postoperatively to ensure structural integrity.

38.11 Postoperative Care

Antibiotic ointment should be applied to the incision for 1 week. Analgesia is critical, and patients should be monitored for pain. Consider overnight admission of patients for monitoring and pain control; during this time, consider intravenous corticosteroids to decrease swelling (generally, 8 mg of dexamethasone administered intravenously). Patients should apply ice to the site constantly. Patients should be reminded to avoid bending, straining, and lifting for 1 week.

References

[1] Turbin RE. Lateral orbitotomy. In: Langer PD, Dunn JP, eds. Basic Techniques of Ophthalmic Surgery. 2nd ed. San Francisco: American Academy of Ophthalmology; 2015:520–527
[2] Nerad JA, ed. Approach to deep lateral lesions: the lateral orbitotomy. In: Techniques in Ophthalmic Plastic Surgery: A Personal Tutorial. New York: Elsevier; 2010:447–450
[3] De Castro DK, Fay A, Wladis EJ, et al. Self-irrigating piezoelectric device in orbital surgery. Ophthal Plast Reconstr Surg. 2013; 29(2):118–122
[4] Melicher JS, Nerad JA, Kim JW. Lateral orbitotomy. In: Levine MR, ed. Manual of Oculoplastic Surgery. Thorofare, NJ: Slack; 2010:297–301

39 Transcranial Orbital Approaches

Wenya Linda Bi and Ian F. Dunn

Summary

Transcranial approaches afford circumferential access and visualization of the optic apparatus and serve an important role in the resection of mass lesions involving the optic nerve, especially those at the posterior third of the orbit, with intracranial extension, or with bilateral involvement. Transcranial approaches to the orbit may be conceived as a series of modular advancements, centered about the superior orbital rim, with stepwise expansion to the lateral orbital rim, zygoma, and frontotemporal calvarium. Selection of the operative approach is dictated by specific features of the lesion itself—location, extension outside the orbit, presumed pathology, vascular supply, and anticipated firmness are some important considerations. Additional concerns include existing neurologic symptoms and suspected neurovascular involvement, cosmetic considerations, and surgeon experience. Decompression of the anterior clinoid and optic canal are critical in preservation or restoration of vision in situations of optic nerve compression. Potential risks include postoperative periorbital swelling, temporary impairment of globe motility and extraocular movements, frontalis weakness, and enophthalmos or exophthalmos. Visual integrity is optimized with avoidance of intraoperative hypotension, rapid cerebrospinal fluid drainage, thermal injury from drilling or coagulation, and aggressive dissection around the optic apparatus.

Keywords: cranio-orbito-zygomatic approach, supraorbital craniotomy, skull base surgery, optic nerve decompression, optic nerve meningioma

The transcranial approach for intraorbital tumors and intracranial tumors with canalicular or intraorbital extension has been long pursued, as eloquently advocated by Walter Dandy.[1] Strikingly, Dandy noted that prevention of brain swelling through improvements in anesthesia allowed the size of the craniotomy to be greatly reduced and that a small bony opening was equally effective as a larger one. This astute observation of transosseous exposure of the lateral and superior orbit transformed circumferential access to the optic apparatus. In particular, Dandy advised the intracranial approach, for facile exploration and extirpation of tumor from any compartment of the orbit, especially those that extend posterior to the orbit.

39.1 Goals

- To provide access to the entire orbit, especially the posterior third, and any lesions with intracranial extension (▶ Fig. 39.1).
- To allow access to bilateral optic nerves with simultaneous access to the intraorbital and intracranial compartments.
- To expose periorbita for exploration of infiltrating tumor.

39.2 Advantages

- Wide access to the full length of the optic nerve, superior orbital fissure, and bony orbit.

- Ability to address pathologies that span the cranio-orbital compartments.
- Vascular control of the proximal ophthalmic system.

39.3 Expectations

- Postoperative periorbital swelling and possible temporary paresis of extraocular movements, depending on the extent of periorbital violation and intraorbital dissection.
- Possible frontalis weakness.
- Possible enophthalmos or exophthalmos may result from intraorbital scarring and reconstruction.

39.4 Key Principles

Selection of the operative approach is dictated by lesion factors, including its location, pathology, vascular supply, and anticipated firmness; existing neurologic symptoms and suspected neurovascular involvement; cosmetic considerations; and surgeon experience. Transcranial approaches to the orbit may be conceived as a series of modular advancements, centered about the superior orbital rim, with stepwise expansion to the lateral orbital rim, zygoma, and frontotemporal calvarial vault (▶ Fig. 39.2). Additionally, the endoscope affords a complementary route to the medial and inferior orbit that may be

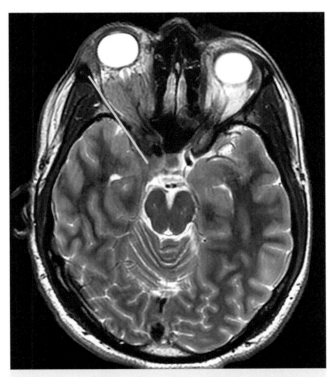

Fig. 39.1 Axial T2 MRI of a right optic nerve sheath meningioma with invasion of the cavernous sinus and retrobulbar orbital space (demarcated by line), leading to proptosis.

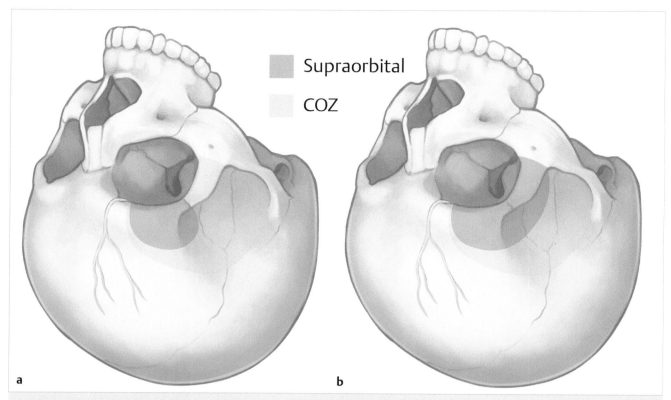

Fig. 39.2 (a) The supraorbital craniotomy allows removal of the superior orbit with variable amounts of the lateral orbital rim. (b) The cranio-orbito-zygomatic approach affords flexible exposure of the full orbit, anterior fossa, middle fossa, with facile extension into the infratemporal fossa and posterior fossa.

considered for select pathologies as a primary modality or to augment the visualization around angles and critical neurovascular structures.

Orbital pathologies which span extraorbital compartments include meningiomas, gliomas, metastatic tumors, hemangiomas, fibrous dysplasia, tumors of the lacrimal gland, vascular malformations, and inflammatory conditions, among others. Of these, meningiomas are the most common and the most varied in their anatomic involvement. Anteriorly based tumors that involve the periorbita and orbit commonly present with proptosis and impairment of motility; posteriorly based tumors manifest classically with painless progressive visual loss. The presence of proptosis in a bone invasive meningioma mandates exploration of periorbita to excise invasive tumor, while visual loss should prompt exploration and decompression of the optic canal.

39.5 Indications

- Exposure of lesions involving both the intraorbital and intracranial compartments.
- Access to the posterior third of the orbit.
- Access to bilateral optic nerves and the optic chiasm, including a long length of the optic nerve sheath.
- When primary orbitotomy provides inadequate access to a lesion.

39.6 Contraindications

- Anticipated poor healing with limited reconstructive options if a wide transcranial incision and exposure is performed.
- Patient concerns regarding temporary or permanent cosmetic sequelae.

39.7 Preoperative Evaluation and Preparation

A contrast-enhanced magnetic resonance imaging (MRI) with dedicated sequences to evaluate the orbit and optic nerves is frequently the most useful preoperative diagnostic test. The relationship of the osseous structures surrounding the optic apparatus, including involvement of the anterior clinoid, superior orbital fissure, or if tumor extends through foramen ovale or rotundum into the infratemporal fossa, is critical to learn prior to surgery, and best appreciated with a thin-cut CT. Formal neuroophthalmology evaluation of visual acuity, fields, and extraocular motility may be merited before and after surgery. Extension of tumor to the sella should also prompt endocrinologic evaluation of pituitary-associated hormone levels.

Expectations should be established regarding anticipated cosmetic results, extraocular movement function, and potential risk to vision prior to surgery. In particular, removal of the orbital rim in transcranial approaches, with or without violation of the periorbita, frequently incurs periorbital edema and limited extraocular motility postoperatively.

39.8 Operative Technique

39.8.1 Craniotomy and Orbitotomy

The cranio-orbital approach can be viewed as a series of stepwise modular extensions, tailored to the extent of the target lesion and goals of surgery (▶ Fig. 39.2).[2] Patient positioning aims to maximize exposure of the tumor extension from the orbit to the intracranial space, while minimizing brain retraction. The patient is positioned supine, with head rotated 15 to 30 degrees to the opposite side. The vertex of the head is dropped toward the floor, such that the zygoma becomes the highest point of the operative field, and tilted slightly to the contralateral shoulder; this allows gentle gravitational pull of the frontal and temporal lobes away from the cranial base and opens the operative corridor.

The skin is sharply incised in curvilinear fashion from 1 cm anterior to the tragus to, or beyond, the midline, just posterior to the hairline. The scalp is retracted forward to expose the superior orbital rim and desired area for craniotomy. Dissection of the pericranium from the scalp allows preservation of a vascularized graft for reconstruction purposes. The ipsilateral border between the pericranium and the insertion of the temporalis fascia is transected and curved toward the contralateral side as posterior as possible. The pedicled pericranium may be harvested prior to the craniotomy and reflected forward, or simply dissected off the bone after a partial release of its posterior boundary and retracted to the side as a "rescue" flap to be harvested fully if desired at the end of the surgery.

Sharp dissection at the orbital rim should be carried deliberately to free the orbital rim from the periorbita, especially at the point of greatest adhesion at the frontozygomatic suture. The superior orbital rim is typically freed from lateral to medial, until the supraorbital nerve is encountered in its groove or notch. This typically demarcates the lateral boundary of the frontal sinus. The lateral orbital rim and zygoma are variably exposed as needed for the desired cranio-orbital approach by dissecting the temporalis muscle inferiorly and/or posteriorly.

A burr hole, known as MacCarty keyhole, placed approximately 1 cm posterior to frontozygomatic suture allows concurrent exposure of periorbita and the frontal dura, bisected by the superior orbital roof. This provides the critical entry point to free both the superior and lateral orbital rims and allows removal of the orbital rim along with the cranial flap in one piece, which is important for cosmetic reconstruction. A two-piece flap refers to a frontal or frontotemporal craniotomy followed by removal of the superior and lateral orbit as a separate piece. Additional bur holes are placed as needed to permit epidural dissection and facile release of the craniotomy flap. One can extend the lateral orbital osteotomy down to the malar eminence to add a fully lateral approach to the orbit to the superior one conferred by the cranial approach. The bony lateral and superior orbit are left once the cranial flap is removed; these can be taken off with a high-speed drill separately or taken with a small rongeur.

The supraorbital craniotomy provides exposure to orbital roof, planum sphenoidale, tuberculum, suprasellar area, and opticocarotid triangle intradurally. The incision for a purely supraorbital craniotomy may be tailored to extend from the level of the superior orbital rim, or the inferior limit of desired orbital rim cut, to above the superior temporal line rostrally. The size of the craniotomy flap is determined by the desired space for brain relaxation for access to any intracranial extension of a mass, with progressive expansion to a pterional or larger frontotemporal craniotomy. Downward deflection of the zygoma through cuts at its insertion with the maxillary prominence and its root provides further space for temporalis muscle displacement and facilitates trajectory to the floor of the middle fossa, along the full extent of the sphenoid wing, and potential access to the posterior fossa; this cranio-orbito-zygomatic (COZ) approach serves as a foundational corridor to the anterolateral skull base, including full access to the orbit.

39.8.2 Considerations of the Optic Nerve and Chiasm

Removal of the anterior clinoid, either extradurally or intradurally, decompresses the lateral aspect of the optic nerve as it enters the optic canal (▶ Fig. 39.3). For bone invasive pathologies, such as meningiomas, an anterior clinoidectomy is critical in the presence of hyperostosis even without overt compressive optic neuropathy, to prevent future visual compromise with tumor progression or recurrence from the bone. Subsequent unroofing of the optic canal through bony removal of planum sphenoidale ridge as well as release of the falciform ligament provides an additional quadrant of decompression for the optic nerve. Care should be taken to identify and preserve the ophthalmic artery and vasa vasorum of the optic nerve during exposure, manipulation, and dissection of any abutting or encircling mass lesions.

39.8.3 Intraorbital Exposure

Exposure of periorbita produces predictable periorbital swelling within the first 48 hours, which may preclude serial assessments of visual acuity and function; placement of a subgaleal drain may mitigate the onset or severity of such periorbital swelling to permit accurate tracking of the visual exam in the early postoperative setting.

Following the orbitotomy, three primary routes offer varying exposure of the intraorbital contents.[3] The medial approach provides a corridor between the superior oblique and levator muscles; the central approach between the superior rectus and levator muscles; and the lateral approach between the levator and the lateral rectus muscles. Manipulation of intraorbital fat to identify extraocular muscles and their innervation during orbital exploration may be abetted by a cotton tip dissector.

The oculomotor (superior and inferior divisions), trochlear, abducens nerves, and ophthalmic division of the trigeminal nerve pass through the superior orbital fissure (SOF) to reach the orbital apex, and conversely, the superior and inferior ophthalmic veins exit through the SOF to reach the cavernous sinus. Care should be taken to avoid violation of these neurovascular structures if exposing the annulus of Zinn, and one can attempt to reconstruct the annulus after dissection.

It is critical to understand the relationship of the optic nerve and ophthalmic arterial supply in a landscape potentially made hostile by the targeted pathology. It is often wise to find normal

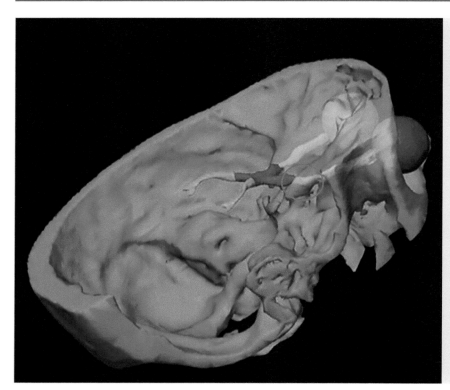

Fig. 39.3 Relationship of the cranial base to optic nerves and chiasm. **(a)** Oblique lateral view of the intracranial skull base with reconstruction of the bilateral globes (*burgundy*), optic nerves (*lavender*), optic chiasm (*blue*), and optic tracts (*green*). The anterior clinoid (encircled) forms the lateral boundary of the optic canal, with continuation as the lateral orbital wall.

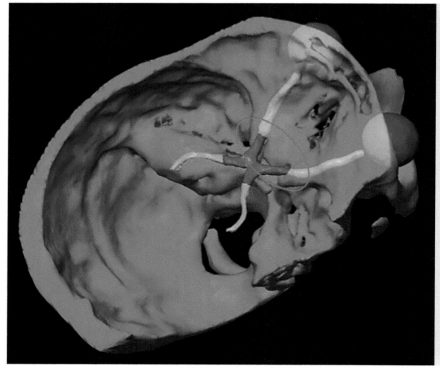

(b) Rostral view of the cranial base and optic apparatus, highlighting the facile exposure of bilateral optic nerves at their entry into the optic canals, the optic chiasm, and sellar and suprasellar space from a transcranial approach.

optic nerve first, and use this as a guidepost for subsequent foray toward the surgical target. While the microscope is a critical tool in this process, it is occasionally helpful to operate under loupe magnification to provide a wider gauge of the operative field.

39.8.4 Reconstruction

Following the goals of surgery using a transcranial approach to the orbit, several potential pitfalls for reconstruction should be considered. Violation of the frontal, sphenoid, or ethmoid sinuses may be repaired with abdominal fat, local muscle, fibrin glue, or, preferably, a vascularized pericranial graft, to minimize the risk of cerebrospinal fluid (CSF) leak. Likewise, if an anterior clinoidectomy was performed, potential exposure of air cells should be sealed with fat, muscle, or fibrin glue. While Dandy specifically noted an absence of pulsating exophthalmos following removal of the orbital roof in his early series on orbital tumors resected from a transcranial approach,[1] either exophthalmos or its converse, enophthalmos, continues to be concerns after transcranial approaches to the orbit. This mainly centers on how the bony superior and lateral orbit are reconstructed before the cranio-orbital bone flap is replaced. If this is removed, it can be re-plated; if it was rongeured, it may be reconstructed with titanium mesh which is easily contoured prior to re-plating of the cranio-orbital flap. There is a wide variability in practice in the reconstruction of the superior and lateral orbital wall, with some opting not to reconstruct at all.

39.9 Tips and Pearls

- Much is written about a one- or two-piece cranial flap; the one-piece has the advantage of cosmesis.
- The MacCarty keyhole (a burr hole) is important to the appropriate exposure of the one-piece cranio-orbital flap.
- Extent of orbitotomy and craniotomy: if one is considering a transcranial approach to the orbit rather than a conventional oculoplastic approach, one should ensure the broad exposure these approaches can provide. A purely orbital lesion may require a smaller frontal craniotomy with superior and lateral orbit included; adding a lateral and inferior trajectory to the orbit can be accomplished by extending the frontal craniotomy in the temporal direction. Pathology extending to extraorbital compartments may require lesion-specific modification.
- Incisions behind the hairline heal very well.
- Preservation of the ophthalmic vasculature is crucial, as is recognition of the normal course of the optic nerve.

- Inspection of the contralateral optic nerve should be conducted in tumors involving the optic nerve at the anterior skull base, to prevent tumor recurrence or functional impairment of the unaffected eye.
- Appropriate reconstruction may mitigate abnormal globe position.

39.10 What to Avoid

- Avoid intraoperative hypotension and rapid CSF drainage, especially if dissecting around the optic nerve sheath.
- Avoid thermal injury to the optic nerve during drilling of the anterior clinoid and roof through continuous irrigation.
- Be vigilant in the detection of neurovascular structures of the orbit during dissection.

39.11 Complications/Bailout/Salvage

- Extraocular motility may be impaired by traction on cranial nerves, especially during dissection of the cavernous sinus, superior orbital fissure, or orbit; manipulation or retraction of extraocular muscles during orbital dissection; and periorbital edema.
- Frontalis weakness may result from manipulation of the temporalis fascia.
- Manipulation, pressure, and ischemia of the optic nerve and apparatus risks visual acuity.

39.12 Postoperative Care

Transcranial approaches to the orbit frequently incur postoperative peri-orbital edema, which is most severe in the initial 48 to 72 hours following surgery and should be anticipated by the patient. Since evaluation of early postoperative visual function is frequently critical when resecting tumor or operating around the optic apparatus, visual acuity and field should be assessed immediately following surgery before the onset of postoperative periorbital swelling.

References

[1] Dandy WE. Results following the transcranial operative attack on orbital tumors. Arch Ophthalmol. 1941; 25(82):191–216

[2] al-Mefty O, Smith RR. Tailoring the cranio-orbital approach. Keio J Med. 1990; 39(4):217–224

[3] Natori Y, Rhoton AL, Jr. Transcranial approach to the orbit: microsurgical anatomy. J Neurosurg. 1994; 81(1):78–86

Part IX

Anophthalmic Socket

IX

40 Enucleation

Prashant Yadav

Summary

Enucleation is a definitive surgery for intraocular tumors, globe perforations where the eye cannot be salvaged, blind painful eyes, and disfigured eyes. The surgery, if performed with implant placement in experienced hands, can give excellent results in terms of eliminating the pathology and achieving good cosmesis.

Keywords: tumors or blind eyes, enucleation (globe removal), orbital implant placement, ocularist, artificial eye

40.1 Goals

The objectives of this surgery are to remove the eye (keeping the integrity of the sclera and ocular structures intact) and to achieve the best cosmetic outcomes in an anophthalmic socket by minimizing socket deformities.

- Completely remove the globe for treatment of tumor, infection, or pain.
- The orbital implant should be of adequate volume and lie in the most natural position in the orbit.
- The orbital implant should have excellent motility in order to transmit the movement to the prosthesis.
- The integrity of the anophthalmic socket is responsible for holding the ocular prosthesis in the sulci for prolonged periods of time. Gravitational forces may displace the prosthesis, so sulcus adequacy is of prime importance.
- The eyelids should have adequate opening and closure with the prosthesis in place.
- An ocular prosthesis in place should look as close to the normal eye as possible.

40.2 Advantages

- Provides dramatic relief to the patient with a painful blind eye commonly due to absolute glaucoma, endophthalmitis, or penetrating trauma. Improved cosmesis with a prosthesis can also provide psychological comfort.
- Although risks are small, minimizes the risks of sympathetic ophthalmia seen in traumatic globes with uveal prolapse.
- Permits a complete histological examination of the eye and optic nerve influencing future treatments particularly in intraocular tumor cases.
- Advanced prosthesis designs allow the surgeon to compensate for the loss of volume after globe removal and custom-made prostheses give excellent cosmetic results which match the contralateral eye.

40.3 Expectations

- Alleviation of pain in the enucleated side (if present).
- Removal of tumor or lesion for histological diagnosis to determine further management.

- Aesthetically acceptable anophthalmic socket with a mobile ocular prosthesis.

40.4 Key Principles

- Clinical evaluation including history, imaging, and detailed consent.
- Careful identification and marking of the eye to be enucleated is crucial on the day of the surgery.
- Adequate preservation of the conjunctiva, Tenon capsule, and extraocular muscles during surgery.
- Choosing the right implant with the best fit for the anophthalmic socket.
- Preservation of fornices on closure to maintain the prosthesis adequately.
- Address any volume deficits like fractures or contracted socket to consider simultaneous volume enhancement to match the contralateral eye.
- Working with an ocularist to make a customized prosthesis for the most natural look.

40.5 Indications

- Intraocular tumors which are not amenable to other therapy: most commonly choroidal melanoma[1] and retinoblastoma.[2]
- Trauma to the globe where globe salvage is not possible. Above tumors, trauma is the most common reason for enucleation in the United States. The surgery can rarely be a primary enucleation if globe repair is not possible. Secondary enucleation can be performed if there is infection or pain. Surgery in the setting of sympathetic ophthalmia has only been demonstrated to be beneficial to remove the inciting eye within 14 days of the onset of sympathetic ophthalmic symptoms/findings. In a comprehensive review of 24,444 enucleation specimens obtained over 55 years, Spraul and Grossniklaus found that trauma had been the cause of enucleation in 40.9% of cases and neoplastic disease had been the cause in 24.2%.[3,4]
- Blind painful eye secondary to absolute glaucoma, neovascular glaucoma, failure of filtration procedures, endophthalmitis and panophthalmitis, corneal ulceration, and perforation.[5]
- Severely disfigured, phthisical eyes without useful vision which may be psychologically distressing to the patient. In these patients, it is critical they understand that surgery may improve the current deformity but may not match the other eye completely. The patient should be counseled about postoperative ptosis, superior sulcus deformity, and enophthalmos.[6]

40.6 Contraindications

- A seeing eye. The importance of a thorough clinical exam, fundus exam, imaging, and visual evoked potentials cannot be understated. Any patient with visual potential should be considered carefully (e.g., intractable pain in an eye with light perception vision).

- Intraocular tumor with extrascleral or orbital involvement and/or metastatic disease (e.g., retinoblastoma with extraocular seeding or choroidal melanoma with extension outside of the globe). These cases may require additional nonsurgical treatment or possible exenteration.
- Extraocular primary tumor with intraocular metastatic disease. It is important to rule out the possibility of a primary neoplasm or metastatic disease elsewhere.[7]

40.7 Preoperative Preparation

- Preoperative evaluation consists of obtaining informed consent and a medical evaluation. Patients must be offered alternative treatments and counseled as to a realistic surgical and cosmetic outcome. This is one of the most important preoperative considerations in surgery for enucleation.
- Taking a thorough history gives the surgeon insight on what may be encountered during surgery. History of scleral buckle surgery, filtering procedures for glaucoma, drug reactions, and conjunctival scarring should be identified prior to surgery. Implants used in the aforementioned surgeries can cause scarring of conjunctiva and Tenon capsule, further shortening of the fornices, as well as postoperative inflammatory reactions. History of anticoagulants and oculofacial trauma is also important.[7]

40.7.1 Clinical Evaluation

The value of a detailed eye examination cannot be understated.
- Vision assessment including light perception and projection of light in a dark room. In the event of doubt, a visual evoked potential maybe considered.
- Examination of the conjunctival fornices and the ocular surface in order to prepare for possible foreshortening with closure and scarring.
- Pupillary reaction, slit-lamp anterior segment evaluation, and integrity of the limbus since areas of scleral thinning may rupture and cause expulsion of ocular contents during nerve resection.
- If there is no view to the posterior to the pupil, a B-scan ultrasound is indicated to rule out intraocular tumors, retroorbital masses, and thickened extraocular muscles. The B-scan also allows a rough estimate of the axial length from which the size of the implant can be calculated. In patients with a history of trauma, a CT scan may be ordered to evaluate the orbital walls and the sinuses.[7]
- Evaluation of the periorbita and the orbit. Volume assessment in relation to the contralateral eye.
- Complete systemic evaluation. Patients with intraocular tumors should be evaluated for metastatic disease before surgery.
- In the operating room, it is important for the surgeon to review the patient's record and examine the patient's eye to ensure that the correct eye is enucleated. Eye should be marked prominently and confirmed with the patient prior to

anesthesia and placement of a shield over the nonoperative eye to avoid accidental injury during surgery.

40.8 Operative Technique

40.8.1 Anesthesia Options

Monitored anesthesia care (MAC), anesthesia (retrobulbar anesthesia with conscious sedation), or general anesthesia may be used. Most physicians prefer general anesthesia as the patient may become uncomfortable despite adequate blocking techniques.

40.8.2 Instrumentation

Instruments are 0.5 forceps and/or Bishop-Harmon forceps, muscle hook, Castroviejo needle driver, bipolar cautery, Kelly or 90-degree clamp, bulldog/serrefine clips, Westcott and Stevens tenotomy scissors, Metzenbaum or enucleation scissors, Wells enucleation spoon, sponges and cotton-tipped applicators, thrombin, local anesthetic, or cocaine (can soak sponges and apply for local hemostasis), malleable retractor, implant and suture materials: 5–0 or 6–0 polyglactin, 4–0 silk.[7]

40.9 Surgical Technique

- An eyelid adjustable wire speculum is placed, and a 360-degree conjunctival limbal peritomy using Westcott scissors is performed. Care is taken to keep the curve of Westcott following the curvature of the limbus to allow smooth separation of the conjunctiva and maximal preservation of the conjunctiva (▶ Fig. 40.1). Keeping the Tenon capsule intact during dissection is of utmost importance. Once the peritomy is done, Stevens tenotomy scissors are used to bluntly dissect in each oblique quadrant. A good technique is to lift the conjunctiva and then gradually separate the blades of the tenotomy scissors to make an adequate pocket. The dissection can be carried out deep just beyond the globe (▶ Fig. 40.2).
- Each of the rectus muscles is localized with the aid of a muscle hook (▶ Fig. 40.3). Minimal cleaning of the tissue at the muscle insertion is carried out so that Tenon fascia is disturbed as little as possible in this area. A good way is to use moistened cotton-tipped applicators to bare the tendon and muscle. Once the rectus muscle is identified, the muscle can be tented off the globe with the help of an assistant and two muscle hooks. This allows a free path to pass the double armed 6–0 polyglactin suture in a whiplock fashion to secure the muscle tendon. This maneuver is important as globe perforation with a needle, especially in intraocular tumors, can cause orbital seeding. Once the suture is secure, the muscle is released from the globe. The suture is then placed in a serrefine clamp.[8]
- The oblique muscles are also identified and released from the globe. Sometimes, the oblique muscles can be hard to identify by a beginner. It is best to sweep the muscle hook lateral to medial to hook the inferior oblique muscle. The trochlea and the origin of inferior oblique are easy to find along the medial orbital rim. Some surgeons tag the inferior oblique muscle

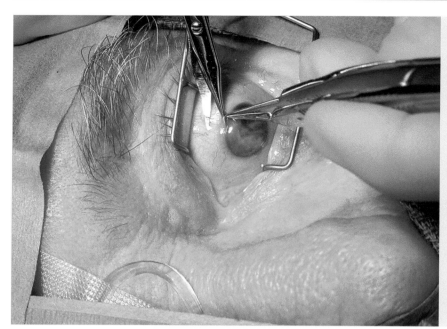

Fig. 40.1 Conjunctival peritomy with Westcott scissors.

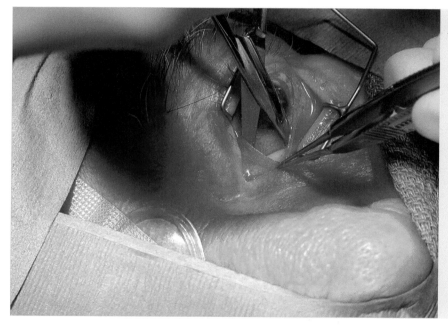

Fig. 40.2 Stevens tenotomy scissors being used to separate the Tenon capsule from the globe.

with a polyglactin suture in similar fashion as is performed with the rectus muscles. It is then used as a hammock to prevent implant migration. The superior oblique is severed and allowed to retract.[8]

- Although the optic nerve can be accessed medially or laterally, the author prefers a lateral approach. A 4–0 silk suture can be attached to the lateral rectus insertion site to allow traction of the globe anteriorly. Others directly grasp the lateral rectus stump itself. Once all the muscles have been isolated, the eyelid speculum is removed. A Wells enucleation spoon is introduced into the field. It slides behind the globe and hugs the optic nerve at its insertion. The spoon is rotated to free any residual Tenon attachments. The globe is gently retracted anteriorly by lifting the spoon. At this point, the lateral rectus is pulled laterally and the curved Metzenbaum scissors introduced. The optic nerve is localized on either side of the intraorbital optic nerve. The nerve is gently strummed with the closed blades of the scissor. Once the depth of nerve to be incised is identified, the lateral rectus is pulled, and the nerve is severed. Pressure is applied to the socket with thrombin- or cocaine-soaked sponges (or simply saline) for 5 minutes to achieve hemostasis. Malleable retractors are then used to gently retract orbital fat away from the optic nerve stump. Actively bleeding vessels are then cauterized under direct visualization (▶ Fig. 40.4).[8]

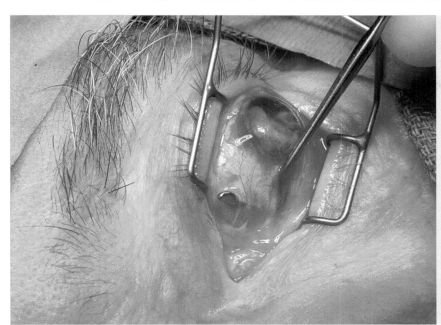

Fig. 40.3 Gass muscle hook lifting the lateral rectus muscle.

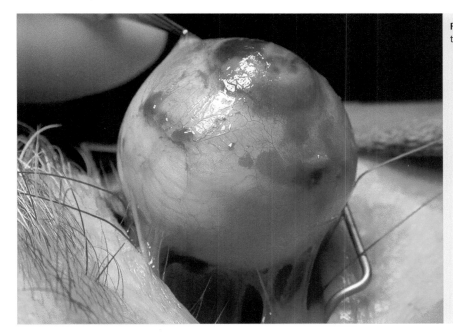

Fig. 40.4 Enucleated globe being removed from the eye socket after severing the optic nerve.

• After hemostasis has been achieved, the implant is prepared. Some surgeons prefer wrapping the implant in donor sclera, while others suture the recti directly onto the implant (► Fig. 40.5). Proper selection of implant volume helps minimize superior sulcus deformity and enophthalmos. Implant size can be used to approximate the capacity of the orbit while taking into account the amount of conjunctiva available. The exact location for implant placement varies among ophthalmic surgeons. Some surgeons prefer to have the orbital implant remain partly within Tenon space and partly behind Tenon (in the intraconal space). Other surgeons prefer placing the implant entirely within the intraconal space. An implant introducer (e.g., Carter sphere introducer; Storz, Bausch & Lomb, Inc., New Jersey) facilitates implant placement while the edges of Tenon fascia are retracted with double-pronged skin hooks (► Fig. 40.6). It is important to avoid dragging anterior Tenon fascia deep with implant placement (a common problem with porous orbital implants). Once the implant is placed into the orbit, surgeons routinely "seat" the implant. To do this, gentle pressure is applied to the anterior implant surface using a cotton-tipped applicator while an Adson toothed forceps is used to unravel any rolled Tenon edge. Additional pressure is applied to the implant with a cotton-tipped applicator while pulling anteriorly on Tenon to place the implant deeper.[8]

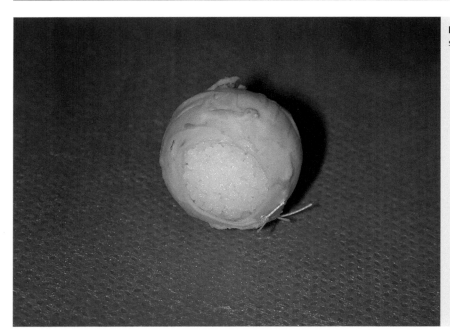

Fig. 40.5 Orbital implant coated with donor sclera.

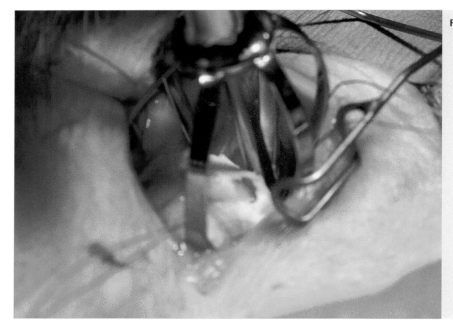

Fig. 40.6 Implant introducer.

- The sutures from the rectus muscles are secured to the anterior portion of the wrapped implant just anterior to their normal anatomic insertion sites. Surgeons generally attach the rectus muscles to the implant so that they are approximately 8 to 10 mm away from the antagonist rectus muscle (▶ Fig. 40.7).[8]
- Anterior Tenon fascia is closed meticulously with a buried 6–0 polyglactin suture in an interrupted fashion. It is extremely important that Tenon not be closed under tension. Conjunctiva is then closed in meticulous fashion taking care not to bury conjunctiva within the wound with a running suture (6–0 polyglactin suture). Closing the anterior Tenon fascia and the conjunctiva is best done with the speculum

under minimum tension. This minimizes button-holing while closing the anterior tissues. At the end, the speculum is removed, a large rigid conformer is placed, and a temporary tarsorrhaphy is performed (▶ Fig. 40.8).

40.10 Tips and Pearls

- Gentle handling of tissues during enucleation is of utmost importance. The conjunctiva, the Tenon fascia, and the rectus muscles can be very friable especially in cases of chronic inflammation. Toothed forceps should be used gently to avoid buttonholes.

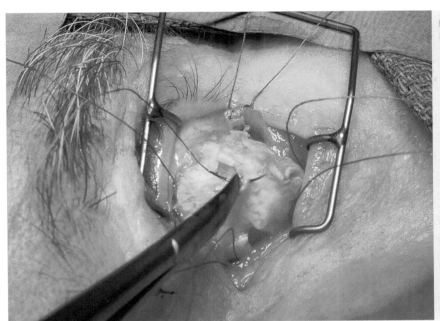

Fig. 40.7 Rectus muscles being sutured onto the implant.

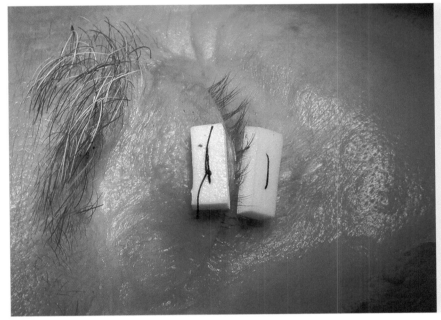

Fig. 40.8 Temporary tarsorrhaphy with silk suture.

- Getting the maximum length of the optic nerve is important in cases of retinoblastoma where the management protocol changes if the cut section has tumor. This component of surgery improves with experience. Some surgeons believe that the use of an optic nerve snare can allow for a longer segment of optic nerve, but the crush involved in the snare may distort histopathological analysis.
- Choosing the right implant for the patient is necessary. Integrated implants like coralline hydroxyapatite (HA) and porous polyethylene, nonintegrated implants like PMMA, and silicone spheres are commonly used.[9,10] Studies have shown the axial length minus 2 mm approximates the implant diameter for optimal volume replacement in emmetropic and myopic individuals. Other authors have suggested a graduated cylinder be used to measure the volume of fluid displaced by an enucleated eye. The volume of the globe minus 2 mL gives the ideal implant size to use. Using individual surgeon-preferred algorithms for implant sizing gives maximum cosmesis.[11,12] Some surgeons suggest that calcific hydroxyapatite implants should be avoided in children with retinoblastoma as iatrogenically introduced calcium can confuse evaluation for recurrence of this tumor and complicate secondary irradiation of the orbit.[13] It is also best preferred to use nonintegrated implants in patients with chronic inflammation. The porous implants may incite a fibroblastic reaction and worsen the inflammation. To

decrease the incidence of this reaction, the surgeon may wrap the porous implant with donor sclera.

- The porous polyethylene (Medpor, Stryker, Portage, MI) tunneled implant is commonly used in enucleation surgery. It can get cumbersome to tunnel the needle on the polyglactin suture into the small openings. It is advisable to flatten the curvature of the needle using a needle holder and this will allow a smooth pass.

40.11 What to Avoid

- Operating on the wrong eye. This is a possibility when there is bilateral tumor involvement as in retinoblastoma. Follow the "time out" protocol. Such an event can be avoided by taking an informed consent, attentiveness of support staff, good communication between the physician and patient, examination of the patient immediately before enucleation, and marking of the eye to be enucleated before anesthesia.[14]
- Not taking an adequate consent and the patient has wrong notions and expectations from the procedure.
- Using the wrong implant and the wrong size of the implant.
- Losing and slippage of the extraocular muscle.
- Not addressing other factors influencing the orbit size, e.g., postradiation socket, orbital wall fractures, and sinus fractures.

40.12 Complications/Bailout/ Salvage

40.12.1 Intraoperative Complications

Intraoperative Hemorrhage

Anticoagulants should be stopped after consulting with the primary care provider. Retrobulbar anesthetic with epinephrine can reduce hemorrhage. If hemorrhage does occur, it can be controlled with packing and pressure applied within the muscle cone or with application of absorbable gelatin sponge (Gelfoam), cocaine, or thrombin. Identifiable bleeding vessels can be cauterized.[15]

Extraocular Muscle Injury or Loss

This can be avoided by careful placement of traction sutures. As described earlier in a whiplock fashion. If a muscle is lost, it can be easily located by grasping Tenon fascia with forceps in the meridian of the muscle in a hand-over-hand fashion until the muscle is found. Temporary removal of implant can facilitate muscle recovery.[14]

40.12.2 Postoperative Complications

Early

Orbital Hemorrhage and Edema

This is not a common phenomenon. When it does occur it is best managed by compression pressure bandage. A large hematoma might require surgical exploration and drainage.[15]

Orbital Infection

It is best avoided by maintaining an aseptic surgical technique, keeping the operating field clean, and a personal preference is to do a vancomycin wash of the socket before closing in cases of endophthalmitis/panophthalmitis. In enucleation being performed for chronic infections, it is best to give a short course of postoperative antibiotics. If an abscess is observed on ultrasound, it is best to remove the implant and drain the abscess.[16] It may also be advisable to perform enucleation and implant placement as a staged procedure to ensure that the infection has cleared prior to placing a foreign body in a potentially infected space.

Conformer Extrusion

This is a common problem seen in the immediate postoperative period. Significant chemosis of the conjunctiva can occur that expels the conformer. In cases of chronic inflammation, shortening of fornices may occur. If the conformer fails to hold, it is best to perform a temporary tarsorrhaphy to prevent permanent shallow fornices that may require a mucous membrane graft (▶ Fig. 40.8).[17]

Late

Deepened Superior Sulcus

This phenomenon is caused by loss of orbital volume from orbital fat atrophy and relaxation of tissues within the orbit. Clinically, it appears as a deep groove between the upper eyelid and orbital rim with enophthalmos and ptosis. Numerous techniques can be used to manage this complication including secondary subperiosteal implant, suturing the levator complex tendon to the periosteum of the superior orbital rim, dermis fat grafting, and injecting filler materials to augment orbital volume.[18,19,20,21]

Fornix Contracture

This complication can occur due to shortening of the posterior lamella, implant extrusion, or trauma and can include complete obliteration of the fornices with inability to retain the prosthesis. It is best prevented by preservation of conjunctiva during surgery, limited conjunctival dissection, and regular conformer use. It is managed with prosthesis modification for mild cases, and fornix reconstruction with mucous membrane graft, hard palate graft, or dermis fat grafts in more severe cases.[17]

Orbital Implant Exposure/Extrusion

Inadequate implant size, shape, and material might increase risk of exposure/extrusion (irregular surfaces create pressure points that might increase exposure rate). Some important causes include anterior placement of implant, inadequate Tenon capsule closure, closure of conjunctiva under tension, poor wound healing (e.g., previous radiation or collagen vascular disease), infection, and foreign body inflammatory response to implant materials. Small defects may close spontaneously under cover of topical antibiotics. Larger defects require tissue grafts placement (donor sclera, allogenic dermis, hard palate, dermis fat, temporalis fascia, and tarsoconjunctival grafts have all been used to give tectonic support). When none of these works, the implant should be removed and replaced.[22,23]

Ectropion

This is commonly due to increased eyelid laxity and skin cicatrix formation. It is best managed by canthal tendon tightening or in severe cases by a skin graft.[24]

Entropion

This may occur due to eyelid laxity or a contracted socket. Cicatricial entropion is best managed by prosthesis modification, skin muscle excision, and, in severe cases, contracted socket repair with mucous membrane grafting.[24]

Ptosis

This is caused by levator muscle disinsertion, superotemporal implant migration, and superior fornix scarring. It is best managed by prosthesis modification, levator surgery, or frontalis suspension in severe ptosis.[25]

Poor Prosthesis Motility

This is seen in lost, restricted, or paretic muscles; inadequate conjunctiva; poor prosthesis fit or inadequate implant volume; or implant migration. Enucleation surgery or the underlying condition requiring enucleation may limit motility due to altered orbital anatomy or trauma to the nerves or muscles. Secondary surgery for correction-limited motility alone is rare. It may be managed by reattachment of muscles, implant exchange or orbital volume enhancement, placement of a peg into the implant for improved prosthesis motility.[26,27]

Giant Papillary Conjunctivitis—Chronic Mucous Discharge

This occurs due to poor prosthesis hygiene and fitting. It is best managed by topical corticosteroids, nonsteroidal anti-inflammatory agents, and artificial tears. If all else fails, prosthesis modification may be considered.[24]

40.13 Postoperative Care

The patient is prescribed antibiotic ointment for a week. It acts twofold by preventing infection and lubricating the ocular surfaces. If placed at the time of surgery, tarsorrhaphy suture should be removed 1 week after surgery. A tight patch for 5 to 7 days works for hemostasis and allows resorption of blood and chemosis. Pain medicines help relieve postoperative discomfort, although opioid medications should be used judiciously due to risk of nausea/vomiting. Strenuous activity can be resumed after 1 to 2 weeks. Once adequate healing has occurred the patient can visit the ocularist for a custom-made prosthesis in 4 to 6 weeks. Polycarbonate lens/safety frame prescription is advised for the fellow eye. Patient should be adequately counseled for prosthesis hygiene, use of lubricants, periodic prosthesis inspection, and prosthesis polishing. The prosthesis may be replaced if it shows extensive wear or poor fit.[7]

References

[1] Shields JA. Current approaches to the diagnosis and management of choroidal melanomas. Surv Ophthalmol. 1977; 21(6):443–463

[2] Shields CL, Shields JA. Recent developments in the management of retinoblastoma. J Pediatr Ophthalmol Strabismus. 1999; 36(1):8–18, quiz 35–36

[3] Spraul CW, Grossniklaus HE. Analysis of 24,444 surgical specimens accessioned over 55 years in an ophthalmic pathology laboratory. Int Ophthalmol. 1998; 21(5):283–304

[4] Erie JC, Nevitt MP, Hodge D, Ballard DJ. Incidence of enucleation in a defined population. Am J Ophthalmol. 1992; 113(2):138–144

[5] Moshfeghi DM, Moshfeghi AA, Finger PT. Enucleation. Surv Ophthalmol. 2000; 44(4):277–301

[6] Custer P, Cook B. The team approach to the anophthalmic patient. Adv Ophthalmic Plast Reconstr Surg. 1990; 8:55–57

[7] Yoon M, MacIntosh PW. Clinical Education/Oculofacial Plastic Surgery Education Center, American Academy of Ophthalmology website 2017. https://www.aao.org/about-preferred-practice-patterns

[8] Jordan DR, Klapper SR. Surgical techniques in enucleation: the role of various types of implants and the efficacy of pegged and nonpegged approaches. Int Ophthalmol Clin. 2006; 46(1):109–132

[9] Perry AC. Integrated orbital implants. Adv Ophthalmic Plast Reconstr Surg. 1990; 8:75–81

[10] Perry AC. Advances in enucleation. Ophthal Plast Reconstr Surg. 1991; 4:173–182

[11] Kaltreider SA, Lucarelli MJ. A simple algorithm for selection of implant size for enucleation and evisceration: a prospective study. Ophthal Plast Reconstr Surg. 2002; 18(5):336–341

[12] Custer PL, Trinkaus KM. Volumetric determination of enucleation implant size. Am J Ophthalmol. 1999; 128(4):489–494

[13] Shah SU, Shields CL, Lally SE, Shields JA. Hydroxyapatite orbital implant in children following enucleation: analysis of 531 sockets. Ophthal Plast Reconstr Surg. 2015; 31(2):108–114

[14] Stone W. Complications of evisceration and enucleation. In: Fasanella RM, ed. Management of Complications in Eye Surgery. Philadelphia, PA: W.B. Saunders; 1957:278–317

[15] Meltzer MA. Complications of enucleation and evisceration: prevention and treatment. Int Ophthalmol Clin. 1992; 32(4):213–233

[16] Lyon DB, Dortzbach RK. Enucleation and evisceration, Eye Trauma. St. Louis, MO: Mosby-Year Book, Inc.; 1991:354–367

[17] Schaefer DP. Evaluation and management of the anophthalmic socket and socket reconstruction. In: Nesi FA, Lisman RD, Levine MR, eds. Smith's Ophthalmic Plastic and Reconstructive Surgery. 2nd ed. St. Louis, MO: Mosby-Year Book, Inc.; 1998:1079–1124

[18] Malhotra R. Deep orbital Sub-Q Restylane (nonanimal stabilized hyaluronic acid) for orbital volume enhancement in sighted and anophthalmic orbits. Arch Ophthalmol. 2007; 125(12):1623–1629

[19] Smerdon DL, Sutton GA. Analysis of the factors involved in cosmetic failure following excision of the eye. Br J Ophthalmol. 1988; 72(10):768–773

[20] Smith B, Lisman RD. Use of sclera and liquid collagen in the camouflage of superior sulcus deformities. Ophthalmology. 1983; 90(3):230–235

[21] Spivey BE, Allen L, Stewart WB. Surgical correction of superior sulcus deformity occurring after enucleation. Am J Ophthalmol. 1976; 82(3):365–370

[22] Su GW, Yen MT. Current trends in managing the anophthalmic socket after primary enucleation and evisceration. Ophthal Plast Reconstr Surg. 2004; 20 (4):274–280

[23] Lee V, Subak-Sharpe I, Hungerford JL, Davies NP, Logani S. Exposure of primary orbital implants in postenucleation retinoblastoma patients. Ophthalmology. 2000; 107(5):940–945, discussion 946

[24] Jung SK, Cho WK, Paik JS, Yang SW. Long-term surgical outcomes of porous polyethylene orbital implants: a review of 314 cases. Br J Ophthalmol. 2012; 96(4):494–498

[25] Riebel O. Plastic surgery on the upper eye-lid after enucleation of the eye. Br J Ophthalmol. 1976; 60(10):726–727

[26] Jordan DR, Chan S, Mawn L, et al. Complications associated with pegging hydroxyapatite orbital implants. Ophthalmology. 1999; 106(3):505–512

[27] Lee SY, Jang JW, Lew H, Kim SJ, Kim HY. Complications in motility PEG placement for hydroxyapatite orbital implant in anophthalmic socket. Jpn J Ophthalmol. 2002; 46(1):103–107

41 Evisceration

Sanjai Jalaj and Bryan J. Winn

Summary

Evisceration is a surgical method for eye removal while preserving the sclera of the eye. This is employed in cases of acute endophthalmitis, phthisis bulbi, or other causes of blind, painful eye without a known or suspected malignancy. Advantages of this surgery over enucleation include preservation of orbital anatomic relationships and a technically faster procedure. Prior to surgery, unless the posterior segment can be visualized, imaging must be acquired. Various techniques of scleral preservation or modification have been described and can be selected based on surgeon preference and patient factors.

Keywords: evisceration, enucleation, anophthalmos, orbital implant, sympathetic ophthalmia

41.1 Description

Evisceration is a technique in which the intraocular contents of the globe are removed without removal of the entire globe itself. This entails removing the vitreous, retina, and uvea, while preserving the sclera and the extraocular muscles that insert onto the sclera. This is in contrast to enucleation in which the extraocular muscles are disinserted and the globe is removed in its entirety.

41.2 Key Principles

- The goal of evisceration is to maintain the nonvisual structure and functions of the adnexa, including providing adequate volume replacement and maintaining motility for maximal cosmetic outcome.
- Evisceration allows the removal of the intraocular source of pathology without complete loss of the structure and function of the globe.

41.3 Expectations

The patient's expectation is twofold: (1) relief of pain in a nonseeing eye and (2) a cosmetically acceptable outcome. The primary advantage of evisceration over enucleation is that the anatomical relationship of the extraocular muscles to the sclera is preserved.[1] This translates to a less complex surgery with anatomic motility giving the patient a higher likelihood of achieving his or her goal of a cosmetically acceptable outcome with relief from pain. In addition, evisceration may be psychologically easier for patients to accept than enucleation.

41.4 Indications

Indications include the following:
- A blind painful eye (often with neovascular glaucoma or infectious endophthalmitis).
- Cosmesis for phthisis bulbi.
- Trauma.

41.5 Contraindications

The only absolute contraindication to evisceration is the presence of an intraocular malignancy because of the risk of incomplete removal of tumor and the risk of tumor spread. Relative contraindications include the following:
- Blind painful eye in which pathologic review is necessary.
- Severe phthisis bulbi or microphthalmos in which there is insufficient sclera to cover an adequately sized implant.
- Large staphyloma that could complicate complete removal of intraocular contents.
- Intraocular infection (endophthalmitis, panophthalmitis) due to theoretical risk of spread of infection to the cerebrospinal fluid space through the cut end of the optic nerve.

41.6 Preoperative Preparation and Considerations

41.6.1 Implant Choice

Implant choices in evisceration essentially break down into two categories: integrated and nonintegrated implants.[2] An integrated implant allows for fibrovascular ingrowth and possible peg placement, whereas nonintegrated implants do not. Nonintegrated implants include inert materials such as acrylic or silicone. They are relatively inexpensive and not prone to infection. Because there is no fibrovascular ingrowth, motility is not directly transmitted to the implant. Furthermore, they have higher rates of migration.

There are a number of materials used for integrated implants. Hydroxyapatite implants have been successfully used for many years. It is the main inorganic calcium phosphate salt that comprises bone. The pores within the material allow for fibrovascular ingrowth conferring increased motility and decreased migration compared to nonintegrated implants. Porous polyethylene (Medpor, Stryker, Kalamazoo, MI) and aluminum oxide bioceramic implants have been developed more recently. Various studies have revealed varying degrees of success of each implant type. A recent meta-analysis by Schellini et al that examined over 3,800 patients revealed no difference in implant exposure between porous polyethylene and hydroxyapatite implants.[2] There was a lower rate of exposure with porous polyethylene compared to bioceramic implants. The choice of implant can be a difficult one and often comes down to surgeon preference, although a few special circumstances, such as pegging or active infection, may help dictate selection.

41.6.2 Pegging

A pegged implant is one in which a sleeved socket is created within the integrated implant such that a prosthesis with a peg can fit into the socket. The advantage of this technique is that motion of the implant is directly transmitted to the prosthesis, potentially improving cosmesis. However, pegged implants have higher risks of side effects such as discharge, exposure, and infection compared to nonpegged implants. Many surgeons feel hydroxyapatite is superior to other materials in terms of the ability to support a peg sleeved socket in the long term. Typically, the peg socket is drilled into the integrated implant during a second procedure about a year after implant placement, once fibrovascular integration of the implant is complete. Therefore, patients can decide if they are pleased with the amount of motility they have without the peg before committing to this procedure. Magnetic resonance imaging with contrast can help confirm fibrovascular integration. However, in evisceration specifically, anecdotal experience has found that pegging confers *too much* movement to the prosthesis, allowing the edges of the prosthesis to become exposed during normal eye movement, detracting from the desired cosmetic outcome.

41.6.3 Endophthalmitis

An important consideration when considering evisceration versus enucleation is the presence of endophthalmitis or panophthalmitis at the time of surgery. Conventional wisdom dictates that placing an implant into a space that was infected would increase the risk of postoperative infection and secondary implant removal. However, numerous studies have demonstrated low complication rates in patients with endophthalmitis who have successfully received a primary, nonporous implant at the time of evisceration.[3,4] In these circumstances, preoperative intravenous antibiotics and postoperative oral antibiotics are indicated. At times, the sclera may become so necrotic and friable due to the inflammation from infection that an evisceration may need to be converted to an enucleation. Again, nonporous implants should be used primarily in these situations.

41.6.4 Malignancy

A criticism of evisceration in comparison to enucleation is that there is a risk of eviscerating an eye with an occult intraocular malignancy. Eviscerating in such circumstances can lead to local and distant spread of disease. In retrospective analyses of evisceration samples, malignancies have been found in 1 to 10% of cases.[5,6,7] Patients ought to be made aware of this risk prior to surgery. In addition, a dilated exam, B-scan ultrasound, CT, or MRI should be performed prior to all eviscerations to identify possible neoplasms before surgery.[8] If one has any suspicion of malignancy or the eye cannot be imaged adequately, evisceration is contraindicated.

41.6.5 Perioperative and Postoperative Antibiotics

Practice patterns have varied in regard to administering antibiotics in cases of eviscerations with implant placement. The use of perioperative and postoperative antibiotics has been a matter of physician preference. However, recent studies have suggested that both perioperative IV antibiotics and postoperative oral antibiotics do not alter the rate of surgical infections.[9] Perioperative antibiotics may be recommended in those with higher risk of infection, such as cases of poorly controlled diabetes, trauma, malnutrition, obesity, smoking, immunosuppression, or prolonged anticipated hospital stay and, of course, in cases of active infection such as endophthalmitis or panophthalmitis.

41.6.6 Choice of Anesthesia

General anesthesia either via endotracheal tube or laryngeal mask airway (LMA) is often employed and allows for maximum patient comfort and lack of awareness during the procedure. However, in high-risk patients or in other circumstances where general anesthesia is less desirable or cannot be performed, monitored anesthesia care (MAC) with a retrobulbar block consisting of a 1:1 mix of 2% lidocaine with epinephrine 1:100,000 and 0.75% bupivacaine with or without hyaluronidase can be used to successfully keep patients comfortable during evisceration or enucleation.[10] When using either type of anesthesia, delivering 0.75% bupivacaine at the end of surgery to the orbit allows for several hours of initial postoperative comfort.

41.7 Operative Technique

- After anesthesia is induced (see above), an eyelid retractor is placed. Subconjunctival local anesthetic is infiltrated to balloon the conjunctiva to facilitate dissection. A 360-degree limbal peritomy is then made with Westcott scissors and then used to undermine conjunctiva and Tenon fascia. It is important to undermine liberally in order to be able to close the wound at the end of the procedure. Care is used to prevent tearing of the conjunctiva.
- A total keratectomy at or just behind the limbus is begun with an 11 or 15-degree blade and completed using Westcott scissors. The entire cornea must be removed to prevent cyst formation should any corneal epithelium be left behind (▶ Fig. 41.1).
- With an evisceration spoon, the contents of the globe are removed. Attempt should be made to remove contents en bloc. This will allow for better histopathologic examination. The spoon is then used to scrape the inner sclera to remove any adherent uvea (▶ Fig. 41.2).
- A cotton swab soaked in absolute ethyl alcohol can be used to denature any of the remaining uveal tissue (▶ Fig. 41.3).
- Relaxing incisions can be made in the sclera in the intermuscular areas at 10:30 and 4:30 to allow for placement of a properly sized implant. A number of other modifications to the posterior sclera can be performed to allow an adequately sized implant. Those techniques are described in the next section.
- Graduated sizing spheres are used to determine the proper size of an implant that will still allow anterior closure of the sclera. Typically, the ideal size is approximately 20 mm. Kaltreider and Lucarelli have suggested an algorithm of axial length of the contralateral eye minus 3 mm for evisceration.[11]
- The implant is then placed within or behind the scleral shell with the aid of a Carter sphere introducer holder. Removal of the eyelid speculum may aid in implant insertion.
- The sclera is closed with interrupted 5–0 or 6–0 polyglactin or polydioxanone sutures. Tenon capsule is then closed in one or two layers with interrupted, buried 5–0 polyglactin sutures. The authors have found that the use of the 8-mm semicircular P-2 needle facilitates this closure. Finally, the conjunctiva can be closed with running 6–0 plain gut sutures.

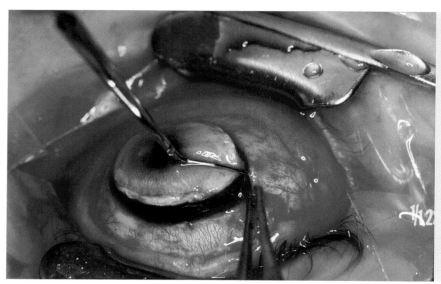

Fig. 41.1 A 360-degree incision is made just posterior to the limbus allowing for complete removal of the cornea. (Courtesy of Bryan S. Sires, MD, PhD.)

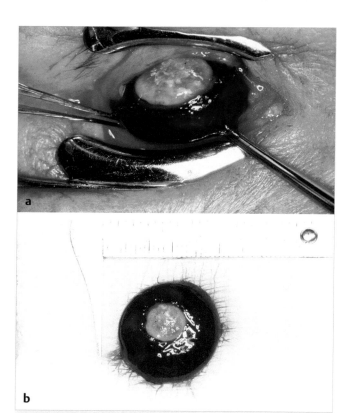

Fig. 41.2 **(a)** Smooth concentric motions of the evisceration spoon allow for complete removal of the uvea. **(b)** An intact uvea facilitates histopathologic evaluation. (Courtesy of Bryan S. Sires, MD, PhD.)

- Antibiotic ointment is placed in the socket, followed by a conformer between the eyelids and conjunctiva. The eyelids are then closed via a temporary tarsorrhaphy to prevent conjunctival prolapse. A pressure patch is placed for 3 days postoperatively.

41.8 Tips and Pearls

- Preoperatively, patients need to be adequately counseled about the process of eye removal. In addition, it is up to the clinician to gauge the mental preparation of the patient to have his or her eye removed because the psychological trauma associated with organ removal is not insubstantial. Evisceration may pose less psychological trauma than enucleation since the entire eye is not being removed.
- It is almost impossible to place an adequately sized implant in evisceration procedures while leaving the sclera intact because of a combination of removing tissues such as cornea and the effect of phthisis. A number of techniques have been described to fit a properly sized implant by modifying the sclera.
  - Technique A: The optic nerve can be excised as well as a circular portion of posterior sclera leaving the implant exposed posteriorly.[12] The advantage here is twofold: it allows increased vascularization of a porous implant as well as creating more space to fit a larger implant. Posterior radial incisions can additionally be made to further increase the available space for an implant (▶ Fig. 41.4).
  - Technique B: Two sclerotomies are created, one from the inferonasal limbus and the other starting from the superotemporal limbus, both extending posteriorly all the way to the optic nerve. The flaps are then disinserted from the optic nerve, the implant is placed, and then the sclera is closed with a few millimeters of overlap anterior to the implant (▶ Fig. 41.5).
  - Technique C: The sclera may be quadrisected into four equal "petals" between the four rectus muscles all the way back to the optic nerve.[13] The optic nerve is then disinserted allowing the quadrisections to be closed over the anterior portion of the implant (▶ Fig. 41.6).
  - Technique D: A 360-degree incision is made at the equator splitting the sclera into anterior and posterior halves.[14] The anterior half is used to cover the implant. Care needs to be used not to damage the extraocular muscles when performing this procedure (▶ Fig. 41.7).

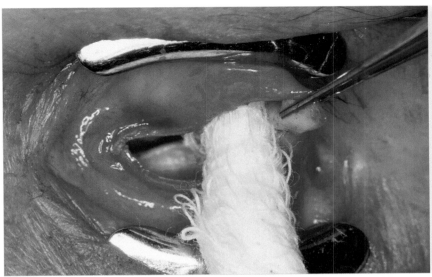

Fig. 41.3 A cotton-tipped applicator soaked in absolute ethyl alcohol is used to denature any residual uvea adherent to the sclera. (Courtesy of Bryan S. Sires, MD, PhD.)

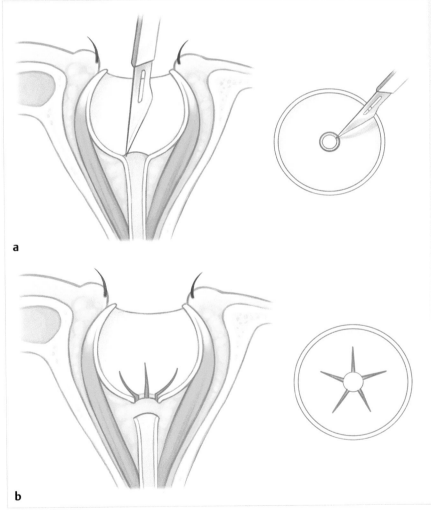

a

b

Fig. 41.4 Technique A. **(a)** The optic nerve is disinserted with an 11 blade and Steven scissors. **(b)** Radial incisions can be made to expand the scleral cavity.

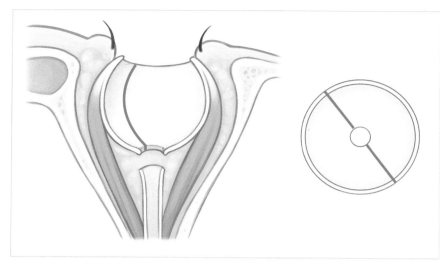

Fig. 41.5 Technique B. *Left*—Anterior view of the globe with inferonasal and superotemporal incision sites marked by the dotted line. *Right*—Internal view of the posterior globe demonstrating the continuation of the anterior to posterior incisions along with a disinserted optic nerve.

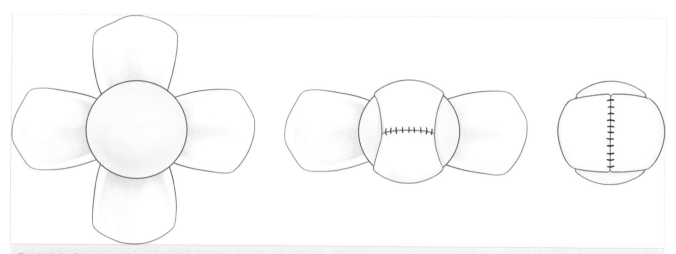

Fig. 41.6 Technique C. Schematic drawing of quadrisected scleral petals. The superior and inferior scleral petals can be closed first. Then the nasal and temporal petals can be closed creating a two-layered closure over the implant.

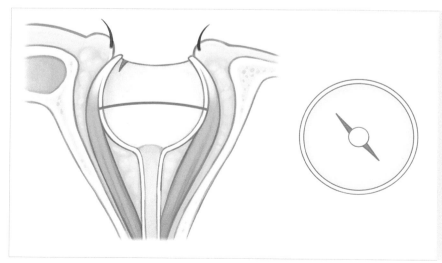

Fig. 41.7 Technique D. Schematic demonstrating a 360-degree equatorial scleral incision along with anterior relaxing incisions.

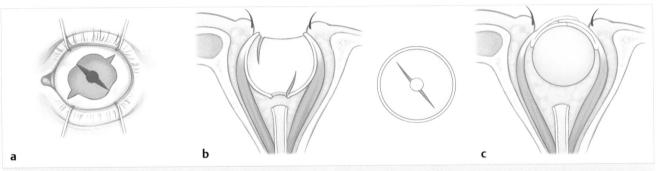

Fig. 41.8 Technique E. **(a)** Frontal view of the anterior and perpendicular posterior sclerotomies. **(b)** Sagittal cross-section of those same sclerotomies. **(c)** Three-layered closure with implant placed completely posterior to the sclera.

- Technique E: The implant can be placed entirely behind the posterior sclera.[15] Two anterior sclerotomies are made in the inferotemporal and superonasal quadrants extending 15 to 20 mm posteriorly. Then two posterior sclerotomies are performed 90 degrees away from the anterior sclerotomies. The superotemporal and inferonasal posterior sclerotomies extend 15 to 20 mm anteriorly from the optic nerve. The optic nerve is disinserted. The two posterior scleral lips are advanced anteriorly and then the implant is placed behind the posterior sclera. This results in three layers of sclera in front of the implant. Each layer should be closed individually (▶ Fig. 41.8).
- Proper closure of Tenon's capsule. Two cotton-tipped applicators can be used to spread the Tenon's capsule closure along the entire length of the wound to identify any areas of incomplete closure and exposure of the sclera. In these areas, additional buried sutures should be placed until no sclera can be visualized.

41.9 Complications/Bailout/Salvage

41.9.1 Conversion to Enucleation

As mentioned earlier, occasionally the surgeon may find the sclera to be too fragile or thin to proceed with evisceration. This is more likely to occur in cases of endophthalmitis/panophthalmitis. In these circumstances, the surgeon should be prepared to switch to an enucleation procedure.

41.9.2 Conjunctival Cysts

Occasionally conjunctival cysts can form if the surgical wound is not closed properly. Cysts are usually not of major consequence, but occasionally they can track posteriorly and be a cause of postoperative proptosis. Superficial cysts can simply be marsupialized. Deep cysts may require temporary removal of the implant to enable excision of all of the embedded conjunctival epithelium.

41.9.3 Chemosis

Postoperative inflammation following evisceration is expected. This may result in chemosis of the conjunctiva preventing the eyelids from closing completely. With chronic exposure of the conjunctiva to air, the chemosis worsens, exposing additional conjunctiva, thus creating a viscous cycle. Chemosis needs to be treated aggressively. Oral steroids and topical steroid/antibiotic ointments may be useful. Placement of a tarsorrhaphy can be curative. The best defense against this is placement of a temporary tarsorrhaphy at the time of surgery.

41.9.4 Surgical Site Infection

Depending on the extent of the infection, antibiotics can be attempted. However, if an infection is persistent or recurrent, the implant itself may need to be removed with delayed secondary replacement.

41.9.5 Sympathetic Ophthalmia

Theoretically, there is a higher risk of sympathetic ophthalmia in the contralateral eye with evisceration than enucleation.[16] The incidence of this condition is so rare that conclusive evidence is lacking. That said, the topic should be included in the informed consent discussion with the patient.

41.9.6 Implant Exposure

Implant exposure is not an uncommon complication.[17,18] These exposures can be repaired with tissue grafts. However, a graft cannot simply be placed over exposed implant material but needs to be placed under vascularized conjunctival tissue. Reports in the literature have described using labial mucosa, dermis fat grafts, temporalis fascia, and periosteal grafts, to name a few, to repair such defects. If unsuccessful, the implant can be removed and exchanged. In certain circumstances, a dermis fat graft may be required to restore both orbital volume and conjunctival surface area after exposed implant removal.

41.9.7 Inadequate Orbital Volume

Despite proper technique and posterior placement of the orbital implant, there may be situations when orbital volume is inadequate, leading to enophthalmos and poor prosthesis movement. In these situations, orbital implant exchange may be attempted, although this may be technically challenging. Implantation of a wedge-shaped implant between the periorbita and orbital floor can increase orbital volume without disturbing the evisceration site.

41.10 Postoperative Care

41.10.1 Conformer Placement and Prostheses

In the postoperative period, a temporary conformer should be placed in the socket for approximately 6 weeks. This keeps the fornices well-formed as the socket heals allowing for the eventual placement of a properly sized, custom prosthesis crafted by an ocularist. The temporary tarsorrhaphy needs to be removed prior to the first visit to the ocularist. Once created and inserted, patients should be encouraged to leave the prosthesis in place, cleaning and maintaining it according to the ocularist's instructions. Patients should be evaluated by an oculoplastic surgeon at least yearly to ensure the health of the socket. Each year the prosthesis should also be polished or resurfaced by an ocularist to limit the risk of conjunctival irritation and inflammation. It is recommended to replace the prosthesis every 5 years. This also may need to be performed if any additional periocular reconstructive surgery is performed. An ill-fitting prosthesis should alert the oculoplastic surgeon to the possibility of some occult conjunctival or orbital process that requires evaluation.

References

[1] Migliori ME. Enucleation versus evisceration. Curr Opin Ophthalmol. 2002; 13(5):298–302

[2] Schellini S, Jorge E, Sousa R, Burroughs J, El-Dib R. Porous and nonporous orbital implants for treating the anophthalmic socket: a meta-analysis of case series studies. Orbit. 2016; 35(2):78–86

[3] Holds JB, Anderson RL. Primary vs delayed implant in evisceration. Arch Ophthalmol. 1989; 107(7):952–953

[4] Tawfik HA, Budin H. Evisceration with primary implant placement in patients with endophthalmitis. Ophthalmology. 2007; 114(6):1100–1103

[5] Makley TA, Jr, Teed RW. Unsuspected intraocular malignant melanomas. AMA Arch Opthalmol. 1958; 60(3):475–478

[6] Novais EA, Fernandes BF, Pacheco LF, et al. A histopathologic review of undiagnosed neoplasms in 205 evisceration specimens. Ophthal Plast Reconstr Surg. 2012; 28(5):331–334

[7] Zimmerman LE. Problems in the diagnosis of malignant melanomas of the choroid and ciliary body. The 1972 Arthur J. Bedell Lecture. Am J Ophthalmol. 1973; 75(6):917–929

[8] Eagle RC, Jr, Grossniklaus HE, Syed N, Hogan RN, Lloyd WC, III, Folberg R. Inadvertent evisceration of eyes containing uveal melanoma. Arch Ophthalmol. 2009; 127(2):141–145

[9] Pariseau B, Fox B, Dutton JJ. Prophylactic antibiotics for enucleation and evisceration: a retrospective study and systematic literature review. Ophthal Plast Reconstr Surg. 2018; 34(1):49–54

[10] Burroughs JR, Soparkar CN, Patrinely JR, Kersten RC, Kulwin DR, Lowe CL. Monitored anesthesia care for enucleations and eviscerations. Ophthalmology. 2003; 110(2):311–313

[11] Kaltreider SA, Lucarelli MJ. A simple algorithm for selection of implant size for enucleation and evisceration: a prospective study. Ophthal Plast Reconstr Surg. 2002; 18(5):336–341

[12] Massry GG, Holds JB. Evisceration with scleral modification. Ophthal Plast Reconstr Surg. 2001; 17(1):42–47

[13] Huang D, Yu Y, Lu R, Yang H, Cai J. A modified evisceration technique with scleral quadrisection and porous polyethylene implantation. Am J Ophthalmol. 2009; 147(5):924–928, 928.e1–928.e3

[14] Georgescu D, Vagefi MR, Yang CC, McCann J, Anderson RL. Evisceration with equatorial sclerotomy for phthisis bulbi and microphthalmos. Ophthal Plast Reconstr Surg. 2010; 26(3):165–167

[15] Jordan DR, Stoica B. Evisceration with implant placement posterior to posterior sclera. Ophthal Plast Reconstr Surg. 2016; 32(3):178–182

[16] Bilyk JR. Enucleation, evisceration, and sympathetic ophthalmia. Curr Opin Ophthalmol. 2000; 11(5):372–386

[17] Custer PL, Trinkaus KM. Porous implant exposure: incidence, management, and morbidity. Ophthal Plast Reconstr Surg. 2007; 23(1):1–7

[18] Jordan DR. Problems after evisceration surgery with porous orbital implants: experience with 86 patients. Ophthal Plast Reconstr Surg. 2004; 20(5):374–380

42 Exenteration

Ann Q. Tran and Catherine J. Choi

Summary

Orbital exenteration involves removal of the entire orbital contents. This radical disfiguring procedure is typically reserved for life-threatening malignancies or severe orbital infection or inflammation not amenable to medical treatment. Appropriate preoperative evaluation and surgical planning is tailored to each patient and the underlying condition. Surgical techniques range from total exenteration to eyelid-sparing and subtotal exenteration. Postexenteration socket reconstruction can be achieved by using a skin graft, myocutaneous advancement flap, dermal substitute, free flap, or a combination thereof. Patients can subsequently be fitted with an oculofacial prosthesis for improved cosmesis and comfort.

Keywords: exenteration, socket reconstruction, prosthesis

42.1 Goals

- To remove the affected tissue for cure of tumor, infection, or inflammation.
- To minimize risk of complication.
- To create a socket that will allow for an oculofacial prosthesis (if desired).

42.2 Advantages

Exenteration is performed as a life-saving procedure in high-grade malignancies involving the orbit for local disease control and to increase overall survival by decreasing the risk of metastasis. For patients with preexisting metastatic disease, exenteration can serve as a palliative measure to improve the quality of life by alleviating intractable pain in cases of significant mass effect or infiltrating disease. Exenteration for invasive orbital infections can decrease overall mortality by preventing or minimizing intracranial spread of the infection.[1,2,3,4]

42.3 Expectations

When discussing the surgical procedure of exenteration and the postoperative recovery, the patient and family members must be prepared for the emotional and psychosocial aftermath of removal of the eye socket and its cosmetic sequelae. Patient's expectations of the aesthetic rehabilitation period including the appearance of the ocular prosthesis and timing of the prosthesis fitting after surgery should be explicitly discussed. Exenteration also does not eliminate the possibility of tumor recurrence or metastatic spread, and the need for continued follow-up should be emphasized. The patient will live with lifelong monocular precautions, including the need for polycarbonate glasses to protect the remaining eye.

42.4 Key Principles

- Exenteration involves removal of all soft-tissue contents of the orbit including the globe, extraocular muscles, periorbita, and ocular adnexa with part or all of the eyelids.
- Depending on the clinical situation, the patient may need total exenteration, eyelid-sparing exenteration, subtotal exenteration, or exenteration in conjunction with additional intracranial or sinus surgeries.
- Primary reconstruction strategies include healing by secondary intention, split-thickness skin graft, myocutaneous advancement flap, dermal substitute, or free flap.

42.5 Indications

- With advancements in medical and surgical care, orbital exenterations occur less frequently than before. Globe-sparing resection, if possible, is always considered first.[2]
- Orbital exenteration is most commonly performed for orbital involvement of malignancies. Due to the anatomic limitations of vital structures being confined within a small space, and the formless nature of orbital fat making reliable identification of tumor margins difficult, complete resection of an infiltrating tumor of the orbit can be challenging. In such cases, exenteration can be the only option to ensure complete resection. Other scenarios include cases in which resection is expected to leave a blind, disfigured eye and ocular adnexa with limited function of the remaining orbital tissues, making exenteration the preferred surgery to achieve the best functional and cosmetic outcome.[1,2,3,4]
- A thorough history and physical examination should be performed, including consideration of the natural history of the tumor, tumor size, stage, histology, visual function, extent of orbital involvement, and the patient's overall health.
- Tissue diagnosis based on permanent histopathology must be confirmed prior to proceeding with exenteration. Under no circumstance should frozen sections be used as a surrogate to decide on exenteration. Frozen sections may be used intraoperatively for margin control during exenteration.[1,2,3,4]
- Examples of primary orbital tumors that may require orbital exenteration: adenoid cystic carcinoma, rhabdomyosarcoma, retinoblastoma, mucoepidermoid carcinoma.[1,2,3,4,5,6,7,8]
- Examples of eyelid or ocular adnexal tumors with invasion into the orbit: melanoma, basal cell carcinoma, squamous cell carcinoma, sebaceous cell carcinoma.[1,2,3,4,5,6,7,8]
- Examples of sinonasal tumors with invasion into the orbit: squamous cell carcinoma, esthesioneuroblastoma.[1,2,3,4,5,6,7,8]
- Exenteration may be indicated in severe life-threatening orbital fungal infections such as mucormycosis and aspergillosis with risk of intracranial extension.[1,2,3,4,5,6,7,8]
- Rare instances of severe periocular necrotizing fasciitis (group A β-hemolytic *Streptococcus*) unresponsive to medical therapy and debridement may undergo exenteration.[9]

- Benign tumors of the orbit or congenital deformities are rarely considered for palliative exenteration, in cases of diffuse disease resulting in irreversible vision loss, uncontrollable pain, or severe disfigurement.[10]
- Severe trauma with extensive involvement of the orbital bone or soft tissues may require an exenteration if attempts to salvage the remaining structures are not successful and not amenable to reconstruction.[11]

42.6 Contraindications

Given the permanent vision loss and facial disfiguration resulting from exenteration, all other alternatives need to be thoroughly discussed with the patient and his or her family. In some elderly, debilitated patients with additional medical comorbidities or limited life expectancy, a realistic discussion regarding the expected benefit of exenteration versus the physical and emotional burden of exenteration must be held. The postoperative wound care regimen can also be a barrier for patients with no family or nursing help. Each patient therefore needs to be considered on an individual basis to make a tailored treatment plan.

42.7 Preoperative Preparation

The patient must undergo a complete ocular examination including vision, motility, globe position, dilated fundus exam, and a thorough eyelid and ocular adnexa evaluation. Preexisting nasolacrimal system obstruction, lymphadenopathy, facial sensory defects, and involvement of adjacent external facial and sinonasal structures should be noted. A definitive pathological diagnosis must be made on permanent histological specimens from a biopsy instead of frozen sections. A metastatic work-up may be indicated depending on the tumor type. Orbital imaging with computed tomography and/or magnetic resonance imaging must be obtained to assess the location and extent of pathology.

If the disease involves the nasal cavity, sinuses, or the intracranial space, the patient should have a preoperative neurosurgery or otolaryngology evaluation to assess if transnasal or transcranial approaches may be required in addition to orbital exenteration. For patients with malignant lesions, medical oncology and radiation oncology are also part of the multidisciplinary team to coordinate neoadjuvant or adjuvant chemotherapy and radiation. For emotional preparation and expectation of possible cosmetic outcomes, patients may also wish to see an ocularist during the preoperative period.

Preoperative planning also includes surgical decision regarding the type of exenteration to be performed. For more posteriorly located tumors without skin or conjunctival involvement, skin-sparing technique can preserve the eyelids, which can be used to line the socket instead of requiring an additional skin graft. Lesions in the anterior orbit, involving the conjunctiva or eyelid skin, may only need a subtotal exenteration and partial excision of the surrounding skin, unless the disease is infiltrative and diffuse in nature (i.e., pagetoid spread of sebaceous cell carcinoma), in which case total exenteration is warranted. Extensive benign lesions can often be managed with an eyelid-sparing exenteration.

42.8 Operative Technique

42.8.1 Incision—Total Exenteration versus Eyelid-Sparing Exenteration

Exenteration is performed under general anesthesia. Injection of local anesthetic with epinephrine (i.e., 2% lidocaine with 1:100,000 epinephrine) to the surrounding eyelids is given for hemostasis. A 4-0 silk suture is typically placed through the eyelid margins as a tarsorrhaphy to help with traction. For total exenteration, a 15 blade or monopolar cutting cautery is used to circumferentially incise the skin outside the orbital rim down to periosteum, 2 to 3 mm outside the arcus marginalis. In an eyelid-sparing exenteration, initial skin incision occurs outside the upper and lower eyelid lash line, down to the pre-orbicularis or pretarsal plane (▶ Fig. 42.1). Dissection in the pre-orbicularis plane decreases the risk of unintended violation of the orbital septum, keeping all orbital contents intact. Dissection in the subcutaneous plane spares the orbicularis muscle providing a more robust vascular supply for eyelid skin and additional skin grafts. A subtotal exenteration spares the soft tissue in the posterior orbit and sometimes the eyelid skin, depending on the extent of the disease being treated.

42.8.2 Dissection

A Freer elevator is used to gently separate the periosteum from the orbital walls from the orbital rim toward the orbital apex. The subperiosteal dissection is taken as posteriorly as needed for subtotal exenteration, or all the way to the orbital apex for total exenteration. Firm attachments will be encountered at the anterior and posterior lacrimal crest, lateral orbital tubercle, trochlea, origin of the inferior oblique muscle, and edges of the superior and inferior orbital fissures. The medial and lateral canthal tendons can be released with sharp dissection. The nasolacrimal sac is transected at the entrance of the nasolacrimal duct. Perforating vessels such as the anterior and posterior ethmoidal arteries must be cauterized and transected. The inferior orbital fissure serves as an important landmark to identify the infraorbital nerve and its perforating vessels. Care is taken when dissecting around the neurovascular bundles such as the supraorbital, supratrochlear, zygomaticofacial, and zygomaticotemporal neurovascular bundles to prevent retraction, making hemostatic control difficult. Other particularly delicate areas include the thin bones of the medial orbital wall and the medial floor where violation should be avoided.

42.8.3 Removal of Orbital Contents

Once the subperiosteal dissection has been carried out as posteriorly as possible by releasing all visible attachments circumferentially, a large hemostat is placed around the apical structures (▶ Fig. 42.2a). The anesthesiologist should be informed at the time of clamping, as some patients can develop a significant bradycardic response. Either enucleation scissors or monopolar cutting cautery can be used to transect the apical tissues above the hemostat (▶ Fig. 42.2b). The orbital contents are delivered *in toto* and sent to pathology for permanent section. A moderate amount of arterial bleed may be seen from the ophthalmic artery, which can be controlled with a surgical vascular clip or

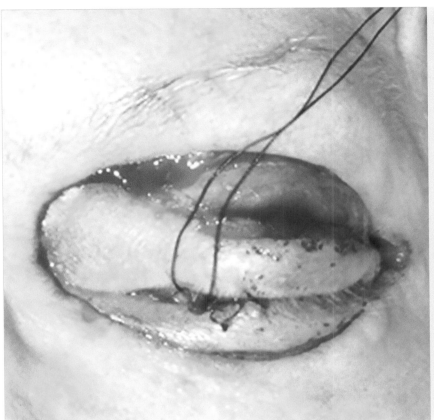

Fig. 42.1 Intraoperative photo demonstrating suture tarsorrhaphy and incision for a partial eyelid-sparing exenteration.

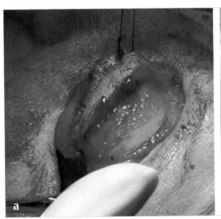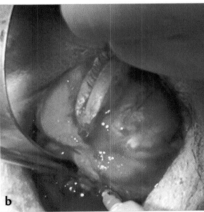

Fig. 42.2 (a) A large hemostat placed around the apical structures of the orbit following complete subperiosteal dissection. **(b)** Monopolar cutting cautery is used to transect the apical tissues above the hemostat.

by clamping and cauterizing thoroughly. If the suspected pathology is thought to involve the orbital apex, careful removal of the remaining stump of apical tissue should be performed with additional biopsies to histologically clear the apical margin. Intraoperative frozen sections can be used to guide margin clearance as needed. If orbital bony erosion is present, concurrent bone resection may be necessary. If the lesion involves the nasolacrimal system, the lacrimal sac is dissected from the lacrimal fossa and the nasolacrimal duct. The anterior wall of the canal should be removed with rongeurs to the entrance of the nose. In some cases, medial maxillectomy may be considered.

42.8.4 Reconstruction of Exenterated Socket

Multiple techniques have been described for primary reconstruction of an exenterated socket. The open cavity techniques range from healing by secondary intention to using a skin graft, myocutaneous advancement flap, or a dermal substitute.[8,12,13,14] The closed cavity technique fills the socket with muscle free flap or orbital fat transfer to the level of the orbital rim. In some instances, bone flaps, synthetic implants, or osseointegration may additionally be utilized.[15] Each reconstruction requires individualized surgical planning.

42.8.5 Healing by Secondary Intention

Healing by secondary intention allows for a shorter operating time and good color match with surrounding skin once healed. The socket is initially packed with iodoform gauze with antibiotic ointment, and the dressing is changed every other day until the socket epithelializes. Granulation over bone starts slowly within the first week with complete epithelialization 3 to 4 months later. While simple, this technique typically results in a shallow socket with a thick or irregular surface, which can mask tumor recurrence. The healing process is also generally less comfortable for the patient, and delays the timing of orbital radiation until the socket is healed.

42.8.6 Placement of Skin Graft

Reconstructing the socket with a skin graft lengthens the surgical time, but shortens the socket healing time, providing a smooth socket surface.[12] Split-thickness skin grafts are more successful than full-thickness skin grafts due to their adherence to the bony surface. Delay in orbital radiation is not required. The anterior or lateral thigh is a common site to harvest a split-thickness skin graft. With a dermatome, a 3- × 5-inch split thickness skin graft 0.3 to 0.5 mm in thickness is harvested. Application of mineral oil decreases friction for easy gliding of the dermatome. The graft may then be processed through a 1:1 or 1:2 ratio mesher, which allows the graft to cover a larger surface area, conforms to the contours of the socket, and allows for drainage of discharge or blood (▶ Fig. 42.3). The graft is sutured to the skin margin around the orbital rim using multiple interrupted and running 7–0 polyglactin sutures. The socket is then covered with antibiotic ointment, and lined with nonadherent dressing (e.g., Telfa). Pressure packing is then fashioned with two to three surgical sponges soaked in antibiotic solution that are then packed into the socket and held in place with horizontal mattress 4–0 silk sutures anchored to adjacent skin. A pressure patch is placed over the orbit and kept for 1 week. The donor site is lined with nonadherent petrolatum gauze dressing (e.g., Xeroform) and dressed with a light gauze wrap. The dressing can be kept on the graft site until it spontaneously falls off, usually in 5 to 7 days.

42.8.7 Use of Dermal Substitute

More recently, the use of dermal substitutes has been introduced for reconstruction of the exenterated socket as a technique with shorter operative time, faster recovery, and fewer complications.[13,14] An acellular biodegradable scaffold matrix of cross-linked bovine tendon collagen and glycosaminoglycan superimposed on a semipermeable layer of silicone membrane (Integra) is used to line the exenterated socket surface.[13,14] The material conforms to the socket contour and demonstrates flexible adherence. The integration of the dermal layer provides rapid granulation over 3 to 4 weeks. By 4 weeks, the layer of silicone is removed, leaving a fully epithelialized surface by 6 to 8 weeks. This reconstructive technique avoids donor site morbidity from skin grafts, but the cost of the material may add expense to the procedure.

42.8.8 Myocutaneous Advancement Flap or Free Flap

In cases where pathology extends beyond the orbit and surgical resection includes the adjacent sinuses or maxilla resulting in a larger area of soft tissue and bony defect, myocutaneous advancement flaps or free flaps are needed for reconstruction.[7,8] One option is transposition of the temporalis muscle and fascia, which can be useful in postradiation cases when vascularity is compromised and skin grafts would otherwise be at risk of failing. Patients will, however, be left with a cosmetically noticeable temporal depression. Other local flaps described include the frontalis, galea-frontalis flap, and the temporoparietal fascial flap. Free flap options include the radial forearm, latissimus dorsi, rectus abdominis, lateral arm, or anterolateral thigh.[7,8] While free flaps can provide effective volume replacement and improved healing, the aesthetic outcome is less natural and subsequent flap debulking may be required. Other disadvantages include long operative times and inpatient monitoring of vascularity. Both myocutaneous advancement flap and free flap reconstruction are also not amenable to oculofacial prosthesis fitting. Lastly, with both techniques, clinically detectable tumor recurrences may be masked, and close surveillance with serial imaging is therefore needed.

42.8.9 Additional Bony Reconstruction

If resected or are otherwise damaged, the orbital floor and medial wall will require reconstruction, as lack of support will otherwise cause the tissue to enter the sinuses and lead to loss of vascularity to support skin grafts. Reconstruction of the orbital floor may require autologous bone grafts or alloplastic

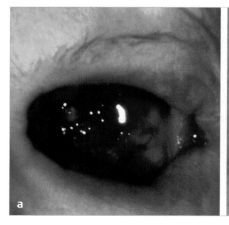
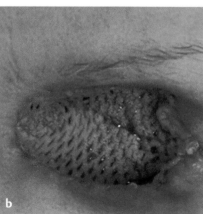

Fig. 42.3 (a) Exenterated socket following removal of orbital contents. (b) A meshed split-thickness skin graft lining the exenterated socket.

implants, such as porous polyethylene with titanium and screws for fixation.[7] Alloplastic implants should be used with caution in irradiated sites as the tissue strength and decreased vascularity increase the risk of failure and infection. Defects in the lateral wall require reconstruction if the entire greater wing of the sphenoid is removed. The orbital roof can be repaired in conjunction with neurosurgery as needed.

42.9 Tips and Pearls

- Intraoperative bleeding is minimized by discontinuing antiplatelet and anticoagulation agents prior to surgery if otherwise medically safe to do so. The primary care physician or cardiology should approve suspension of the medications.
- Hemostasis should be achieved by using any combination of bipolar or monopolar cautery, bone wax for perforating vessels, vascular ligation clips, or pro-hemostatic agents (such as Surgicel, an oxidized cellulose polymer). Avoid cutting into the supraorbital or infraorbital fissures, as the cut end of orbital vessels can retract deep into the fissure and become difficult to isolate while bleeding. Attachments at the fissures should be transected across at or above the plane of the bony edges.
- Moderate amount of arterial bleeding can be encountered after transecting the apical structures. It is difficult to achieve stepwise hemostasis during this process due to limited access and visualization. It is therefore recommended that the removal of orbital contents be completed expeditiously while the assistant suctions the blood, and allows for appropriate hemostasis under direct visualization in order to minimize the total blood loss. The ophthalmic artery often needs to be clamped, followed by thorough cauterization or ligation.
- Application of firm packing inside the socket and a sturdy pressure patch are essential in decreasing the risk of postoperative bleeding.
- Postoperative infection is uncommon. The risk is minimized with a course of oral antibiotics for 1 week following surgery and frequent dressing changes.
- The area of interest adjacent to the tumor or infection should be addressed last during dissection. This allows for subperiosteal dissection along normal bone and orbital structures to proceed first without complications and improve access for the remaining area of interest. In cases of malignancy, care should be taken to preserve intact periorbita to serve as a natural barrier for tumor cells and to theoretically prevent "seeding" the dissection bed of the orbit. Meticulous dissection should be carried out with expectation of possible bony dehiscence or erosion in the area of pathology.
- Good awareness of orbital anatomy is essential for clean dissection. It is imperative for the surgeon to know when to apply pressure and perform sharp dissection (i.e., along the thick bones of the lateral orbital rim and lateral canthal tendon) as opposed to gentle dissection along the very thin bones of the medial orbital wall and the medial floor. It is not uncommon to unintentionally unroof a small piece of bone adherent to periosteum if not approached with care. Overly aggressive use of monopolar cautery for hemostasis on thin bone can also create full-thickness burn to the bone and should be avoided. Such bony violations may lead to

cerebrospinal fluid (CSF) leak or persistent sino-orbital fistulas as discussed later.
- It is essential to have proper retraction by a skilled assistant throughout the procedure. Much of the dissection as well as removal of orbital contents can be expedited by effective retraction and countertraction.

42.10 What to Avoid

- Avoid violating the periorbita during dissection.
- Avoid causing fractures in the medial wall and the orbital floor.
- Avoid cutting into the supraorbital and infraorbital fissures while transecting the apical structures.

42.11 Complications/Bailout/Salvage

42.11.1 Hematoma

Poor hemostasis with hematoma formation beneath the skin graft can lead to graft failure or delayed healing. The hematoma should be evacuated, and areas of necrosis may need debridement. Small areas can be left to granulate, while larger areas may require secondary graft placement. Meshing the skin graft can avoid hematoma formation by allowing for spontaneous drainage. Steps to ensure good hemostasis should be taken as discussed earlier.

42.11.2 Postoperative Infection

With appropriate surgical technique and postoperative wound care, surgical site infection is rare. It is more common for crusting related to granulation tissue formation to be mistaken for an infection. If visibly purulent discharge is present, Gram stain and cultures are obtained to guide antibiotic therapy. Any necrotic tissue should be debrided and the socket treated with povidone-iodine solution wet-to-dry dressing with close monitoring. In cases of exenteration performed for invasive fungal infection, more extensive repeat surgical debridement may be warranted.

42.11.3 Cerebrospinal Fluid Leak

Inadvertent penetration of dura through the orbital roof, cribriform plate, or greater wing of the sphenoid can result in a CSF leak. While a rare complication, it can result in meningitis if untreated. Virtually all CSF leaks into open spaces (e.g., paranasal sinus and empty orbit) require treatment, compared to leaks into confined spaces (e.g., orbit filled with tissue). Small leaks may close spontaneously or with conservative treatments including bed rest, head elevation, and lumbar drainage. Larger leaks may require direct repair of the dura with use of a tissue adhesive or tissue grafts. Neurosurgery consultation may be required.

42.11.4 Sino-orbital Fistula

Fistulas to the adjacent sinuses may occur through bony defects in the orbital walls. The bony defects can be a result of bony erosion from the pathology being treated, or from aggressive dissection. If the fistula is small and asymptomatic, patients can be observed. If the fistula is large, patients may experience chronic discharge from the sinus mucus membrane and difficulty with phonation. Such cases require additional skin graft or vascularized flap for repair. It should be noted that postoperative orbital radiation increases the risk of fistula formation.

42.11.5 Paresthesias/Sensory Loss

Patients typically have permanent facial paresthesia due to disruption of sensory nerves and return of sensation cannot be predicted. The infraorbital nerve can be injured from dissection along the infraorbital canal or inferior orbital fissure. Disruption of the V1 branch of the trigeminal nerve results from severing of the supraorbital, supratrochlear, infratrochlear, and ethmoidal nerves. Disruption of the V2 branch of the trigeminal nerve occurs with severing of the zygomaticotemporal or zygomaticofacial branches. Patients should be adequately counseled preoperatively.

42.11.6 Recurrence

Tumor recurrence from incomplete surgical excision or from residual areas of microscopic disease can occur (▶ Fig. 42.4). Clean surgical margins can decrease this risk, but do not prevent the risk of metastasis or recurrence in the future. Continued surveillance is therefore required for all patients.

42.12 Postoperative Care

A pressure patch is placed at the end of exenteration and removed 5 to7 days later. Care should be taken not to dislodge the skin graft while removing the sponge packing from inside the socket. A wet-to-dry dressing with a 4×4 gauze soaked in a 50:50 mixture of 10% povidone-iodine solution and hydrogen peroxide is initiated twice a day to remove dried blood and keratin debris. The frequency of the dressing change is gradually decreased to daily, then every other day until approximately 2 to 3 months when the socket becomes completely epithelialized. If exenteration was performed for a malignancy, patients are often started on adjuvant radiation during this postoperative period, which can delay the wound healing process. A combination of dressing change, antibiotic ointment, and topical emollient can be used to treat the periorbital radiation dermatitis. Follow-up visits occur weekly for the first month, then monthly thereafter.

Once the socket has completely epithelialized, the patient can obtain a custom-fitted oculofacial prosthesis from an ocularist. An impression of the orbit is made with a plaster cast, followed by a clay mold that can be sculpted to mimic the contour and appearance of the other eye. Silicone prosthesis is then made using the mold and painted. The use of glasses with thicker frame may camouflage the silicone–skin interface and provide additional support. The prosthesis can be directly attached to the frame, or affixed to skin separately with an adhesive. Some patients prefer osseointegrated prostheses in which titanium posts are implanted into the orbital rim and magnetic attachments are used to hold the prosthesis in place with improved retention, comfort, and ease of placement (▶ Fig. 42.5).[15] All

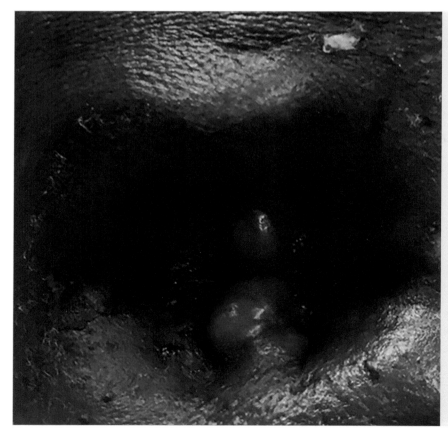

Fig. 42.4 Patient with a history of eyelid-sparing exenteration for invasive squamous cell carcinoma presenting with large nodular growths, concerning for recurrence.

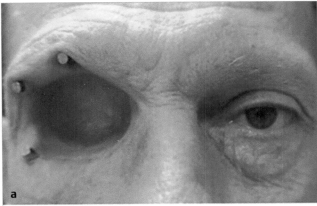

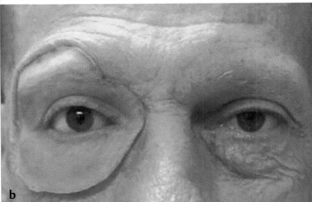

Fig. 42.5 **(a)** A well-healed right socket following total exenteration, placement of split-thickness skin graft, and osseointegrated titanium posts. **(b)** Magnetic oculofacial prosthesis with excellent cosmetic outcome.

types of prosthesis should be maintained and cleaned every 6 months to ensure excellent fit, comfort, and longevity.

References

[1] Bartley GB, Garrity JA, Waller RR, Henderson JW, Ilstrup DM. Orbital exenteration at the Mayo Clinic. 1967–1986. Ophthalmology. 1989; 96(4):468–473

[2] Shields JA, Shields CL, Demirci H, Honavar SG, Singh AD. Experience with eyelid-sparing orbital exenteration: the 2000 Tullos O. Coston Lecture. Ophthal Plast Reconstr Surg. 2001; 17(5):355–361

[3] Levin PS, Dutton JJ. A 20-year series of orbital exenteration. Am J Ophthalmol. 1991; 112(5):496–501

[4] Kiratli H, Koç İ. Orbital exenteration: institutional review of evolving trends in indications and rehabilitation techniques. Orbit. 2018; 37:179–186

[5] Nagendran ST, Lee NG, Fay A, Lefebvre DR, Sutula FC, Freitag SK. Orbital exenteration: the 10-year Massachusetts Eye and Ear Infirmary experience. Orbit. 2016; 35(4):199–206

[6] Ben Simon GJ, Schwarcz RM, Douglas R, Fiaschetti D, McCann JD, Goldberg RA. Orbital exenteration: one size does not fit all. Am J Ophthalmol. 2005; 139(1):11–17

[7] Tse D. Color Atlas of Oculoplastic Surgery. 2nd ed. Lippincott Williams & Wilkins; 2012

[8] Zhang Z, Ho S, Yin V, et al. Multicentred international review of orbital exenteration and reconstruction in oculoplastic and orbit practice. Br J Ophthalmol. 2018

[9] Elner VM, Demirci H, Nerad JA, Hassan AS. Periocular necrotizing fasciitis with visual loss pathogenesis and treatment. Ophthalmology. 2006; 113(12):2338–2345

[10] Rose GE, Wright JE. Exenteration for benign orbital disease. Br J Ophthalmol. 1994; 78(1):14–18

[11] Thach AB, Johnson AJ, Carroll RB, et al. Severe eye injuries in the war in Iraq, 2003–2005. Ophthalmology. 2008; 115(2):377–382

[12] Mauriello JA, Jr, Han KH, Wolfe R. Use of autogenous split-thickness dermal graft for reconstruction of the lining of the exenterated orbit. Am J Ophthalmol. 1985; 100(3):465–467

[13] Rafailov L, Turbin RE, Langer PD. Use of bilayer matrix wound dressing in the exenterated socket. Orbit. 2017; 36(6):397–400

[14] Ozgonul C, Diniz Grisolia AB, Demirci H. The use of Integra® dermal regeneration template for the orbital exenteration socket: a novel technique. Ophthal Plast Reconstr Surg. 2017

[15] Nerad JA, Carter KD, LaVelle WE, Fyler A, Brånemark PI. The osseointegration technique for the rehabilitation of the exenterated orbit. Arch Ophthalmol. 1991; 109(7):1032–1038

43 Dermis Fat Graft

Victoria Starks and Suzanne K. Freitag

Abstract

In the surgical management of the anophthalmic socket, dermis fat grafts serve an important function. The dual nature of this compound graft provides volume augmentation to the socket (fat) as well as a scaffold for conjunctiva to increase the surface area of the socket (dermis). Additionally, dermis fat grafts promote orbital growth when used in children. Complications include fat atrophy, ulceration, graft hirsutism, keratinization, and infection. The surgical technique is straightforward; however, there is a second surgical site at the donor site.

Keywords: dermis fat graft, orbital implant, anophthalmic socket, orbital volume augmentation

43.1 Goals

- To increase orbital soft-tissue volume as well as conjunctivalized surface area in the anophthalmic socket. If there is volume deficiency in the orbit with an orbital implant already present, the dermis fat graft may be placed on top of the implant. If an exposed or infected orbital implant is present, this implant is first removed, and the dermis fat graft is used to replace the lost volume from the implant.
- To optimize the fit and cosmesis of an ocular prosthesis.
- To promote orbital bone development in pediatric anophthalmic sockets, as the graft has the potential to expand paralleling the child's growth, unlike a static sized synthetic implant.[1,2,3,4]
- To reconstruct the anophthalmic socket in special circumstances: previous orbital implant exposure or infection, multiple prior surgeries, and in settings where the cost or access to alloplastic implants precludes their use.
- To augment eyelid or anterior orbit volume in cases of superior sulcus deformity or lower lid fat atrophy from a variety of atrophic or pathologic processes.

43.2 Advantages

Harvesting and transplanting a dermis fat graft is a fundamental oculoplastic surgery skill. There are numerous indications, which will be discussed in detail later. Dermis fat grafts may be used as a primary implant, to augment a preexisting implant, or as a secondary implant. One unique advantage of the dermis fat graft is augmentation of the "bulbar" surface area of the anophthalmic socket, necessary for the creation of adequate fornices. If there is inadequate conjunctiva and Tenon's capsule to create a watertight closure without tension over an orbital implant, the risk of implant exposure and infection is significant. Additionally, if closure is forced under tension, the conjunctiva will be recruited from the fornices, which as a result become too shallow to retain a prosthesis. In such instances, the surgeon can use a dermis fat graft to replace orbital volume with the dermis segment appropriately sized to fill the defect on the "bulbar" conjunctival surface.

Although dermis fat grafts in adults undergo predictable mild atrophy, in children there can be growth of the graft and occasional hypertrophy. This is a useful feature of the dermis fat graft because placing it in the anophthalmic socket of a child can stimulate growth of the bony orbit that would not occur with a static sized implant. This bony expansion may minimize disfiguring facial asymmetry.

Alloplastic orbital implants have been adopted by the majority of ophthalmic plastic surgeons for primary implants after enucleation or evisceration in the United States. However, in developing nations, there may be a lack of availability of such implants. Dermis fat grafts are a cost-effective means of reconstructing the anophthalmic socket and optimizing the patient's appearance. Dermis fat grafts add sufficient volume to the orbit and permit use of an ocular prosthesis despite the lack of alloplastic orbital implants.

43.3 Expectations

- Atrophy of roughly 15% of the graft volume, more in cases of poor recipient bed conditions including previous multiple surgeries or radiation therapy.[1,5,6,7,8,9,10,11,12]
- Epithelialization of the dermis in 8 to 10 weeks for primary grafts; 12 to 16 weeks for secondary grafts or traumatized sockets.[7]

43.4 Key Principles

The dermis fat graft is a composite graft that provides both dermis, a scaffold for surface epithelialization, and fat for volume augmentation. Free fat grafts in the orbit were largely abandoned due to significant and unpredictable atrophy. The inclusion of dermis allows for better vascularization and survival of the graft than seen in free fat grafts. Graft vascularization is key to preventing atrophy. To promote vascularization, one must avoid excessive handling of the graft, cautery to the recipient bed, and optimize systemic patient factors.

43.5 Indications

- Secondary implant after implant exposure, extrusion, or infection.
- Secondary implant to augment orbital volume on top of a preexisting implant.
- Primary orbital implant in pediatric anophthalmic patients.
- Primary implant in traumatized sockets that are unlikely to retain an alloplastic implant due to insufficient conjunctiva for closure.
- Primary orbital implant if alloplastic implants are not available.
- Volume augmentation for superior sulcus deformity or other volume deficiencies.

43.6 Contraindications

- Patient unwilling or unable to undergo orbital surgery with a second surgical site (donor site).
- Active orbital infection.
- Previous radiation to the socket is a relative contraindication.

43.7 Preoperative Preparation

To set expectations, the patient and surgeon agree on the donor site prior to surgery. The most common sites include the anterior aspect of the flank, the buttock, or the abdomen. There are various considerations with each donor site. When harvesting from the flank or the abdomen, the intraoperative positioning is simple because both the donor site and the orbit can be accessed in the supine position. However, the healed incision will result in a scar that may be visible in a bathing suit. It should be noted to avoid the right flank in patients who still have their appendix, as postdermis fat excision scarring could complicate appendectomy surgery. The flank incision should be thoughtfully placed to avoid the waistband of clothing. Harvesting from the buttock allows better cosmetic concealment of the scar; however, the incision may cause discomfort when sitting. The superolateral quadrant of the buttock is the ideal site of harvest to minimize the risk of injury to the sciatic nerve. For young children, the donor site is also placed superiorly on the buttock to avoid contamination in the diaper.

A dermis fat graft is frequently used to replace an infected orbital implant. In such cases, prior to surgery, the surgeon must ensure treatment and resolution of any orbital infection which would compromise the survival of the graft.

43.8 Operative Technique

General anesthesia is preferred. Generally, a supine position allows the donor and recipient sites to be accessed simultaneously. If the flank is the intended site of graft harvesting, the supine position is adequate. If the buttock is the intended site of graft harvesting, one leg is crossed over the midline and secured (▶ Fig. 43.1). Local anesthetic with a mixture of bupivacaine and lidocaine with 1:100,000 epinephrine is injected below the conjunctiva along the previous midline horizontal incision of the anophthalmic socket as well as at the donor site.

Additionally, local anesthetic can be used to hydrodissect the epidermis from the dermis at the donor site. The patient is prepped and draped at both sites.

The orbit is prepared first. After placement of an eyelid speculum, the conjunctiva is incised along the horizontal meridian, typically through the line of previous closure. Preexisting implants are explanted, if planned. If an epithelialized capsule remains after implant removal, it should be either excised to allow expansion and vascularization of the dermis fat graft or incised to deepen the recipient site. The defect in the conjunctiva is measured as a guide for sizing the donor dermis. Minimal cautery should be used in the recipient bed to optimize vascularization of the graft.

Attention is then turned to harvest the dermis fat graft. The skin is marked in an ellipse, which is oversized by 20% compared to the conjunctival defect. The epidermis must then be completely removed. This can be performed with a blade or preferably with a dermabrader. If excising the epidermis with a blade, the skin markings should be first incised to the level of the dermis, and then the epidermis removed by placing the blade parallel to the body surface and shaving the epidermis in one continuous plane. When using a dermabrader, the skin must be held taut. Greater stability can be achieved if the skin markings are not incised prior to this step. Dermabrasion is performed by continuously moving the rotating burr (4 mm diamond bur) over the epidermal surface until there is diffuse punctate hemorrhage indicating the dermis has been reached. Meticulous removal of all epidermal elements is essential to prevent keratinization (▶ Fig. 43.2).

A 15 blade is then used to extend the incision through dermis into the fat. Using scissors, such as a curved Stevens, an appropriate-sized graft of the fat underlying the dermis is then excised. The scissors should first be pointed outward from the edges of the dermis, as the fat component should be much wider than the dermis (▶ Fig. 43.3). The surgeon should carefully inspect while dissecting to avoid damage to nerves or vessels. If the graft is to be the sole anophthalmic socket implant, a sphere of fat with a diameter of approximately 25 mm is desirable. If the implant is to fit over a preexisting implant, then the volume and shape of the fat graft can be adjusted for the individual patient.

Once an adequately sized graft is obtained, it is placed into the recipient bed. The harvested fat should be oversized compared to the volume deficit. An adequate graft should be

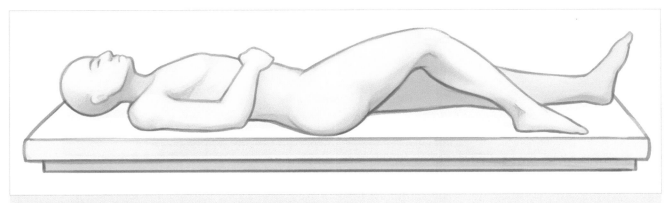

Fig. 43.1 Patient positioning to access the orbit and buttock simultaneously.

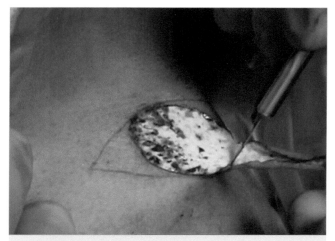

Fig. 43.2 The epidermis is excised from the face of the dermis fat graft with a blade. A dermabrader may also be used.

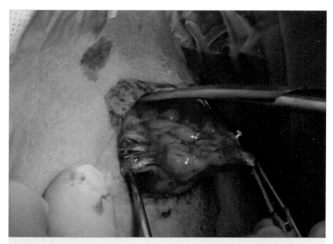

Fig. 43.3 Technique of harvesting the dermis fat graft such that the diameter of the fat exceeds the diameter of the dermis.

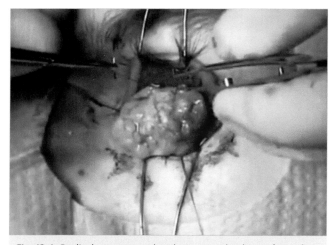

Fig. 43.4 Cardinal sutures are placed to secure the dermis fat graft to the conjunctiva while the fat is gently coaxed into the orbit.

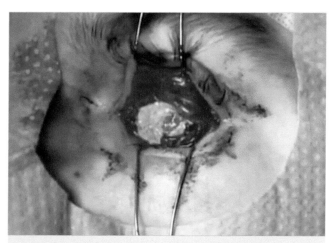

Fig. 43.5 The dermis fat graft secured within the orbit.

challenging to completely fit in the orbit. If the amount of fat implanted is too small, with the expected 15% fat graft atrophy, the final volume will be inadequate. The dermis is secured to conjunctiva with cardinal sutures at the four poles of the dermis with interrupted 5–0 polyglactin sutures (▶ Fig. 43.4). 5–0 polyglactin suture is then placed between the cardinal points and the surgeon continually gently reposits the fat into the recipient bed between each suture (▶ Fig. 43.5). Antibiotic ointment and a rigid conformer are placed in the socket. The conformer should maintain the fornices without placing excessive pressure on the graft. A temporary tarsorrhaphy with 4–0 silk suture is placed followed by a pressure patch.

The donor site is closed with interrupted buried 4–0 polyglactin sutures. A similar size suture is placed in a continuous running fashion to close the skin. The donor site is dressed with antibiotic ointment, and a nonadherent dressing covered with a moisture-resistant adhesive dressing.

In patients who are not anophthalmic, a dermis fat graft can be used to augment volume in a deep superior sulcus or hollow lower eyelid. The composite graft can be placed on the periosteum such that the fat component faces anteriorly or below skin and orbicularis muscle with the dermis directed anteriorly. The dermis may be anchored with 6–0 polyglactin suture to the periosteum or the capsule of the preaponeurotic fat.

43.9 Tips and Pearls

- Sizing the graft: Some atrophy (about 15%) of the volume of the graft fat is expected; thus, the graft is oversized. It would be difficult to fit the graft into the orbit. A graft diameter of approximately 25 mm is an approximate goal.
- A dermis fat graft can be placed over an existing implant to add more volume. The graft can be positioned to address the areas of volume deficit, e.g., superiorly in the orbit for a superior sulcus deformity.
- An inhospitable socket, such as in a patient who has undergone multiple surgeries or radiation therapy, will cause the graft to incorporate slowly, atrophy significantly, and in

rare cases necrose. However, these contracted sockets with limited surface area often cannot retain an alloplastic implant and a dermis fat graft may be the only option.

43.10 What to Avoid

It is important to avoid incomplete epidermis removal on the dermal surface of the graft. Retained epidermis can form cysts below the conjunctiva once the graft is conjunctivalized. While such cysts can usually be excised in the office, in some cases large cysts may require a return to the operating room. Incomplete removal of epidermis can also lead to keratinization or cilia formation of the graft. Keratin forms white plaques on the conjunctival surface causing irritation and discharge which may limit wearing a prosthesis. Graft ciliary growth may also lead to irritation and may be disturbing to the patient.

Good surgical technique is essential to reduce graft atrophy. Excessively large grafts, overhandling of the graft, or excessive cautery in the orbit may increase atrophy of graft fat.

43.11 Complications/Bailout/Salvage

- Graft atrophy: best avoided by the methods described earlier.
- Graft hypertrophy: more commonly observed in children younger than 4 years, also observed in adults who sustain significant weight gain. Debulking can be performed by opening the incision at the perimeter of the dermis and carefully debulking fat.
- Conjunctival cysts or granulomas: best avoided by careful epidermis removal at the time of graft harvest. Most can be excised under local anesthesia in the office.
- Delayed epithelialization or ulceration of the dermis: a dermal ulcer may be removed by excising and closing the adjacent dermis.
- Postoperative infection: intraoperative antibiotics and systemic antibiotics for 1 to 2 weeks postoperatively are used to prevent this complication. Preoperative treatment of preexisting orbital infection is required.
- Graft hirsutism: may be treated with epilation if detected prior to epithelialization of the dermis. Cilia below the conjunctiva often do not need to be addressed as the follicle usually degrades.
- Keratinization of the socket: large areas of keratin may be excised down to dermis and left to reepithelialize.

- Donor site dehiscence: strict activity limitations are stressed for the early postoperative period to prevent dehiscence. Significant dehiscence must be repaired.

43.12 Postoperative Care

Proper hygiene of the donor site is essential, especially in patients wearing diapers. In children, a watertight occlusive dressing (e.g., Tegaderm) is placed over the donor site, and the dressing is replaced after each soiled diaper change. A course of oral antibiotics is recommended in all patients to prevent infection.

At the recipient site, a pressure patch and temporary tarsorrhaphy are removed after 5 to 7 days. The conformer should be maintained at all times to protect the fornices from contraction until a custom ocular prosthesis is made. If the conformer falls out, patients are advised to replace the conformer after rinsing it with tap water within 24 hours. The graft must be completely conjunctivalized before an ocular prosthesis can be worn.

References

[1] Guberina C, Hornblass A, Meltzer MA, Soarez V, Smith B. Autogenous dermis-fat orbital implantation. Arch Ophthalmol. 1983; 101(10):1586–1590

[2] Heher KL, Katowitz JA, Low JE. Unilateral dermis-fat graft implantation in the pediatric orbit. Ophthal Plast Reconstr Surg. 1998; 14(2):81–88

[3] Tarantini A, Hintschich C. Primary dermis-fat grafting in children. Orbit. 2008; 27(5):363–369

[4] Hauck MJ, Steele EA. Dermis fat graft implantation after unilateral enucleation for retinoblastoma in pediatric patients. Ophthal Plast Reconstr Surg. 2015; 31(2):136–138

[5] Smith B, Bosniak S, Nesi F, Lisman R. Dermis-fat orbital implantation: 118 cases. Ophthalmic Surg. 1983; 14(11):941–943

[6] Aguilar GL, Shannon GM, Flanagan JC. Experience with dermis-fat grafting: an analysis of early postoperative complications and methods of prevention. Ophthalmic Surg. 1982; 13(3):204–209

[7] Bosniak SL. Avoiding complications following primary dermis-fat orbital implantation. Ophthal Plast Reconstr Surg. 1985; 1(4):237–241

[8] Lee MJ, Khwarg SI, Choung HK, Kim NJ, Yu YS. Dermis-fat graft for treatment of exposed porous polyethylene implants in pediatric postenucleation retinoblastoma patients. Am J Ophthalmol. 2011; 152(2):244–250.e2

[9] Shore JW, McCord CD, Jr, Bergin DJ, Dittmar SJ, Maiorca JP, Burks WR. Management of complications following dermis-fat grafting for anophthalmic socket reconstruction. Ophthalmology. 1985; 92(10):1342–1350

[10] Martin PA, Rogers PA, Billson F. Dermis-fat graft: evolution of a living prosthesis. Aust N Z J Ophthalmol. 1986; 14(2):161–165

[11] Bosniak SL. Complications of dermis-fat orbital implantation. Adv Ophthalmic Plast Reconstr Surg. 1990; 8:170–181

[12] Guberina C, Hornblass A, Smith B. Pitfalls of autogenous lipodermal implantation to the orbit. Ophthal Plast Reconstr Surg. 1987; 3(2):65–70

Part X

Miscellaneous

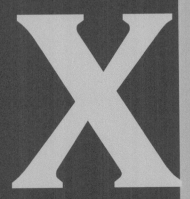

44 Temporal Artery Biopsy

Juan C. Jiménez-Pérez

Summary

Temporal artery biopsy is a simple office procedure that can allow the physician to diagnose a life-threatening condition. Giant cell arteritis treatment should never be postponed waiting for the biopsy or its result. If the condition is suspected, oral steroid treatment should be initiated immediately. Biopsy can be safely done as long as anatomy is known and certain landmarks are avoided. This chapter reviews the knowledge needed to perform the procedure safely and with confidence.

Keywords: temporal artery biopsy, giant cell arteritis, oral steroid

44.1 Description

Temporal artery biopsy (TAB) is a simple procedure to obtain an artery specimen to diagnose giant cell arteritis (GCA). This systemic disease is an inflammatory vasculopathy causing segmental necrotizing reaction in the vessel wall of medium-to-large size arteries characterized by a predominance of mononuclear cell infiltrate or a granulomatous process with multinucleated giant cells.[1] GCA is known to have skip lesions, areas that are uninflamed between other areas of inflammation. Therefore, a negative TAB result cannot be used to rule out GCA. While there are criteria for clinical diagnosis of GCA, the definitive diagnosis is based on a positive histopathologic specimen.

44.2 Key Principles

- Intimate knowledge of the temple anatomy is crucial for successful surgery without complication. In most cases, the parietal branch can be biopsied safely. Although its presence within the hairline may interfere with visualization of the surgical site, it generally heals well with low risk of alopecia, creating a favorable invisible biopsy site.
- Meticulous preoperative mapping of the course of the artery is critical.
- A sufficient length of artery should be biopsied for the highest likelihood of a representative sample. In general, a 3-cm length is sufficient.
- Due to the presence of skip lesions, the artery to be biopsied should be made based on symptoms (indicating laterality) and clinical findings (painful, enlarged, tender, pulseless arteries). If clinical suspicion for GCA is high, a negative biopsy should be followed by an additional biopsy.

44.3 Anatomy

The superficial temporal artery is one of the terminal branches of the external carotid artery and supplies the face and scalp. It begins at the level of the parotid gland and passes over the zygomatic arch. About 3 to 5 cm above this bone, it divides into the frontal and parietal branches. It runs posterior to the superficial temporal vein and anterior to the auriculotemporal nerve.

Importantly, it lies within the superficial temporal fascia along with the temporal branch of the facial nerve; so, care should be taken not to injure these structures.

44.4 Expectations

This procedure can be performed in the office setting in less than 30 minutes. Local anesthesia alone is generally sufficient for patient comfort. Although the risk of postoperative hemorrhage and facial nerve damage exists, it can be minimized by proper site selection (avoiding the "danger zone"), blunt dissection in the area of the facial nerve, and clear exposure of the surgical site.

44.5 Indications

Biopsy is warranted based on clinical suspicion. GCA can cause a myriad of ophthalmic findings including arteritic ischemic optic neuropathy, retinal artery occlusion, choroidal ischemia, cotton-wool spots, and cranial nerve palsies. The American College of Rheumatology established diagnostic criteria for GCA.[1]

1. Age ≥ 50 years at disease onset.
2. New onset of localized headache.
3. Temporal artery tenderness or decreased temporal artery pulse.
4. Elevated erythrocyte sedimentation rate ≥ 50 mm/hour by Westergren method.
5. Positive TAB.

The presence of three or more of these criterias has been reported to have a sensitivity of 93.5% and specificity of 91.2%. The presence of jaw claudication has the highest predictive value for a positive TAB.[2]

44.6 Contraindications

There are no absolute contraindications to biopsy. Some authors recommend caution in patients using steroids for greater than 2 weeks, as the interpretation of the histopathologic result may be confounded. Positive results still can be found even after 6 weeks of using steroids, but the percentage of these results decreases.[3] Current use of blood thinners can increase the risk of perioperative bleeding,[4] although a delay in biopsy is not recommended due to the devastating consequences of a missed or delayed diagnosis. Bleeding can be stopped by ligating bleeding vessels or applying pressure to the area.

44.7 Preoperative Preparation

- Risk, benefits, and alternative are explained to the patient, and informed consent is obtained.
- Start by palpating both superficial temporal arteries looking for area of tenderness and nodularity; the side that has ocular manifestations or symptoms is recommended for biopsy.

- Place the patient in supine position with the head looking away from the affected side.
- Then, using a marking pen, trace the artery and confirm the course and area with the Doppler ultrasound. Biopsy of the parietal branch is recommended. Length should be 3 cm or more (▶ Fig. 44.1).
- Inject local anesthesia (1:1 of 2% lidocaine with 1:100,000 epinephrine mixed with 0.5% bupivacaine) adjacent to the marking to avoid intra-arterial infiltration.
- Although always not needed, consider trimming overlying hair with scissors to improve visualization. Shaving the area is generally not needed. Application of ointment or gel lubricant (as used for the Doppler ultrasound) is needed to retain hair away from the surgical field.

- Sterile preparation of the surgical field using Betadine 10% solution. Drape the area with sterile towels leaving the face exposed to allow patient to breathe without any problem.

44.8 Operative Technique

- Using a Bard Parker 15 blade, incise the premarked area of skin all the way down to the subcutaneous fat. Avoid deeper incision due to risk of lacerating the artery. Place blade beveled in the plane of the hair shafts to avoid transecting the bulb and causing alopecia.
- Then, bluntly dissect the fat plane perpendicular to the incision to spread wound open using a curved Steven tenotomy scissors or a curved hemostat (▶ Fig. 44.2).

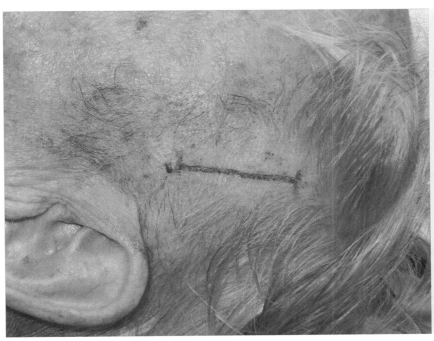

Fig. 44.1 After confirming the course of the superficial temporal artery with a Doppler ultrasound, a "best fit line" is drawn as a straight line within the hair-bearing scalp. *Note*: it is superior to the pinna. If hair is in the way, it can be shaved, cut short with scissors, or matted away from the incision using ointment. (Photo courtesy of Michael K. Yoon, MD.)

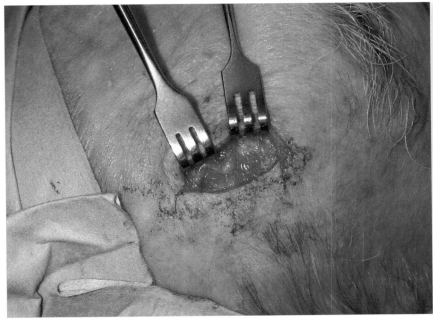

Fig. 44.2 After incision through the skin, the subcutaneous fat should be bluntly dissected by spreading. This will then reveal the underlying superficial temporal artery. Note its tortuous course, although this can be variable. (Photo courtesy of Michael K. Yoon, MD.)

- Continue until the superficial temporal fascia is visualized. The superficial temporal artery will be located within the fascia. Continue blunt dissection, this time parallel to each side of the vessel along the entire incision.
- The proximal aspect of the artery is suture ligated using a 4–0 silk suture leaving the ends of the suture long. Then, pull the long ends of the tied suture toward the distal end allowing further exposure of the proximal end of the artery. Tie a second 4–0 silk suture about 3 to 4 mm apart. The same double suture ligation is done at the distal end. Make sure no collaterals are present, if present also ligate with 4–0 silk suture (▶ Fig. 44.3).
- At this point, using a Westcott scissor cut the artery between the tied suture at the proximal and distal end. Carefully retract the artery from either side, bluntly dissecting away any adventitial tissue. Place the specimen in formalin. Adequate hemostasis should be achieved with additional bipolar cauterization if needed.
- Place a single interrupted 5–0 plain gut suture centrally to align the incision. Then, close the remaining incision with 5–0 plain gut suture in a running fashion. Remove the drapes and clean the area. Place antibiotic ointment over the incision (▶ Fig. 44.4).

44.9 Tips and Pearls

- Know the anatomy (specifically temporal region layers) and the course of the facial nerve.
- If possible, biopsy the parietal branch of the superficial temporal artery to avoid the facial nerve.[5]

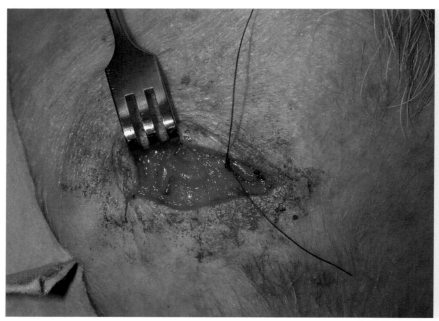

Fig. 44.3 After isolating the artery, 4–0 silk sutures are placed around the artery to ligate it. (Photo courtesy of Michael K. Yoon, MD.)

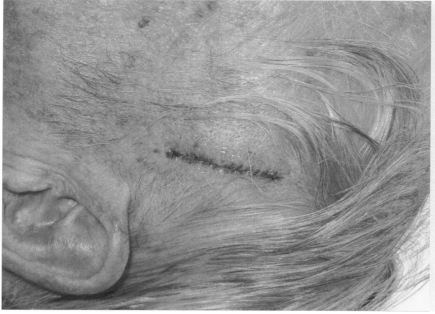

Fig. 44.4 The incision can be closed with a running 5–0 plain gut suture. (Photo courtesy of Michael K. Yoon, MD.)

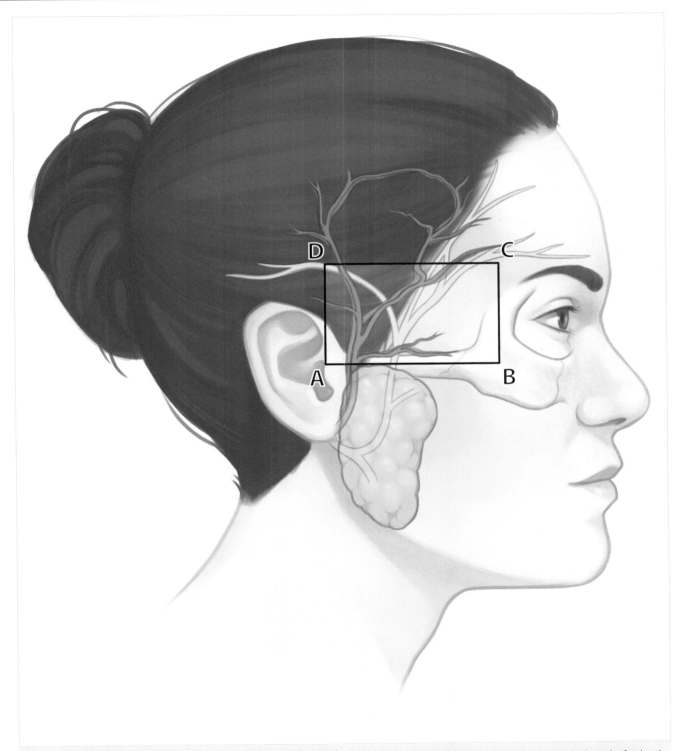

Fig. 44.5 Temporal danger zone. In yellow we appreciate the facial nerve as it emerges from the parotid gland and travels superiorly to the forehead. In red we see the superficial temporal artery as it divides in the frontal branch anteriorly and parietal branch posteriorly. (**A**) the tragus of the ear, (**B**) the junction of the zygomatic arch and lateral orbital rim, (**C**) the area 2 cm superior to the superior orbital rim, and (**D**) the point superior to the tragus and in horizontal alignment with (**C**).

- There is no indication to perform bilateral simultaneous TAB.[6] Contralateral biopsy is recommended in cases where initial biopsy was negative, but clinical suspicion remains high.
- Confirm location using Doppler ultrasound.
- Aim to obtain at least 2 cm artery specimen.[7]
- GCA is a sight-threatening medical emergency that requires prompt recognition and treatment.[8] Do not delay initiation of steroid treatment of suspected patients while awaiting biopsy.
- A positive histopathologic result can be suspected when a thick, nodular, tortous, pale artery with little bleeding is encountered intraoperatively and an apparently occluded lumen is encountered.[9]
- Maintain meticulous technique as deviations from principled surgery increase the risk of complication.

44.10 What to Avoid

Sharp dissection should be avoided to decrease chance of lacerating the artery or the facial nerve. As previously mentioned, avoid biopsy of the frontal branch of the superficial temporal artery as the branch of the facial nerve may mirror its course. Specifically avoid the "danger zone" which is an area bounded by (A) the tragus of the ear, (B) the junction of the zygomatic arch and lateral orbital rim, (C) the area 2 cm superior to the superior orbital rim, and (D) the point superior to the tragus and in horizontal alignment with (C) (▶ Fig. 44.5).[10]

44.11 Complications, Bailout, and Salvage

In the hands of a trained experience surgeon, biopsy is safe. The most common complication that can happen during the biopsy is bleeding. Minor bleeding is controlled with application of pressure. Some cases may require bipolar cautery. Rarely, a slipped ligature or unrecognized large arterial branch may require placement of another ligature. An uncommon complication is a hematoma. If minor, it can be managed with a pressure dressing around the head to avoid progression. But if it enlarges rapidly, it should be evacuated immediately and the source of bleeding must be identified and ligated. Consider oral antibiotics in the presence of a hematoma, as the risk of infection within this unperfused mass is increased.

Other uncommon complications are wound dehiscence and infection. These are more likely to occur in cases of poor compliance of patient with postoperative instructions.

Lastly, but not least, facial nerve palsy causes permanent disability from incision in the known course of the frontal branch of the facial nerve.[5,11] These pareses often do not recover substantially.[5]

44.12 Postoperative Care

Patient should keep area clean and avoid getting any direct water to the area for the first 48 hours. Patient should avoid rubbing the stitches due to risk of wound dehiscence. Also, should avoid heavy lifting or strenuous exercise for 2 weeks after the procedure. Use antibiotic ointment three times a day over the incision for a week to decrease the risk of infection.

References

[1] Hunder GG, Bloch DA, Michel BA, et al. The American College of Rheumatology 1990 criteria for the classification of giant cell arteritis. Arthritis Rheum. 1990; 33(8):1122–1128

[2] Hayreh SS, Podhajsky PA, Raman R, Zimmerman B. Giant cell arteritis: validity and reliability of various diagnostic criteria. Am J Ophthalmol. 1997; 123(3): 285–296

[3] Ray-Chaudhuri N, Kiné DA, Tijani SO, et al. Effect of prior steroid treatment on temporal artery biopsy findings in giant cell arteritis. Br J Ophthalmol. 2002; 86(5):530–532

[4] Achkar AA, Lie JT, Hunder GG, O'Fallon WM, Gabriel SE. How does previous corticosteroid treatment affect the biopsy findings in giant cell (temporal) arteritis? Ann Intern Med. 1994; 120(12):987–992

[5] Yoon MK, Horton JC, McCulley TJ. Facial nerve injury: a complication of superficial temporal artery biopsy. Am J Ophthalmol. 2011; 152(2):251–255.e1

[6] Boyev LR, Miller NR, Green WR. Efficacy of unilateral versus bilateral temporal artery biopsies for the diagnosis of giant cell arteritis. Am J Ophthalmol. 1999; 128(2):211–215

[7] Breuer GS, Nesher R, Nesher G. Effect of biopsy length on the rate of positive temporal artery biopsies. Clin Exp Rheumatol. 2009; 27(1) Suppl 52:S10–S13

[8] Rahman W, Rahman FZ. Giant cell (temporal) arteritis: an overview and update. Surv Ophthalmol. 2005; 50(5):415–428

[9] Cetinkaya A, Kersten RC, Brannan PA, Thiagarajah C, Kulwin DR. Intraoperative predictability of temporal artery biopsy results. Ophthal Plast Reconstr Surg. 2008; 24(5):372–376, discussion 377

[10] Scott KR, Tse DT, Kronish JW. Temporal artery biopsy technique: a clinico-anatomical approach. Ophthalmic Surg. 1991; 22(9):519–525

[11] Bhatti MT, Goldstein MH. Facial nerve injury following superficial temporal artery biopsy. Dermatol Surg. 2001; 27(1):15–17

45 Aberrant Eyelash Management

Ashley A. Campbell and Roxana Fu

Summary

Aberrant eyelash management is indicated when significant ocular surface discomfort and/or evidence of corneal damage is present. Prior to choosing a management option, the underlying etiology for aberrant eyelashes should be evaluated and addressed. Existing infections or inflammations should be treated prior to surgical intervention, if possible, as surgery may exacerbate the eyelash problem. There are many different techniques that can be considered in the management of aberrant eyelashes. The choice of technique often depends on the etiology, the extent of the aberrant lashes on the eyelid, the location of the misdirected lashes, and the patient's preference.

Keywords: trichiasis, distichiasis, epilation, hyfrecation, cryotherapy, trephination, entropion

45.1 Goals

The goal of managing aberrant lashes, or trichiasis, is to prevent lashes from touching the cornea which can lead to corneal irritation and/or damage. Trichiasis is defined as lashes that are in the normal position, yet are pointing in an abnormal direction (▶ Fig. 45.1). This is distinct from distichiasis, which refers to lashes growing in an abnormal position, usually posterior to the normal lash line in the area of the Meibomian gland orifices.

45.2 Advantages

Aberrant lashes can be extremely uncomfortable for patients as well as potentially harmful to the ocular surface. Any technique to manage aberrant eyelashes has the advantage of removing lashes that touch the ocular surface.

45.3 Expectations

Management of aberrant lashes is fraught with difficulty. It is important to tell patients that it will likely take more than one procedure to eradicate the lashes, and even any intervention may not be completely successful.

45.4 Key Principles

One of the most important things to consider when managing aberrant lashes is to establish what is causing the lashes to turn inward. The most common causes for aberrant lashes are cicatricial processes from acute inflammation (viral, chemical burns, trauma, radiation, surgery, or cryotherapy) and chronic inflammation (blepharitis, trachoma, ocular cicatricial pemphigoid [OCP], Stevens-Johnson syndrome [SJS], topical medications, and tumor). Entropion can also lead to aberrant lashes; yet, this is often simply addressed by fixing the malposition of the eyelid. Failure to establish the etiology of aberrant lashes can undermine any intervention. For example, undiagnosed

OCP can lead to blindness if the patient is not initiated on immunosuppressants as well as worsen the surgical result.

45.5 Indications

Significant ocular surface discomfort and/or evidence of corneal damage from aberrant lashes are indications for intervention.

45.6 Contraindications

Management for aberrant lashes should not be undertaken until the etiology has been determined. Ocular lubrication and bandage contact lenses can be used in the interim to prevent corneal damage and help ease discomfort. Current infections or inflammations should be treated prior to surgical intervention, if possible, as surgery may exacerbate the eyelash problem.

45.7 Preoperative Preparation

Preoperative preparation includes a careful history to elicit previous eyelid trauma, surgery, foreign travel, history of oral or skin lesions suggestive of herpetic infection, history of prior radiation in the periocular area, use of glaucoma medication, or the use of any cosmetic eyelash preparations. A complete ophthalmic examination should also be performed focusing on the location and type of abnormal eyelash growth. Attention should be paid to the inferior fornix for evidence of active conjunctival inflammation, cicatrized conjunctiva, or tarsal fibrosis. It should be noted whether there are any eyelid lesions causing lash distortion which could suggest a cutaneous neoplasm. The cornea should be evaluated for any superficial punctate keratopathy, thinning, cellular infiltrates, or scarring. If an infectious process is suspected, appropriate culture should be performed. Suspicious eyelid lesions should be biopsied. A conjunctival biopsy should be performed if OCP is suspected. If a patient has a diagnosis of OCP or other severe ocular surface inflammation, perioperative immunosuppression (e.g., oral steroids) should be considered after consultation with the treating subspecialist (cornea or uveitis).[1]

45.8 Operative Technique

- There are many different techniques that can be considered in the management of aberrant eyelashes. The choice of technique often depends on the etiology, the extent of the aberrant lashes on the eyelid, the location of the misdirected lashes, and the patient's preference. No technique is 100% effective.
- Manual epilation: This can be performed at the slit lamp with just topical anesthesia. This is minimally invasive, but does necessitate frequent office visits as it only takes 1 to 2 months for the lashes to grow back. Some also feel that this can accelerate lash growth.
- Radiofrequency or electrolysis: Radiofrequency or electrolysis is useful when there are few aberrant lashes on a single lid or

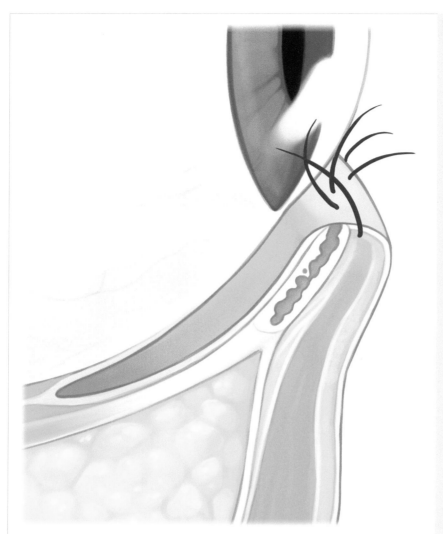

Fig. 45.1 Schematic drawing of aberrant lashes touching the ocular surface.

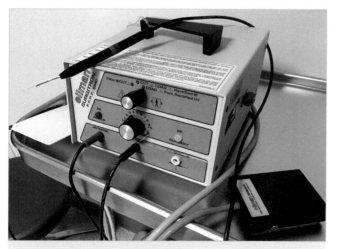

Fig. 45.2 Ellman Surgitron unit with super fine tip needle attached to probe.

multiple lids. In both instances, energy is delivered to the hair follicle on a fine-tip probe. Electrolysis delivers electrical energy to an individual hair follicle. A radiofrequency device, such as the Ellman Surgitron (Ellman International Manufacturing, Hewlett, NY; ▶ Fig. 45.2), can be used to selectively deliver energy at 3.8 MHz (radio wave) to the hair follicle. Radiofrequency devices deliver more focused energy with less collateral tissue damage than electrolysis units (such as a Bovie electrosurgical unit). After local anesthesia is infiltrated into the eyelid, a fine wire-tip electrode is inserted into the hair shaft parallel to the direction of the abnormal eye lash, approximately 2 to 3 mm in depth. The Ellman is set on "cut" or "coag" (i.e., coagulation) starting at level 4 and can be adjusted upward to a maximum of 8. The electrical current is applied until bubbles are noted at the hair follicle opening. At that point, the aberrant lash should either come out on its own (i.e., with withdrawal of the probe) or be easily removed with forceps. Each lash must be treated separately. It is often useful to use a slit lamp or an operating microscope to adequately visualize the lashes. If necessary, treatment can be repeated after several weeks. Recurrences are common, and often a few retreatments are needed.[2]

- Argon laser ablation: Argon laser is used to apply focal tissue coagulation within the follicle with minimal surrounding tissue damage. After local anesthetic is injected, the patient is positioned in an argon laser headrest. A laser-safe corneal protective shield is placed over the eye. The eyelid is everted and the argon laser beam is directed parallel to the direction of the aberrant eyelash. The spot size is set to 100 to 200 μm with a pulse duration of 0.5 seconds with a low power setting of 1 watt. Repeated pulses are applied to a depth of 2 to 3 mm. As with hyfrecation, recurrences are common and often at least three treatments are required. Hypopigmentation and dimpling of the lid margin can occur.[3]

- Cryoepilation: Cryosurgery has the ability to treat multiple eyelash follicles at once. The eyelid can be manually distracted from the globe or a corneal protector can be placed. After injection of local anesthesia, the cryotherapy probe is applied at the base of the affected eyelashes, either on the eyelid skin or the palpebral conjunctiva. Various cryotherapy devices have been described, with application times ranging from 20 to 25 seconds to 30 to 45 seconds, allowing the tissue to reach −20 °C. A microthermocouple needle probe can be used to monitor the tissue temperature. It is placed within the orbicularis oculi muscle 3 mm away from the cilia base. During application, ice crystals allow the probe to adhere to the tissue surface and will disengage as the probe temperature rises. A second application is then completed. Hypopigmentation, eyelid notching, and prolonged pain and edema may occur. Eyelid necrosis is associated with treatment below −30 °C.

- Trephination: The eyelash follicle can be removed in its entirety with a microtrephine. Various microtrephines have been described, including a diameter as small as 0.81 mm. The eyelid is injected with local anesthesia and is manually stabilized with forceps. The affected eyelash is introduced into the lumen of the microtrephine, and the instrument is then used to core out the base of the eyelash, including its follicle and a minimal cuff of surrounding tissue, to a depth about 2 mm. Success rates have been described similar to electrolysis. As with electrolysis, a slit lamp or operating microscope is recommended for improved visualization. Eyelid scarring is a potential complication.[4]

- Full-thickness wedge resection: For focal areas of trichiasis or distichiasis, a full-thickness wedge resection can be considered. After local anesthetic is infiltrated, the area can be incised in a pentagonal fashion. Partial-thickness tarsal sutures are placed with 6–0 polyglactin or silk suture. The tarsus at the margin is closed in a similar manner or with vertical mattress suture placement to more effectively evert the edges (▶ Fig. 45.3). The eyelash line and skin are closed with the surgeon's choice of external suture. Eyelid scarring or notching are potential complications, although rare.

- Lid splitting with anterior lamella recession: When the entire horizontal extent of the eyelid is affected, recession of the lash line with lid splitting is considered. After injection of local anesthesia, the gray line of the eyelid margin is incised along the horizontal extent of the affected eyelid. Sharp-tip Westcott scissors are used to dissect off the anterior lamella,

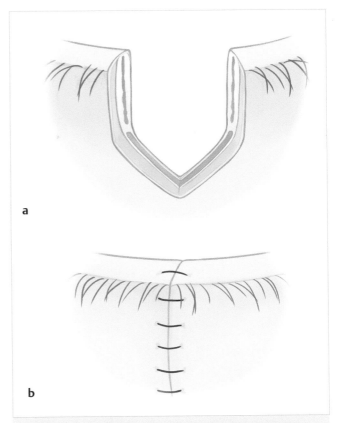

a

b

Fig. 45.3 (a) Pentagonal wedge resection for localized trichiasis. (b) Repair with a partial thickness suture placed through the tarsus followed by interrupted sutures at the margin, lash line, and skin.

exposing the anterior tarsus. Recession of the anterior lamella is facilitated by full-thickness incisions of the anterior lamella at the medial and lateral aspects of the dissection. The eyelash line can be treated with destructive procedures as previously described, or removed entirely. The anterior lamella is sutured in place, 2 mm from the posterior margin, with multiple horizontal mattress sutures that are placed in a partial-thickness fashion through the tarsus and full-thickness through the anterior lamella (▶ Fig. 45.4). The patient should be informed of the permanent change in appearance of the eyelid margin, so this procedure should therefore be reserved for refractory cases.

- Tarsal fracture (Weis procedure): Another consideration for trichiasis affecting the entire eyelid is a horizontal blepharotomy with rotation of the eyelid margin. The eyelid is anesthetized and an eyelid plate is placed behind the eyelid. A full-thickness incision is made 3 to 4 mm from the eyelid margin, along the full horizontal width of the tarsus. Double-armed absorbable 5–0 suture is used to rotate the margin outward by approximating the proximal marginal skin edge, to the distal posterior tarsal edge. This is repeated across the horizontal extent of the incision, and the skin is closed with the surgeon's choice of external suture (▶ Fig. 45.5). A permanent change in eyelid appearance is possible. Overcorrection can occur and be treated with massage or cautery to the palpebral conjunctiva.

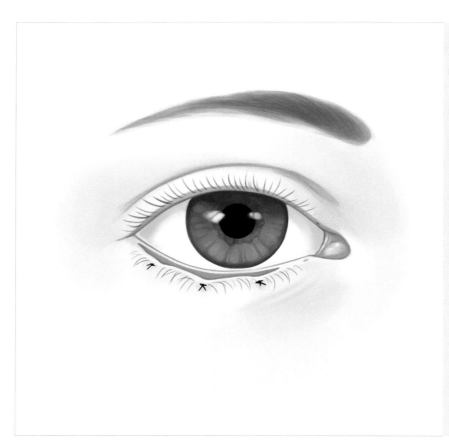

Fig. 45.4 Anterior lamella recession with multiple horizontal mattress sutures in place.

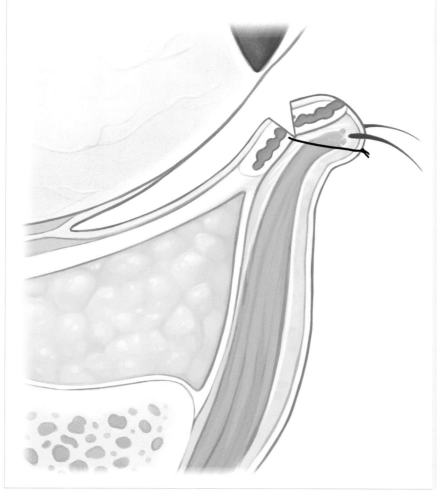

Fig. 45.5 Tarsal fracture (Weis procedure) with full-thickness incision made through the tarsus 3–4 mm below the lid margin and horizontal mattress sutures placed to rotate the lash line outward.

- Modified tarsotomy: This procedure is similar to the Weis procedure, yet is less destructive with excellent cosmetic and functional results. The eyelid is anesthetized and a 4–0 silk traction suture is placed through the margin. This lid is then everted over a cotton-tipped applicator. A Supersharp blade is used to make a full-thickness tarsal incision 2 mm proximal to the lid margin. The length of the incision should extend 2 mm beyond the area of cicatrization. Relaxing incisions are made medially and laterally toward the lid margin. Dissection is performed between the tarsal place and the orbicularis oculi muscle to the lid margin. As in the Weis procedure, rotational horizontal mattress sutures are then placed with double-armed 6–0 Vicryl sutures from the proximal tarsus through the skin just above the lash line. This is repeated across the horizontal extent of the incision.[5]
- Eyelash extirpation with mucous membrane grafting: Lid splitting with eyelash extirpation and mucous membrane grafting is an option for recurrent or severe cicatricial entropion from SJS or OCP. In this technique, the anterior and posterior lamellae are divided, and the eyelash line is excised at a depth sufficient to remove the eyelash follicles. Mucous membrane can be obtained from either the lower lip mucosa, buccal mucosa, or hard palate. The mucous membrane is then sewn into position onto the raw anterior surface of the posterior lamella along the eyelid margin (▶ Fig. 45.6). The advantage of the hard palate is that it is more durable with little shrinkage, compared to that of the lower lip mucosa. Another advantage of this procedure is that recurrence is rare and other eyelid pathology, such as conjunctival keratinization, is addressed. The disadvantages are postoperative discomfort of the donor site until re-epithelialization and change of eyelid appearance. Thus, this procedure should be reserved for severe cases.[6]

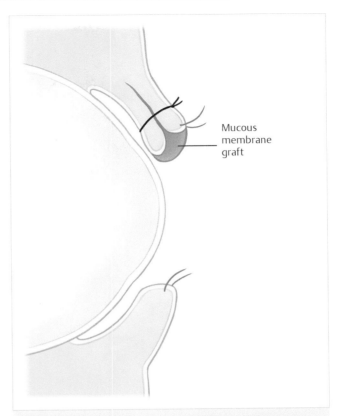

Fig. 45.6 Lid splitting with mucous membrane grafting between the anterior and posterior lamella.

45.9 Tips and Pearls

After determining the etiology, the preoperative discussion and management of expectations are essential prior to any treatment. Even with the most extensive approaches, patients should understand treatment is an ongoing, tailored process likely requiring multiple interventions.

In cases of SJS, OCP, or other chronic inflammatory/autoimmune processes, consultation with a rheumatologist or ocular surface specialist is essential. Surgery can incite an inflammatory response, making perioperative immunosuppression necessary in some cases.

The number of overall procedures performed on an eyelid should be considered and limited. The accumulation of scar tissue and interrupted blood supply can result in a fibrotic, inelastic eyelid.

45.10 What to Avoid

It is important to avoid incorrect procedure selection that does not address the underlying etiology of the aberrant lashes. For example, electroepilation is likely not appropriate in cases where a cicatricial entropion is present and multiple lashes touch the corneal surface.

It is important to avoid damage to the eye during any of these procedures. Using protective devices, such as eyelid plates (e.g., Jaffe eyelid plate) or a corneal shield, can be helpful.

45.11 Complications/Bailout/ Salvage

The most common complication is recurrence, with an estimated 50% recurrence rate, although this varies based on the underlying etiology and treatment technique employed. Many patients also require repeated treatments, particularly for radiofrequency and hyfrecation. Patients can develop eyelid notches and scars with radiofrequency, hyfrecation, and cryoepilation.

45.12 Postoperative Care

Postoperative care after hyfrecation, argon laser, or cryotherapy should include an antibiotic and/or steroidal drop or ointment with ice application to the eyelids. Patients familiar with the procedure can be seen again weeks after the treatment for possible retreatment. Postoperative care after incisional surgery should include ice packs, antibiotic ointment, and rest. Patients should be seen at postoperative week 1. If sutures are present, they may be removed at this time.

References

[1] Nerad JA. Techniques in Ophthalmic Plastic Surgery. Cincinnati, OH: Elsevier Inc.; 2010

[2] Kezirian GM. Treatment of localized trichiasis with radiosurgery. Ophthal Plast Reconstr Surg. 1993; 9(4):260–266

[3] Al-Bdour MD, Al-Till MI. Argon laser: a modality of treatment for trichiasis. Int J Biomed Sci. 2007; 3(1):56–59

[4] McCracken MS, Kikkawa DO, Vasani SN. Treatment of trichiasis and distichiasis by eyelash trephination. Ophthal Plast Reconstr Surg. 2006; 22(5):349–351

[5] Chi M, Kim HJ, Vagefi R, Kersten RC. Modified tarsotomy for the treatment of severe cicatricial entropion. Eye (Lond). 2016; 30(7):992–997

[6] Silver B. The use of mucous membrane from the hard palate in the treatment of trichiasis and cicatricial entropion. Ophthal Plast Reconstr Surg. 1986; 2(3):129–131

46 Tarsorrhaphy (Temporary and Permanent)

Seanna Grob, Emily Charlson, and Jeremiah P. Tao

Summary

This chapter describes both the temporary and permanent options to join the upper and lower eyelids. Tarsorrhaphy may be indicated to protect the ocular surface, forestall eyelid retraction after surgery, or to maintain a conformer or prosthesis. Temporary tarsorrhaphies include different suture techniques, both adjustable and nonadjustable, that can be performed quickly and may be vital for treatment of acute ocular surface exposure. Permanent tarsorrhaphy options include intermarginal adhesions and minor flaps, when long-term management of corneal exposure is necessary. Even after a tarsorrhaphy is placed, continued monitoring is required to ensure appropriate ocular surface protection.

Keywords: tarsorrhaphy, temporary tarsorrhaphy, permanent tarsorrhaphy, suture tarsorrhaphy, intermarginal adhesions, Frost suture, tarsoconjunctival onlay flap

46.1 Goals

A tarsorrhaphy is the temporary or permanent joining of the upper and lower eyelids. Surgical closure of the eyelids is most frequently indicated to protect the cornea and ocular surface in the setting of exposure from lagophthalmos or eyelid malposition. Other indications include maintenance of a conformer or ocular prosthesis in the anophthalmic socket, and counter traction (e.g., Frost suture tarsorrhaphy) after eyelid surgery especially in the setting of a graft. A tarsorrhaphy may be placed medially or laterally for partial coverage and to preserve the central visual axis, or centrally to completely cover the eye when necessary.

46.2 Advantages

A tarsorrhaphy is a powerful and relatively simple, usually reversible technique to provide immediate protection to the ocular surface. It is usually expedient and can often be completed in the office or at bedside with local anesthesia and no sedation. There are many tarsorrhaphy variations, including temporary and permanent, as well as partial and complete. A partial tarsorrhaphy closes the lateral and/or medial portion of the eyelids maintaining a central opening to preserve the visual axis and space for ocular examination. A complete tarsorrhaphy ensures closure of the entire palpebral aperture for maximal protection. An adjustable suture is a temporary measure that allows for repeated opening and closing of the eyelids that afford ocular examination and medication administration.[1] A Frost suture tarsorrhaphy provides counter traction postoperatively to forestall or correct eyelid malposition after some types of eyelid surgery.

46.3 Expectations

Tarsorrhaphies can provide symptomatic relief, improved corneal protection, and expedited healing due to exposure.

Suturing the eyelids together can be distressing for some patients and cosmetically unacceptable for others.

46.4 Key Principles

A successful tarsorrhaphy achieves the appropriate amount of eyelid closure. The decision for a temporary versus permanent tarsorrhaphy is based on the desired duration of ocular surface coverage. Tarsorrhaphies with or without bolsters should bring the upper and lower eyelids in tight apposition to cover the corneal surface or in cases of anophthalmia, to prevent extrusion of the conformer or prosthetic eye.[2] During the placement of a tarsorrhaphy, care should be taken to avoid damage that may cause scarring or trichiasis.

46.5 Indications

A tarsorrhaphy is indicated to protect and promote healing of the ocular surface in the setting of corneal exposure, infection, or poor healing. Other applications are to forestall eyelid retraction immediately following eyelid surgery (i.e. Frost suture tarsorrhaphy), as well as to help maintain a conformer, symblepharon ring, or an ocular prosthesis in the anophthalmic socket.

Temporary suture tarsorrhaphy is indicated when immediate protection of the cornea is needed due to inadequate eyelid closure. Suture tarsorrhaphy may be particularly useful when corneal sensation is impaired since the absence of pain or discomfort that normally induces volitional eyelid closure increases the risk for corneal damage and infection. Acting as a natural bandage, a tarsorrhaphy can promote healing of ocular surface disorders including persistent epithelial defects, corneal thinning, or postinfectious sterile corneal ulcers. When used for these indications, a temporary tarsorrhaphy can be customized to protect the affected area. Lastly, a tarsorrhaphy can stretch tissue to counteract wound contraction after eyelid surgery, especially when a skin graft or flap is utilized.

In cases where ocular exposure is expected to be long-standing (months to years), a permanent tarsorrhaphy can be considered. Generally, these are placed laterally and for persistent lagophthalmos from facial nerve palsy or in patients with central nervous system causes for poor or absent blink. Although the term "permanent" is used with these tarsorrhaphies, opening the eyelids in a reversal procedure is possible.

46.6 Contraindications

Tarsorrhaphies have a few contraindications and are readily reversed if needed. An active infected corneal ulcer is a relative contraindication for complete tarsorrhaphy since ongoing visualization of the ocular surface is necessary; however, a partial tarsorrhaphy may be beneficial for ulcer treatment in some cases. Once ulcers have been sterilized with antibiotic treatment, a tarsorrhaphy may be placed to encourage epithelial healing. Although not a definitive contraindication, placing a complete tarsorrhaphy over the only seeing eye in a monocular patient may be quite debilitating, although it may be necessary to preserve vision in the one functional eye. Similarly, bilateral, complete tarsorrhaphies are undesirable. In these cases, other modalities such as scleral contact lenses or amniotic membrane devices (e.g., Prokera) may be utilized to prevent occlusion of the visual axis.

46.7 Preoperative Preparation

Most types of tarsorrhaphy can be completed at the bedside, office, or operating room. Local anesthesia is administered in the upper and lower pretarsal eyelid in the location of suture placement. The area is then prepped and draped to maintain a sterile field.

Also important is a discussion with the patient or the health care proxy regarding the type of tarsorrhaphy that will be placed, specifically the appearance of the eyelid and how the vision will be affected by the tarsorrhaphy.

46.8 Operative Technique

46.8.1 Temporary Tarsorrhaphy

Nonsurgical Options

There exist several nonsurgical options for a temporary tarsorrhaphy. The least invasive options include closing the eyelids using adhesive (e.g., tape or Steri-Strips) with or without a pressure patch. However, this may require frequent replacement that could be uncomfortable or compromise the skin, and there is a risk of a corneal abrasion if the eyelid opens under the patch. Botulinum toxin can be injected into the upper eyelid to target the levator palpebrae superioris causing ptosis of the upper eyelid and improved eyelid closure.[4,5] This option can provide easy access for examination and administration of eye drops and will last weeks to months; however, the induced ptosis blocks the visual axis and may affect the superior rectus muscle causing vertical diplopia. A temporary tarsorrhaphy can also be created using cyanoacrylate glue, which can last approximately 1 to 15 days, averaging 1 week.[6] Care must be taken to avoid accidental application of glue to the ocular surface.

46.8.2 Suture Tarsorrhaphy

A temporary suture tarsorrhaphy can be used in patients who require only temporary closure of the eyelids or as a bridge until a definitive treatment (permanent tarsorrhaphy or other eyelid procedure) can be performed. Although most cases of idiopathic facial nerve palsy (i.e., Bell palsy) recover spontaneously without significant damage to the cornea, if significant exposure exists, suture tarsorrhaphy may be an ideal temporary solution.

After the upper and lower eyelids are injected with local anesthesia, a suture tarsorrhaphy can be achieved with a 4–0 or 5–0 monofilament nylon, polypropylene, or silk suture in a horizontal mattress fashion with or without bolsters to protect the skin (▶ Fig. 46.1). The suture passes should be placed with care so that the suture is not exposed through the posterior lamella or interpalpebral zone that could result in corneal abrasion. A lateral suture tarsorrhaphy can be placed in cases where partial eyelid closure and preserving the visual axis are desired. This can be helpful in patients who are dependent on the affected eye or in patients in whom a lateral tarsorrhaphy provides a sufficient amount of eyelid closure to treat the corneal exposure or issue. A medial suture tarsorrhaphy similarly preserves the visual axis and can be helpful with eyelid malposition in this zone; however, care must be taken to avoid damage to the canalicular apparatus.

46.8.3 Frost Suture Tarsorrhaphy— Lower Eyelid Suspension Suture

The Frost suture is a lower eyelid suspension suture that is placed at the end of a surgical procedure involving the lower eyelid to help prevent postoperative ectropion and retraction.[7,8,9] A Frost suture is commonly placed using a 4–0 silk suture in a horizontal mattress fashion and then the suture tails are left long and secured to the forehead with the sutures passed through the brow skin or with adhesive tape (▶ Fig. 46.2). This helps keep the lower eyelid on stretch in the immediate postoperative period. This is often done after a skin graft is placed on the lower eyelid for cicatricial ectropion repair. This allows the skin graft to be kept in good apposition to the underlying tissue and vascular supply. A pressure patch over the lower eyelid or a bolster is also usually placed to keep the skin graft

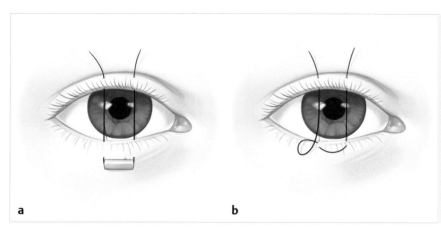

Fig. 46.1 (a,b) Suture tarsorrhaphy with and without a bolster.

a　　　　　　b

tightly apposed to the recipient bed. Similarly, if a skin graft is placed on the upper eyelid, the traction suture tarsorrhaphy can be left long and taped inferiorly to the cheek to keep the upper eyelid on stretch.

46.8.4 Adjustable Drawstring Tarsorrhaphy

The drawstring adjustable suture tarsorrhaphy utilizes rubber or soft plastic bolsters along with a 5–0 or 6–0 polypropylene

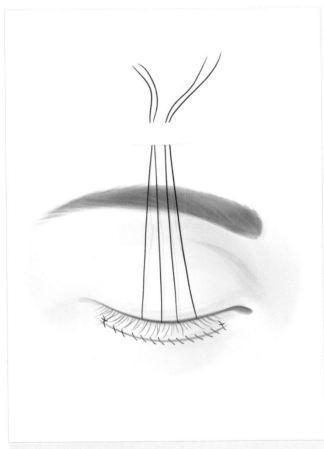

Fig. 46.2 Frost suture tarsorrhaphy.

suture passed through the upper and lower eyelid margins.[1] This technique provides complete closure of the eyelids while still providing easy access to the eye for placement of eye drops and for clinical examination.

The bolster is fashioned by cutting a Foley catheter or other medical tubing into two semicircular strips (▶ Fig. 46.3). One of these strips is then cut into two 2-cm sections and the other into a 1-cm section. The 1-cm bolster acts to close the polypropylene suture drawstring over one of the 2-cm sections. The advantages of the bolsters are to protect the eyelid skin and also assist with eyelid eversion, so the eyelashes do not damage the ocular surface.

A double-armed polypropylene suture is passed completely through one of the 2-cm bolsters about 2 mm from the end. The same needle is then passed 3 to 4 mm from the nasal upper eyelid margin into the tarsus and out through the eyelid margin at the gray line. The needle then should enter the lower eyelid margin in the same location and exit the lower eyelid approximately 2 to 3 mm inferior to the margin. The other end of the double-armed suture is then passed similarly through the lateral aspect of the bolster and upper and lower eyelids. Both needles are then passed through the second 2-cm bolster that will be positioned over the lower eyelid margin. Tightening of the suture at this point should then allow the eyelids to close.

In order to create the drawstring, the two suture arms are then passed through the 1-cm bolster. Then the needles are removed and the suture ends are tied together leaving approximately 2 to 3 cm of suture slack to allow for adjustment of the tightness. The suture can now be pulled to draw the 2-cm bolsters against the eyelids and close the eye. The 1-cm bolster is then pulled against the lower eyelid 2-cm bolster to secure the tarsorrhaphy and keep the eyelids closed. To open the tarsorrhaphy, the smaller bolster is just pulled away from the larger bolster to allow for opening of the eyelids to examine the eye or administer eye drops. The suture and bolsters can be cleaned with dilute povidone iodine as needed.

Other temporary and adjustable tarsorrhaphy techniques have been described in the literature with or without bolsters or tubes.[10,11,12] Dortzbach and coworkers[10] described a technique of using plastic tubes sutured to the upper and lower eyelid margins. Passing a suture through the upper and lower eyelid tubes and securing the suture accomplish eyelid closure.

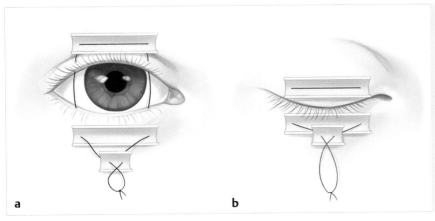

Fig. 46.3 (a,b) Adjustable drawstring tarsorrhaphy.

a   b

46.8.5 Permanent Tarsorrhaphy

Intermarginal Adhesions

A permanent tarsorrhaphy achieves lasting closure of the lateral and/or medial canthal angles. Adherence of the upper to lower eyelid margin is permanent unless surgically or traumatically dehisced.

There are various methods of intermarginal adhesion tarsorrhaphy. After administering local anesthesia, the upper and lower eyelid margins are incised at the gray line with a no. 15 blade, denuded of epithelium with the blade or scissors. The tarsal borders of the upper and lower eyelid margins are approximated using interrupted 5–0 polyglactin mattress sutures. The skin can be closed with interrupted sutures or a temporary mattress suture tarsorrhaphy can be placed to reinforce the adhesion tarsorrhaphy (▶ Fig. 46.4). Skin flaps with excision of the eyelashes in the location of the tarsorrhaphy can also be created in both medial and lateral permanent tarsorrhaphies.[13] The limitations of intermarginal adhesions include poor cosmesis and alteration of the eyelid margin, including keratinization of the margin, madarosis, and trichiasis.

Tarsoconjunctival Onlay Flap

After administering local anesthesia, a 5–0 (or larger caliber) silk or polyglactin suture is passed through the upper eyelid margin to aid in upper eyelid eversion over a cotton-tipped applicator or Desmarres retractor.[14] The tarsoconjunctival flap is marked on the lateral posterior lamella using a surgical marking pen or methylene blue approximately 4 mm superior to the eyelid margin and extending into the lateral fornix. A horizontal incision with a no. 15 blade extends medially from the lateral canthus approximately 4 to 8 mm depending on the desired amount of eyelid closure. A no. 15 blade and Westcott scissors are used to elevate and create the tarsoconjunctival flap. Then the lateral lower eyelid is incised at the gray line using a no. 15 blade from the lateral canthus medially measuring the same length as that of the superior flap. The margin epithelium of the lower eyelid posterior lamella is then denuded using a blade or scissors. The leading edge of the flap from the upper eyelid is secured to the exposed tarsus on the lower eyelid margin using interrupted mattress 5–0 polyglactin sutures (▶ Fig. 46.5). If there is significant laxity to the lower eyelid, a horizontal shortening procedure such as a lateral tarsal strip can be performed

immediately after the tarsoconjunctival flap is secured. The benefit of this procedure is the added elevation of the lower eyelid, akin to pant suspenders, for the lower eyelid. In the presence of a strong Bells reflex, there is additional desirable lower eyelid elevation upon eyelid closure due to movement of the upper fornix, where the flap originates.[14] This procedure can also be easily reversed without significant disruption of the upper eyelid margin. Eyelash and margin scarring problems are less significant on the lower eyelid margin possibly due to the shorter, finer eyelashes.[14]

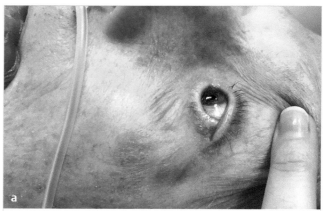
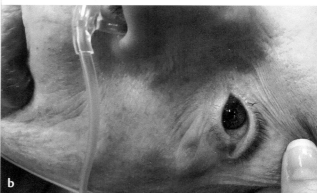

Fig. 46.5 (a,b) Clinical photographs showing a lateral tarsoconjunctival onlay flap in a patient with corneal exposure from a seventh nerve palsy.

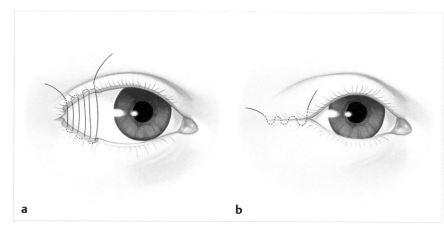

Fig. 46.4 Permanent tarsorrhaphy by intermarginal adhesions both **(a)** before and **(b)** after the sutures are tied.

Tarsoconjunctival flaps can also be designed to achieve "pillar" tarsorrhaphies.[15] In this procedure, thin tarsoconjunctival strips are derived from the upper eyelid just at the medial and lateral corneoscleral limbus and are secured to the lower eyelid. Pillar flaps are very effective in achieving lower eyelid elevation and central eyelid closure, but may be limited by poor cosmesis due to the visible tissue bands in the interpalpebral zone.

46.9 Tips and Pearls

The choice of tarsorrhaphy depends on the patient, the status of the ocular surface, the need for a temporary versus more permanent solution, and even the status of the opposite eye. It is important to ensure appropriate closure of the eye to protect the corneal surface and prevent permanent scarring, perforation, or other causes of permanent vision loss. Often a temporary tarsorrhaphy can be placed initially. If the condition becomes more lasting, then permanent tarsorrhaphy options can be considered. Postoperative monitoring is key as some patients may require a larger, wider, tighter, or more complete tarsorrhaphy. Some patients may also require additional surgery, such as lower eyelid retraction repair with or without grafts, an upper eyelid weight implant, or facial reanimation surgery, if indicated, in the setting of irreversible facial paralysis. Follow-up is also important as the tarsorrhaphy can be reversed if the condition improves.

46.10 What to Avoid

The most important thing to avoid when considering a tarsorrhaphy is further damage to the ocular surface. Usually the cornea is damaged or at risk at baseline. Exposed tarsorrhaphy sutures and misdirected eyelashes are iatrogenic causes for worsening of the ocular surface condition.

46.11 Complications

Complications of tarsorrhaphy placement include bleeding, infection, scarring, dehiscence, visual field obstruction, and even claustrophobia or anxiety due to partial or complete vision obstruction. Scarring of the eyelid margin or disruption of the normal eyelid architecture may lead to trichiasis, further eyelid malposition, or irregularity of the eyelid margin. Other complications include suboptimal eyelid closure leading to progression of corneal disease. Patients may complain of impaired depth perception and difficulty seeing with one eye closed or partially closed. The extent of these different tarsorrhaphies can be titrated with further closure or opening of the eyelids depending on each patient's need. Often, the difficulty with tarsorrhaphy is finding a balance between sufficient eyelid closure to allow for healing and protection of the cornea with preservation of functional use of the eye.

46.12 Postoperative Care

Postoperative management for a tarsorrhaphy follows standard oculofacial surgery protocols. Ice packs can be used intermittently (the authors recommend 20 minutes on/off) for the first 48 hours while awake to aid with pain control, hemostasis, and swelling. Physical activity should be limited temporarily and usually for the first week. An ophthalmic antibiotic ointment is often applied two to four times a day for the first 5 to 7 days after the procedure.

An important aspect of postoperative care is continued monitoring of the ocular surface. Sometimes the tarsorrhaphy is not sufficient and additional eyelid closure is required to prevent worsening of the corneal disease.

References

[1] Kitchens J, Kinder J, Oetting T. The drawstring temporary tarsorrhaphy technique. Arch Ophthalmol. 2002; 120(2):187–190

[2] McInnes AW, Burroughs JR, Anderson RL, McCann JD. Temporary suture tarsorrhaphy. Am J Ophthalmol. 2006; 142(2):344–346

[3] Wagoner MD, Steinert RF. Temporary tarsorrhaphy enhances reepithelialization after epikeratoplasty. Arch Ophthalmol. 1988; 106(1):13–14

[4] Kirkness CM, Adams GG, Dilly PN, Lee JP. Botulinum toxin A-induced protective ptosis in corneal disease. Ophthalmology. 1988; 95(4):473–480

[5] Wuebbolt GE, Drummond G. Temporary tarsorrhaphy induced with type A botulinum toxin. Can J Ophthalmol. 1991; 26(7):383–385

[6] Donnenfeld ED, Perry HD, Nelson DB. Cyanoacrylate temporary tarsorrhaphy in the management of corneal epithelial defects. Ophthalmic Surg. 1991; 22 (10):591–593

[7] Connolly KL, Albertini JG, Miller CJ, Ozog DM. The suspension (Frost) suture: experience and applications. Dermatol Surg. 2015; 41(3):406–410

[8] Desciak EB, Eliezri YD. Surgical Pearl: temporary suspension suture (Frost suture) to help prevent ectropion after infraorbital reconstruction. J Am Acad Dermatol. 2003; 49(6):1107–1108

[9] Murphy MT, Bradrick JP. Technique for fixation of the Frost suture. J Oral Maxillofac Surg. 1995; 53(11):1360–1361

[10] Rapoza PA, Harrison DA, Bussa JJ, Prestowitz WF, Dortzbach RK. Temporary sutured tube-tarsorrhaphy: reversible eyelid closure technique. Ophthalmic Surg. 1993; 24(5):328–330

[11] Hallock GG. Temporary tarsorrhaphy "zipper". Ann Plast Surg. 1992; 28(5): 488–490

[12] Dryden RM, Adams JL. Temporary nonincisional tarsorrhaphy. Ophthal Plast Reconstr Surg. 1985; 1(2):119–120

[13] Codner MA, McCord CD. Eyelid & Periorbital Surgery. 2nd ed. Boca Raton, FL: CRC Press; 2016

[14] Tao JP, Vemuri S, Patel AD, Compton C, Nunery WR. Lateral tarsoconjunctival onlay flap lower eyelid suspension in facial nerve paresis. Ophthal Plast Reconstr Surg. 2014; 30(4):342–345

[15] Tanenbaum M, Gossman MD, Bergin DJ, et al. The tarsal pillar technique for narrowing and maintenance of the interpalpebral fissure. Ophthalmic Surg. 1992; 23(6):418–425

Index

Note: Page numbers set **bold** or *italic* indicate headings or figures, respectively.